W. NORMAN SCOTT, M.D.

Chief of Joint Implant Service
Associate Attending Orthopaedic Surgeon
Lenox Hill Hospital, New York, New York

Arthroscopy of the Knee

Diagnosis and Treatment

1990

W.B. SAUNDERS COMPANY
Harcourt Brace Jovanovich, Inc.

Philadelphia   London   Toronto   Montreal   Sydney   Tokyo

W. B. SAUNDERS COMPANY

Harcourt Brace Jovanovich, Inc.
The Curtis Center
Independence Square West
Philadelphia, PA 19106-3399

Library of Congress Cataloging-in-Publication Data

Arthroscopy of the knee: diagnosis and treatment/[edited by] W. Norman
   Scott.

      p.   cm.

   ISBN 0-7216-8032-1

   1. Knee—Endoscopic surgery. 2. Arthroscopy I. Scott, W. Norman.

   [DNLM: 1. Arthroscopy. 2. Joint Diseases—diagnosis. 3. Knee Joint—
surgery. WE 870 A7868]

   RD561.A78 1990   617′.5820754—dc19

   DNLM/DLC

   for Library of Congress   89-5951
                                                      CIP

Editor: Edward H. Wickland, Jr.
Designer: W. B. Saunders Staff
Production Manager: Carolyn Naylor
Manuscript Editor: Wynette Kommer
Illustration Coordinator: Lisa Lambert
Indexer: George Vilk

ARTHROSCOPY OF THE KNEE: DIAGNOSIS AND TREATMENT   ISBN 0–7216–8032–1

Printed in the United States of America.

Last digit is the print number: 9   8   7   6   5   4   3   2   1

To my deceased parents, Joan and Walter, my first teachers, as a small token of visible appreciation for *"just"* being such loving parents, providers of opportunity, and role models: Thanks

CONTRIBUTORS

Albert B. Accettola, Jr., M.D.
Adjunct Assistant Professor, New York University School of Education, Health, Nursing and Arts Professions, New York, New York; Attending, Staten Island Hospital; Adjunct Attending, Richmond Memorial Hospital and Saint Vincent's Medical Center of Richmond, New York
Arthroscopic Diagnosis and Treatment of Intra-Articular Fractures

Michael Alexiades, M.D.
Orthopedic Fellow, The Hospital for Special Surgery, affiliated with the New York Hospital–Cornell University Medical College, New York, New York
The Evolution of Arthroscopy

James P. Bradley, M.D.
Clinical Fellow, Kerlan-Jobe Orthopedic Clinic, Inglewood, California
Arthroscopic Diagnosis and Treatment of Patellofemoral Disorders

Joseph J. Combs, Jr., M.D.
Assistant Professor of Internal Medicine and Rheumatology, Mayo Medical School; Staff Consultant in Rheumatology, Rochester Methodist and St. Mary's Hospitals, Rochester, Minnesota
Arthroscopic Diagnosis and Treatment of Symptomatic Plicae

Peter J. Fowler, M.D., FRCS (C)
Professor, Department of Surgery, Division of Orthopaedic Surgery, and Head, Section of Sport Medicine, University of Western Ontario; Active Staff, University Hospital, London, Ontario
Arthroscopic Anatomy

Andrew G. Franks, Jr., M.D., FACP
Clinical Associate Professor, New York University School of Medicine; Senior Attending Rheumatologist, Lenox Hill Hospital; Associate Attending Rheumatologist, Hospital for Joint Diseases, New York, New York
Synovial Fluid Characteristics

Marc J. Friedman, M.D.
Assistant Clinical Professor of Surgery, UCLA School of Medicine, Los Angeles; Southern California Orthopedic Institute, Van Nuys, California
Arthroscopic Diagnosis and Treatment of Cruciate and Collateral Ligament Injuries

Jonathan L. Glashow, M.D.
Chief Resident, Orthopedic Surgery, Lenox Hill Hospital, New York, New York
Diagnostic Imaging of the Knee

Ronald P. Karzel, Jr., M.D.

Southern California Orthopedic Institute, Van Nuys, California
Arthroscopic Diagnosis and Treatment of Cruciate and Collateral Ligament Injuries

Richard Katz, M.D.

Clinical Instructor in Radiology, Cornell Medical College/New York Hospital; Assistant Radiologist, Memorial Sloan Kettering Hospital, New York, New York
Diagnostic Imaging of the Knee

Michael A. Kelly, M.D.

Assistant Professor of Orthopedic Surgery, College of Physicians and Surgeons, Columbia University; Attending Orthopedic Surgeon, Columbia Presbyterian Medical Center, New York, New York
Arthroscopic Diagnosis and Treatment of Loose Bodies

Patricia A. Kolowich, M.D.

Senior Staff, Henry Ford Hospital, Center for Athletic Medicine, Detroit, Michigan
Arthroscopic Diagnosis and Treatment of Meniscal Disorders

Stephen J. Lombardo, M.D.

Associate Clinical Professor of Orthopedic Surgery, University of Southern California Medical Center Los Angeles; Staff, Centinela Hospital Medical Center, and Daniel Freeman Hospital, Inglewood, California
Arthroscopic Diagnosis and Treatment of Patellofemoral Disorders

Christopher M. Magee, M.D.

Attending Orthopedic Surgeon and Chief, Orthopedic Section, Washington Adventist Hospital, Takoma Park, Maryland
Arthroscopic Diagnosis and Treatment of Loose Bodies

George Pianka, M.D.

Chief Orthopedic Resident, Lenox Hill Hospital, New York, New York
Arthroscopic Diagnosis and Treatment of Symptomatic Plicae

H. Keith Pinchot, M.D.

Director, Ambulatory Anesthesia and Assistant Attending Anesthesiologist, Hospital for Special Surgery, Cornell University Medical College, New York, New York
Anesthetic Considerations in Arthroscopy

James A. Rand, M.D.

Associate Professor of Orthopedic Surgery, Mayo Medical School; Consultant in Orthopedic Surgery, Mayo Clinic; Rochester Methodist Hospital and St. Mary's Hospital, Rochester, Minnesota
Arthroscopic Diagnosis and Management of Articular Cartilage Pathology

John P. Reilly, M.D.

Adjunct Attending, Staten Island Hospital; Lenox Hill Hospital Assistant Adjunct Attending, and Richmond Memorial Hospital, New York
Arthroscopic Diagnosis and Treatment of Intra-Articular Fractures

Thomas D. Rosenberg, M.D.
Associate Clinical Professor of Orthopedic Surgery, University of Utah, School of Medicine; Clinical Staff, LDS Hospital and Holy Cross Hospital, Salt Lake City, Utah
Arthroscopic Diagnosis and Treatment of Meniscal Disorders

Morton Schneider, M.D.
Consultant Medical Staff in Diagnostic Radiology, Lenox Hill Hospital, New York, New York
Diagnostic Imaging of the Knee

W. Norman Scott, M.D.
Associate Attending Orthopedic Surgeon and Chief of the Implant Service, Lenox Hill Hospital, New York, New York
Diagnostic Imaging of the Knee

Giles R. Scuderi, M.D.
Orthopedic Surgeon to the Outpatient Department, The Hospital for Special Surgery, affiliated with The New York Hospital–Cornell University Medical College, New York; Orthopedic Surgeon, South Nassau Communities Hospital, Oceanside, New York
The Evolution of Arthroscopy

Nigel E. Sharrock, M.B., Ch.B.
Clinical Assistant Professor of Anesthesiology, Cornell University Medical College and Director, Department of Anesthesiology, Hospital for Special Surgery, New York, New York
Anesthetic Considerations in Arthroscopy

Vincent J. Vigorita, M.D.
Associate Professor of Pathology, State University of New York Health Sciences Center at Brooklyn; Director of Laboratories, Lutheran Medical Center, Brooklyn; Visiting Scientist, The Hospital for Special Surgery, New York, New York
Synovial Disorders

Kelly G. Vince, M.D., FRCS (C)
Consultant, Rancho Los Amigos Medical Center, Downey; Kerlan-Jobe Orthopedic Clinic, Centinela Hospital, Inglewood, California
Osteochondritis Dissecans of the Knee

Robert M. Wilson, M.D.
Associate Attending, Cedars Sinai Medical Center, Los Angeles, California
Arthroscopic Anatomy

Russell E. Windsor, M.D.
Assistant Professor of Surgery (Orthopedics), New York Hospital–Cornell University Medical Center; Assistant Attending Orthopedic Surgeon, Hospital for Special Surgery and New York Hospital, New York, New York
Arthroscopic Diagnosis and Treatment of the Septic Knee

PREFACE

In view of the technologic advances in arthroscopy in the last 15 years, it is somewhat hazardous to publish a textbook on the subject. The perpetual lag inherent in the publication of a scientific text jeopardizes its contribution to the "state of the art." It was with this understanding that the contributors to this book attempted and, I believe, succeeded in presenting a timely discussion of the arthroscopic diagnosis and treatment of knee disorders.

In Chapter 1, Drs. Scuderi and Alexiades present an inherently incomplete, albeit thorough, section on the evolution of arthroscopy. Undoubtedly, projects on the horizon will require an update within the next few years. Although the emphasis of this text is on arthroscopy of the knee, it is imperative, I believe, to chronicle other types of diagnostic modalities to keep a perspective of the options available to the individual assessing knee disorders. Drs. Glashow, Katz, and Schneider have done an excellent job in displaying the role of radiologic modalities. Their emphasis on magnetic resonance imaging (MRI) is especially helpful and timely for all orthopedists. Similarly, Drs. Sharrock and Pinchot's "anesthesia for orthopedists" allows us to discuss intelligently the options with patients.

Anatomically, Drs. Franks, Wilson, and Fowler discuss topics that are not affected by technology and are the basis for developing an understanding for treating knee disorders. The remainder of the book is purposefully divided into anatomic sections illustrating the normal and subsequent deviations. Although sometimes repetitious, each of the authors has reviewed the basic anatomy, and I have encouraged the repetition since anatomy is the "mother of learning."

The ubiquitous structure visualized in the knee is the synovium, and Dr. Vigorita describes the various pathologic conditions that might be encountered. An extension of the synovium, the plica, is generously illustrated by Drs. Pianka and Combs, who share a broad experience of observations and present understanding of what constitutes a pathologic plica.

The treatment of meniscal injuries undoubtedly became the most popular aspect of arthroscopy because of diminished patient morbidity. Drs. Rosenberg and Kolowich use drawings and photographs of the various tears to illustrate those that can be treated by resection or repair. The types of tears are standard, but the technology has allowed new approaches to repair, and the authors mention the current techniques while keeping an eye to the future.

Understanding of articular cartilage pathology has been enhanced by arthroscopy. Dr. Rand illustrates the characteristics of normal articular cartilage and its subsequent degeneration. Dr. Vince's chapter on osteochondritis dissecans, the most comprehensive treatise I've seen, dovetails nicely, allowing the reader to appreciate the transition from normal to abnormal articular cartilage. Drs. Kelly and Magee illustrate how to remove loose bodies, which often are composed of articular cartilage. No discussion of articular cartilage would be complete without a discussion of patellofemoral disorders and Drs. Lombardo and Bradley are quite helpful in putting this difficult problem in perspective.

Ligamentous injuries of the knee often can be addressed with arthroscopic assistance. Drs. Karzel and Friedman are to be congratulated for attempting to summarize what is presently the most tumultuous aspect of knee surgery, the role of arthroscopy and anterior cruciate reconstruction.

One of the newest, albeit undefined, roles of arthroscopy is in the treatment of the septic knee. Dr. Windsor develops the present indication, which undoubtedly will be refined with increasing experience.

Similarly, new horizons, to be better defined, exist with the arthroscope and intra-articular fractures. Drs. Reilly and Accettola show us the technique. Time will manifest the indications.

Arthroscopy is probably the most significant diagnostic procedure in all aspects of knee pathology. Its surgical applications are beginning to be appreciated. As we begin the nineties we are enthusiastic about its usefulness, thanks to the many contributors to the science.

I express my appreciation to all the contributors, and I hope that this volume will in some small way further the education of students, residents, and orthopedists and thus make a contribution to the diagnosis and treatment of knee disorders.

W. Norman Scott

CONTENTS

1 The Evolution of Arthroscopy 1
Giles Scuderi and Michael Alexiades

2 Diagnostic Imaging of the Knee 11
Jonathan L. Glashow, Richard Katz, Morton Schneider and
W. Norman Scott

3 Anesthetic Considerations in Arthroscopy...37
Nigel E. Sharrock and H. Keith Pinchot

4 Synovial Fluid Characteristics 43
Andrew G. Franks, Jr.

5 Arthroscopic Anatomy 49
Robert M. Wilson and Peter Fowler

6 Arthroscopic Diagnosis and Treatment of
Meniscal Disorders 67
Thomas D. Rosenberg and Patricia A. Kolowich

7 Arthroscopic Diagnosis and Treatment of
Symptomatic Plicae.........................83
George Pianka and Joseph Combs

8 Synovial Disorders..........................97
Vincent J. Vigorita

9 Arthroscopic Diagnosis and Management of
Articular Cartilage Pathology 113
James A. Rand

10 Arthroscopic Diagnosis and Treatment of
Cruciate and Collateral Ligament Injuries ..131
Ronald P. Karzel, Jr., and Marc J. Friedman

11 **Arthroscopic Diagnosis and Treatment of Patellofemoral Disorders** **155**
Stephen J. Lombardo and James P. Bradley

12 **Osteochondritis Dissecans of the Knee** **175**
Kelly G. Vince

13 **Arthroscopic Diagnosis and Treatment of Loose Bodies** **193**
Michael A. Kelly and Christopher M. Magee

14 **Arthroscopic Diagnosis and Treatment of the Septic Knee** **207**
Russell E. Windsor

15 **Arthroscopic Diagnosis and Treatment of Intra-Articular Fractures** **215**
John P. Reilly and Albert B. Accettola, Jr.

Index **233**

Giles Scuderi
Michael Alexiades

The Evolution of Arthroscopy

As we learn arthroscopic technique, it is valuable to know the evolution of the arthroscope and its historical application. Originally, endoscopic techniques were developed to look into the bladder and body cavities. After this application arthroscopy progressed to the knee and other synovial joints.

Modern endoscopy began when Bozzini (1773–1809) of Frankfurt devised his "lichtleiter" or light conductor in 1806[25,29,38] (Fig. 1–1). The original instrument was a bifid tube attached to a light chamber. The light source was a candle that reflected light into a body cavity by means of a concave mirror and speculum. Through the back of the instrument there was a small aperture, so that the cavity could be visualized. Bozzini mainly used his device to examine the vagina and rectum. This primitive device was presented to the Joseph Academy of Medical Surgery in Vienna in 1806; the Academy considered it merely a toy and of no importance in the examination of the urologic system.

A few years later, Pierre S. Segalos (1792–1875) in France utilized the same principle of light conduction as Bozzini had, but instead of a concave mirror he used a conical one to introduce the light into the urethra and the interior of the urinary bladder. The procedure was demonstrated to the Royal French Academy, but the illumination was poor and the instrument found little acceptance.[25,29]

A.J. Desormeaux (1815–1882) introduced the cystoscope in 1853 and became the first surgeon to gain acceptance of his endoscopic instrument as a valuable diagnostic and therapeutic tool in urology.[25,29] The light source, called a "gazogene lamp," used a mixture of turpentine and alcohol (Fig. 1–2). A concave perforated reflector directed the light down a series of silver tubes and mirrors. The surgeon looked through an eyepiece into the bladder and urethra. Publication of Desormeaux's work established the value of the cystoscope.

In 1867, J. Andrew improved the light source with the development of a magnesium filament that produced a strong white light. This was the best external light source at the time. Julius Bruch, a Breslau dentist, was the first to introduce the light source into a body cavity. He inserted a platinum filament into the rectum, illuminating the urinary bladder, which he inspected through a speculum. A great disadvantage was the heat generated by the lamp.[25,29]

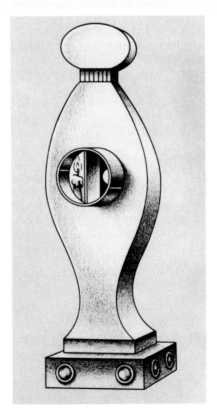

Figure 1–1
The Bozzini lichtleiter. (Reproduced with permission from The Upjohn Company and Joyce JJ III: History of arthroscopy. *In* O'Connor RL (ed): Arthroscopy: A Scope Publication. Kalamazoo, MI, The Upjohn Company, 1977.)

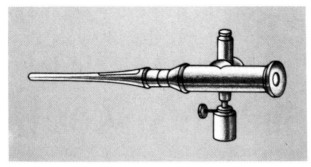

Figure 1—2
The Desormeaux gazogene endoscope. (Reproduced with permission from The Upjohn Company and Joyce JJ III: History of arthroscopy. *In* O'Connor RL (ed): Arthroscopy: A Scope Publication. Kalamazoo, MI, The Upjohn Company, 1977.)

The German physician Max Nitze (1848–1906) recognized the difficulties with an externally reflected light source and in 1876 designed an instrument with a combined light source, reflector, and scope (Fig. 1–3). The instrument consisted of a platinum loop encased in a goose quill, which introduced light directly into the bladder. A flow of water along the instrument protected the tissues, and an improved lens system provided better visualization. He demonstrated his instrument before the Vienna Medical Society of Saxony in October 1879, but was heavily criticized for his "fire and water" invention.[25,29]

With Edison's invention in 1880 of the incandescent lamp, a filament in a glass tube, a more effective light source became available for use with the cystoscope. By 1886, Leopold Van Dittel (1815–1898), a Viennese surgeon, incorporated a mignon lamp into his cystoscope. Nitze, in association with the instrument maker Joseph Leiter (1830–1892), designed a cystoscope that not only had improved illumination but also a better angle of view and a larger field of vision. In 1890, R. Kutner and Nitze introduced the photocystoscope and took the first endoscopic photographs of the bladder. The Zeiss Company in 1907 improved optics with the Amici prism. This produced

a vertical and sharper image. Before this improvement the image was always inverted. Not until the turn of the century did the cystoscope become an important urologic tool.[25,29]

While enormous progress was being made in endoscopic evaluation of the urologic system, Professor Kenji Takagi (1883–1963) of the University of Tokyo adapted endoscopy to the knee joint. He must be considered the father of arthroscopy. Using a #22 French cystoscope, he examined a cadaveric knee joint in 1918. The first "arthroscope" he designed, in 1920, was 7.3 mm in diameter. It contained no lens system but had an incandescent bulb at the tip (Fig. 1–4). The large diameter of the scope made it impractical for examination of the knee joint, but nevertheless he was successful in examining a tuberculous knee. Impressed with the clear view that he was able to achieve with the arthroscope, Takagi concentrated on reducing its diameter. By 1931, he had achieved a diameter of 3.5 mm; subsequent models were even smaller and required a lens system to magnify the images. The original impetus had been to diagnose tuberculosis of the knee, and by the mid 1930s Takagi was able to perform synovial biopsies with a 4-mm (#12) arthroscope. He later introduced a 5-mm (#13) arthroscope that incorporated a forward, oblique, and side viewing lens. In 1936, Takagi took the first reported color photographs of the knee joint, using a 6-mm arthroscope.[43,44]

Independently of Professor Takagi, Eugene Bircher of Switzerland in 1921 used a Jacobeus laparothoracscope to examine the knee joint. He published the results of 20 arthroscopic examinations in 1922. What stimulated Bircher's interest in "arthro-endoscopy" was the disappointing experience with clinical and radiologic diagnosis of knee lesions. Bircher performed arthroscopy under strict aseptic technique.

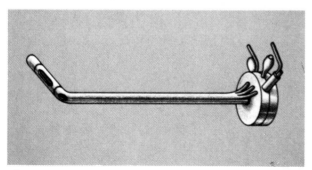

Figure 1—3
The Nitze endoscope. (Reproduced with permission from The Upjohn Company and Joyce JJ III: History of arthroscopy. *In* O'Connor RL (ed): Arthroscopy: A Scope Publication. Kalamazoo, MI, The Upjohn Company, 1977.)

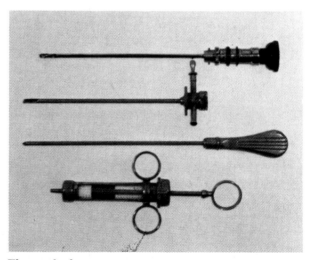

Figure 1—4
The first Takagi arthroscope. (Reproduced with permission from The Upjohn Company and Joyce JJ III: History of arthroscopy. *In* O'Connor RL (ed): Arthroscopy: A Scope Publication. Kalamazoo, MI, The Upjohn Company, 1977.)

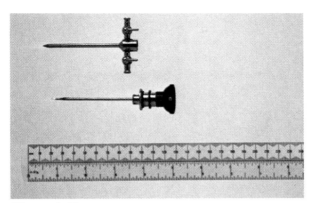

Figure 1–5
The Burman arthroscope. (Reproduced with permission from The Upjohn Company and Joyce JJ III: History of arthroscopy. *In* O'Connor RL (ed): Arthroscopy: A Scope Publication. Kalamazoo, MI, The Upjohn Company, 1977.)

He soaked the arthroscope in 96 percent alcohol for 2 to 3 minutes before and after each procedure. Between cases he stored the arthroscope in a chamber of formalin fumes. The knee joint was distended with oxygen and carbon dioxide, yet he found his examination to be hampered by the cruciate ligaments. In his publications Bircher reported that "arthro-endoscopy" was superior to all other methods of knee joint examination,[1] but he was unable to photograph the interior of the knee joint. In 1925, Philip Kreucher became the first American to report on the use of the arthroscope to diagnose meniscal lesions.[30]

In the early thirties, at the Hospital for Joint Diseases in New York, Drs. Mayer, Finkelstein, and Burman published a number of significant monographs on the subject of arthroscopy.[2–6,12] Dr. Michael Burman (1901–1975) used an arthroscope designed by Mr. R. Wappler that had a trochar 4 mm in diameter, a telescope 3 mm in diameter, and a lamp incorpo-

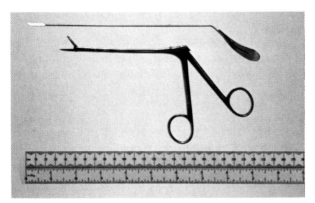

Figure 1–6
Arthroscopic instruments for the Burman arthroscope: knife (top) and forceps (bottom). (Reproduced with permission from The Upjohn Company and Joyce JJ III: History of arthroscopy. *In* O'Connor RL (ed): Arthroscopy: A Scope Publication. Kalamazoo, MI, The Upjohn Company, 1977.)

rated into the shaft, and allowed constant irrigation (Figs. 1–5 and 1–6). In a classic manuscript published in the Journal of Bone and Joint Surgery in 1931, Burman reported his experience with arthroscopy of joints other than the knee.[2] Most of his time was spent investigating tubercular or sarcoid-like disorders of the knee, and he was able to perform punch biopsies of these lesions. In 1936, he published a paper with Drs. Finkelstein and Mayer on the use of punch biopsy in the diagnosis of tuberculosis.[4] Dr. Burman was active in promoting arthroscopy as an important diagnostic tool and exhibited his work at a meeting of the American Medical Association in Cleveland in 1934, at the Third Annual Meeting of Orthopedic Surgeons in New York City in 1935, and at the New York Academy of Medicine in 1936.[38]

In Germany, studies on arthroscopy of the knee were published by Sommer in 1937[42] and Vaubel in 1938.[46] Sommer used the Grave arthroscope and felt that it was a valuable tool in the diagnosis of tuberculosis. He believed that arthroscopy of the knee could be repeated several times without inconvenience to the patient. Vaubel advised arthroscopic examination of the knee for many disorders in order to avoid exploratory arthrotomy.

Interest in arthroscopy revived after World War II, when in 1955 in the French literature E. Hurter described arthroscopy as a "new" method of examining joints.[8] R. Imbert in 1956 and 1957 published further papers in France on the subject of arthroscopy.

Dr. Masaki Watanabe, a pupil of Takagi resuming his mentor's work, developed better instruments and a more reliable lighting system. He also continued Takagi's numbering system for the arthroscope. Until 1959, arthroscopy of the knee joint, including the first surgical arthroscopy, used a #13 arthroscope. Working through trial designs #14 to #20, Dr. Watanabe and Dr. Takeda designed the #21 arthroscope (Fig. 1–7) and described its use in 1960.[50] The Watanabe #21 arthroscope had a diameter of 6.5 mm, a field vision of 100 degrees, and a tungsten light source. It is generally considered that most Americans developed their arthroscopic skill initially with the #21 arthroscope.

The first arthroscopic surgery was performed by Dr. Watanabe on March 9, 1955, when a partially necrotizing xanthomatous giant cell tumor was removed from a patient's knee joint. On February 22, 1961, an osteochondral loose body was extracted arthroscopically after a patellar dislocation, and the first partial meniscectomy was performed by Dr. Watanabe on May 4, 1982.[47,49] Watanabe's original work was published in the *Atlas of Arthroscopy* in 1957, with the second edition (1969) based on 800 cases using the #21 arthroscope.[51] Not yet finished, in 1973 Watanabe presented a preliminary report on the "Selfoc Needlescope," a fiberoptic instrument with a diameter of 2.2 mm and 1.7 mm (Figs. 1–8 and 1–9), useful in the examination of small synovial joints.[49]

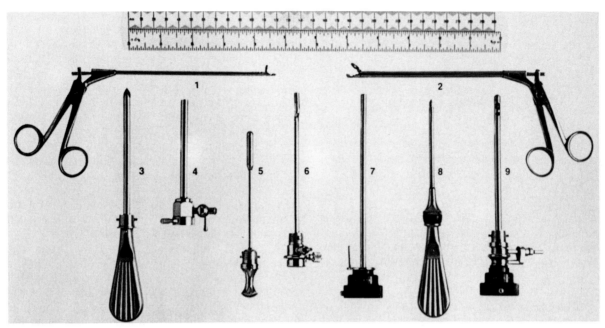

Figure 1—7
The Watanabe No. 21 arthroscope and arthroscopic instruments: biopsy forceps (1,2); trocar (3); sheath (4); obturator (5); bulb carrier (6); direct viewing scope (7); accessory trocar (8); right angle scope (9). (Reproduced with permission from The Upjohn Company and Joyce JJ III: History of arthroscopy. *In* O'Connor RL (ed): Arthroscopy: A Scope Publication. Kalamazoo, MI, The Upjohn Company, 1977.)

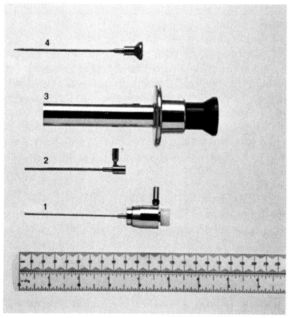

Figure 1—8
The Watanabe Selfoc 2.2-mm arthroscope: objective lens (1); sheath (2); magnifying lens (3); obturator (4); (Reproduced with permission from The Upjohn Company and Joyce JJ III: History of arthroscopy *In* O'Connor RL (ed): Arthroscopy: A Scope Publication. Kalamazoo, MI, The Upjohn Company, 1977.)

The needlescope marked the beginning of the virtual explosion in arthroscopy of the 1970s and 1980s. The tremendous technologic and surgical advances were matched only by the ever-increasing interest of the orthopedic surgeon. In 1968, only 13 surgeons in the United States and Canada owned arthroscopes; by the early 1980s, over 98 percent of orthopedic surgeons used arthroscopy.[27]

Among the few practicing arthroscopists in America in the early 1970s, Robert Jackson was a most active contributor to the field.[28] He presented a review of 200 cases at the combined meeting on arthroscopy in Sydney, Australia, in 1970,[23] and he started to teach courses at the American Academy of Orthopedic Surgeons in 1968.[23] That same year Casscells reviewed 150 arthroscopic cases.[7]

The needlescope of Watanabe that became commercially available in 1972 marked the first in a series of technical innovations that made arthroscopy more worthwhile and popular. In 1973, the first course in arthroscopic surgery in the United States was given at the University of Pennsylvania, chaired by J. Joyce and attended by 75 people.[28] The following year Watanabe was elected the first president of the International Arthroscopy Association.[28] Also at that meeting, closed-circuit television was used for the first time as a teaching tool. J. McGinty gave the first AAOS course in knee arthroscopy utilizing video monitoring in 1975 and later introduced the use of television in performing arthroscopy[32] (Fig. 1–10).

Back in 1972, Lanny Johnson performed his first

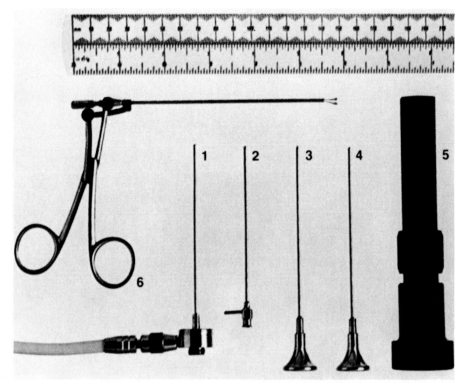

Figure 1–9
   The Watanabe 1.7-mm arthroscope: objective lens (1); sheath (2); trocar (3); obturator (4); magnifying lens (5); biopsy forceps (6). (Reproduced with permission from The Upjohn Company and Joyce JJ III: History of arthroscopy. *In* O'Connor RL (ed): Arthroscopy: A Scope Publication. Kalamazoo, MI, The Upjohn Company, 1977.)

knee arthroscopy using local anesthesia and by 1975 had accumulated 400 such cases.[26] Bircher and Clayton were also advocates of local anesthesia.[27]

In 1974, Richard O'Connor introduced the first rod lens type of operating arthroscope, which has an offset eyepiece to allow for the passage of surgical instruments; this changed the course of arthroscopy, from a diagnostic to a surgical procedure.[23,27,37,41] In 1974, O'Connor removed the first osteochondritic loose body via the arthroscope.[27,37]

In the ensuing few years, O'Connor and H. Ikeuchi of Japan popularized the role of arthroscopy to include meniscectomy and meniscal repairs.[22,37,41] McGinty published their results of total and partial meniscectomies during this time.[33] Arthroscopic meniscal repair introduced by Ikeuchi was further developed by Clancy, Hennings, Mulhollan, and others.[9,11,19] Hennings showed that intrasubstance tears did not heal as well as peripheral tears.[18] As surgical techniques developed in the mid and late 1970s, so did instrumentation. Wolf and Storz developed arthroscopes that supersede the #21 arthroscope of Watanabe because of superior optics and durability. By the late 1970s, the 30-degree, 4-mm arthroscope was the standard[27] (Fig. 1–11). In addition to im-

provements in the arthroscope, the surgical instruments improved. The original instruments were borrowed from neurosurgeons and gynecologists and quickly were developed into newer probes, baskets, and punches with various angles and configurations specifically for knee arthroscopy (Figs. 1–12 and 1–13). New surgical blades were developed for arthroscopic use that are stronger and resist breakage (Fig. 1–14).

Meniscal surgery was not the only surgical technique developed in the 1970s. In 1975, pinning of osteochondritic lesions and in 1978, bone grafting via arthroscopy were developed.[17] In 1976, shelf excisions became quite popular.[18] In that same year Johnson, in conjunction with Dyonics Corporation, introduced the first motorized shaver instruments (Fig. 1–15), which led to the arthroscopic treatment of patellofemoral disorders and degenerative arthritis.[27] The following year Watanabe introduced the first artificial knee joint for arthroscopic teaching purposes.[48]

This time period saw the development of various surgical approaches for knee arthroscopy. From the single portal approach, the development of multiple safe portal approaches was a great aid to operative

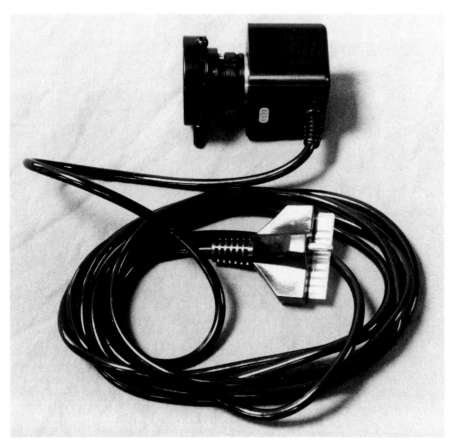

Figure 1–10
Arthroscopic microchip camera.

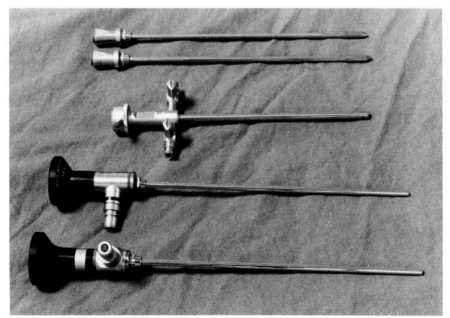

Figure 1–11
Wolf 4-mm 30-degree arthroscope, obturator, and trocars.

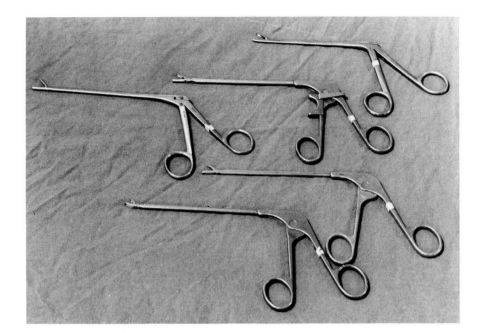

Figure 1–12
Arthroscopic instruments.

arthroscopy. Whipple popularized the polypuncture approach.[52] Gillquist developed the transpatellar tendon approach[26] and Johnson the posteromedial and posterolateral approaches.[15,27] Robert Metcalf popularized posteromedial triangulation, and Patel introduced the proximal approach for the anterior horn of the lateral meniscus.[27]

In 1978, many orthopedists showed lateral retinacular releases to be a worthwhile procedure in treating patellar subluxation.[18,34] Medial retinacular repair for acute dislocation via the arthroscope was developed by Yamamoto,[27] and Austin introduced arthroscopic patellar realignment.[27]

Other arthroscopic procedures developed in the late 1970s and early 1980s include tibial plateau fracture management by Caspari,[27] debridement and synovectomy in arthritic knees,[27] and arthroscopic debridement of septic knees.[18,31]

In 1980 and 1981, Mulhollan and Patel described the complications of arthroscopic surgery, revealing that arthroscopy of the knee is not a benign procedure but must be treated with respect.[36,39]

In 1981, Fox introduced the use of the electrocautery for arthroscopic lateral retinacular release. Whipple, Caspari, Smith, and Nanet investigated the use of lasers in arthroscopic knee surgery.[53,54]

The late 1970s and early 1980s began the era of arthroscopic ligament surgery. Takeda and associates reported on ligament reconstruction under arthroscopic control in 1977.[45] Chandler performed the first anterior cruciate ligament repair. This was followed by Drez performing an arthroscopic reconstruction of the anterior cruciate ligament with fascia lata graft and Dandy performing the first artificial ligament reconstruction using a carbon fiber ligament.[31,34] Presently, arthroscopic ligament recon-

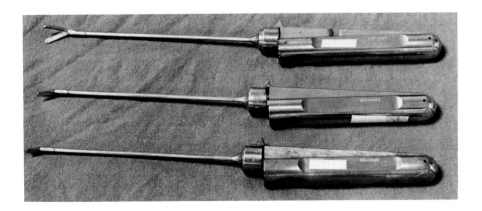

Figure 1–13
Arthroscopic instruments.

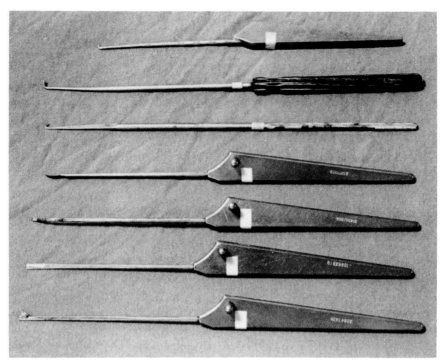

Figure 1–14
Arthroscopic probes and knives.

struction has become popular with the use of autogenous grafts and allografts as well as synthetic artificial ligaments.[13,35,40] Arthroscopic ligament reconstruction has come into its own. With the multitude of techniques, instrumentation, and optics, much of the surgical treatment for knee disorders, once performed open, can now be done entirely arthroscopically. Further refinement in techniques and new and improved instrumentation will be the foundation for the future of arthroscopy.

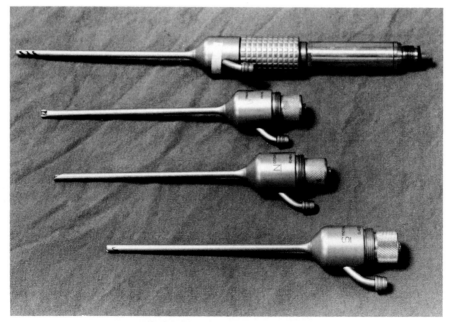

Figure 1–15
Arthroscopic motorized shavers.

References

1. Bircher E: Die Arthroendoskopie. Zentralbl Chir 48:1460, 1921.
2. Burman MS: Arthroscopy, the direct visualization of joints: An experimental cadaver study. J Bone Joint Surg 13A:669, 1931.
3. Burman MS, Finkelstein H, Mayer L: Arthroscopy of the knee joint. J Bone Joint Surg 16A:225, 1934.
4. Burman MS, Finkelstein H, Mayer L: The punch biopsy in the diagnosis of tuberculosis of the knee joint. Am Rev Tuberc 34:5, 1936.
5. Burman MS, Mayer L: Arthroscopic examination of the knee joint. Report of cases observed in the course of arthroscopic examination, including instances of sarcoid and multiple polypoid fibromatosis. Arch Surg 32:846, 1936.
6. Burman MS, Mayer L: Arthroscopy in the diagnosis of meniscal lesions of the knee joint. Am J Surg 43:501, 1939.
7. Casscells SW: Arthroscopy of the knee joint: A review of 150 cases. J Bone Joint Surg 53A:287, 1971.
8. Casscells SW: The early days of arthroscopy in the United States. Arthroscopy 3(2):71–73, 1987.
9. Clancy W, Graf B: Arthroscopic meniscal repair. Orthopedics 6:1125, 1983.
10. Dandy DJ: Arthroscopic Surgery of the Knee. Edinburgh, Churchill-Livingstone, 1981.
11. DeHaven KE: Peripheral meniscal repair as an alternative to meniscectomy. J Bone Joint Surg 63B:463, 1981.
12. Finkelstein H, Mayer L: The arthroscope: A new method of examining joints. J Bone Joint Surg 13A:583, 1931.
13. Fox JM: Arthroscopic insertion of the prosthetic Goretex ligament. In Friedman MJ, Ferkel RD, (eds): Prosthetic Ligament Reconstruction of the Knee. Philadelphia, WB Saunders, 1988, pp 59–64.
14. Fox JM et al: Electrosurgery in orthopedics. Part 1: Principles. Contemp Orthop 8:21, 1984.
15. Gillquist J: Arthroscopic Surgery of the Knee. International Arthroscopic Association Course. Long Beach, CA, Dec 1980.
16. Glinz W: Arthroscopic partial meniscectomy. Helv Chir Acta 47:115, 1980.
17. Guhl JF: Arthroscopic treatment of osteochondritis dissecans. Clin Orthop 167:65–74, 1982.
18. Guhl JF: Evaluation and development of operative arthroscopy, 1974 to present. Orthopedics 6:1104–1109, 1983.
19. Hamberg P, Gillquist J, Lysholm T: Suture of new and old peripheral meniscus tears. J Bone Joint Surg 65A:193, 1983.
20. Hughston JC: A simple meniscectomy. J Sports Med 3:179, 1975.
21. Hurter E: L'arthroscopie, nouvelle methode d'exploration du Genou. Rev Chir Orthop 41:763, 1955.
22. Ikeuchi IT: Paper presented at International Arthroscopy Association Meeting. Copenhagen, Denmark, July 1975.
23. Jackson RW: Memories of the early days of arthroscopy, 1965–1975. Arthroscopy 3(1):1–3, 1987.
24. Jackson RW, Abe I: The role of arthroscopy in the management of disorders of the knee: An analysis of 200 consecutive examinations. J Bone Joint Surg 54B:310, 1972.
25. Jackson RW, Dandy DJ: The history of arthroscopy. In Arthroscopy of the Knee. New York, Grune and Stratton, 1976, pp 1–8.
26. Johnson LL: Arthroscopy of the knee using local anesthesia. A review of 400 patients. J Bone Joint Surg 58A:736, 1976.
27. Johnson LL: Arthroscopic Surgery. St. Louis, CV Mosby, 1986.
28. Joyce JJ: History of the Arthroscopy Association of North America. Arthroscopy 3(4):265–268, 1987.
29. Joyce JJ, Jackson RW: History of Arthroscopy. In AAOS Symposium on Arthroscopy and Arthrography of the Knee. St. Louis, CV Mosby, 1974, pp 1–8.
30. Kreuscher PH: Semilunar cartilage disease: A plea for early recognition by means of the arthroscope and early treatment of this condition. Illinois Med J 47:290, 1925.
31. Mason L: Paper presented at International Arthroscopy Association Meeting. Rio de Janeiro, Sept 1981.
32. McGinty JB: Closed circuit television in arthroscopy. Int Rev Rheumatd 1976, Special Ed, pp 45–49.
33. McGinty JB, Geuss LF, Marvin RA: Partial or total meniscectomy. J Bone Joint Surg 59A:763, 1977.
34. Metcalf RW: An arthroscopic method for lateral release of the subluxating or dislocating patella. Clin Orthop 67:9–18, 1982.
35. Mott WH: Semitendinous anatomic reconstruction for cruciate ligament insufficiency. Clin Orthop 172:9, 1983.
36. Mulhollan JS: Paper presented at Annual Meeting of the American Academy of Orthopedic Surgeons. San Francisco, June 1980.
37. O'Connor RL: Arthroscopy. Philadelphia, JB Lippincott, 1977.
38. Parisien JS, Present DA: Dr. Michael S. Burman, pioneer in the field of arthroscopy. Bull Hosp Joint Dis Orthop Inst 45:119, 1985.

39. Patel S: Paper presented at the Annual Meeting of the American Orthopedic Society of Sports Medicine. Lake Tahoe, NV, 1981.

40. Rusch RM, Nelson EF, and Noel D: Intergraft anterior cruciate ligament reconstruction: Arthroscopic technique. *In* Friedman MJ, Ferkel RD (eds): Prosthetic Ligament Reconstruction of the Knee. Philadelphia, WB Saunders, 1988, pp 59–64.

41. Shahriaree H: O'Connor's Textbook of Arthroscopic Surgery. Philadelphia, JB Lippincott, 1984.

42. Sommer R: Die Endoskopie des Kniegelenkes. Zentralbl Chir 64: 1692, 1937.

43. Takagi K: Practical experience using Takagi's arthroscope. J Jap Orthop Assoc 8:132, 1933.

44. Takagi K: The arthroscope. J Jap Orthop Assoc 14:359, 1939.

45. Takeda S, Mori Y, Maeda Y: Reconstruction of the anterior cruciate ligament under arthroscopic control. Arthroscopy 2:41, 1977.

46. Vaubel E: Die Arthroskopie (Endoskopie des Kniegelenkes): Ein Beitrag zur Diagnostik der Gelenkkrankheiten. *In* Jurgens R (ed): Der Rheumatismus. Vol IX. Dresden, Theodore Steinkopt, 1938.

47. Watanabe M: Arthroscopic diagnosis of the internal derangements of the knee joint. J Jap Orthop Assoc 42:993, 1968.

48. Watanabe M: Arthroscopy: The present state. Orthop Clin North Am 10:505–522, 1979.

49. Watanabe M, Bechtol RC, Nottage WM: History of arthroscopic surgery. *In* Shahriaree, H (ed): O'Connor's Textbook of Arthroscopic Surgery. Philadelphia JB Lippincott, 1984, pp 1–6.

50. Watanabe M, Takeda S: The number 21 arthroscope. J Jap Orthop Assoc 34:1041, 1960.

51. Watanabe M, Takeda S, Ikeuchi H: Atlas of Arthroscopy. 2nd ed. Tokyo, Igaku Shoin Ltd, 1969.

52. Whipple TL, Borsett FH: Arthroscopic examination of the knee. Polypuncture technique with percutaneous intra-articular manipulation. J Bone Joint Surg 60A:444, 1978.

53. Whipple TL, Caspari RB, Meyers JF: Laser energy in arthroscopic meniscectomy. Orthopedics 6:1165, 1983.

54. Whipple TL, Caspari RB, Meyers JF: Arthroscopic laser meniscectomy in a gas medium. Arthroscopy 1:2, 1985.

2

Jonathan L. Glashow
Richard Katz
Morton Schneider
W. Norman Scott
Diagnostic Imaging of the Knee

Diagnosis of soft tissue injuries in and about the knee is a challenging problem. Physical examination and plain radiographs during initial evaluation are essential, but not always exact, in ascertaining an accurate clinical diagnosis. Historically, minimally invasive roentgenographic procedures have had mixed results. Single- and double-contrast arthrography and postarthrographic high-resolution computed tomography (CT) scans have been fairly accurate, but their limitations and disadvantages in relation to arthroscopy are profound. Still in its infancy, magnetic resonance imaging (MRI) has demonstrated great potential for evaluating knee joint disorders. Advantages include excellent soft tissue delineations without the need for contrast medium or exposure to ionizing radiation. Although diagnostic arthroscopy is exceptionally accurate, it is not always indicated; thus, it behooves the knee surgeon to be thoroughly familiar with the various imaging techniques.

ARTHROGRAPHY

Arthrography of the knee was first performed nearly a century ago; only recently has it become a safe, simple, radiographic examination widely available to the orthopedic surgeon.[13,14,32,39,59] The initial knee arthrograms reported by Werndorff and Robinson came only 10 years after the discovery of the x-ray by Roentgen.[26] Gas arthrography was popularized during the 1920s and 1930s but later lost acceptance when reports of near-fatal pulmonary emboli were published.[26,39] Later in the 1930s iodinated

contrast materials were tried, but they were discontinued after they proved too toxic.[26] Not until the 1940s were water-soluble contrast materials introduced, and Lindbloom established the safety and reliability of arthrography using the single positive contrast technique.[26] In the past 35 years, advances in arthrography have been made mostly in the knee. Double-contrast horizontal beam arthrography was first made popular in the 1960s by Freiberger.

The fluoroscopic double-contrast spot filming technique proved advantageous for the examination of menisci and articular cartilage and is currently in use today.[13,14,26] Knee arthrography is the most frequently performed arthrogram; it requires precise attention to detail and technical skill. Although double-contrast arthrography is the study of choice for menisci, articular cartilage, and the cruciate ligaments, single-contrast arthrograms are occasionally made for the examination of synovial abnormalities or loose bodies.[5,13,14]

MENISCI

The normal medial meniscus is larger posteriorly than anteriorly and is attached to the capsule along its entire periphery. Viewed in vertical cross-section, the medial meniscus is triangular with the apex directed centrally. The base of the triangle is formed by the capsular attachment of the meniscus, and the sides of the triangle by the articular surfaces of the meniscus (Fig. 2–1). The arthrogram demonstrates a thin layer of positive contrast coating the meniscus, surrounded by air. No contrast medium enters the

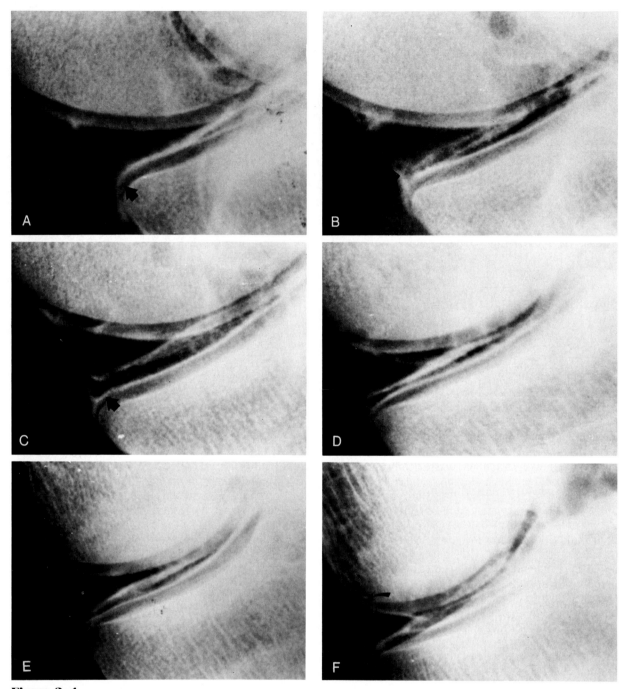

Figure 2–1
  On double-contrast arthrogram, sequential views of a normal medial meniscus from posterior to anterior (*A–L*). No air or contrast is seen within the substance of the meniscus. The tibial attachment can be seen outlined with air and contrast (*A,B,C*) (arrows). The posterior segment is wider than the anterior segment. The meniscocapsular junction is seen well at the mid and posterior portions filled with positive contrast (*F,G*).

body of the meniscus or the meniscocapsular junction. The lax capsular attachments of the meniscus, starting at the meniscosynovial junction, form shallow troughs, or recesses. These recesses are well visualized on vertical section (Fig. 2–1*A,B,C*). Contrast material at the meniscocapsular attachment may be projected overlying the meniscus and must

not be misinterpreted for oblique or horizontal meniscal tears. It is often quite difficult to make this distinction, which is a frequent cause of false-positive diagnosis of a horizontal or oblique meniscal tear.[25]
  Knee arthrography is of great value in the evaluation of meniscal tears. Tears may be classified as ver-

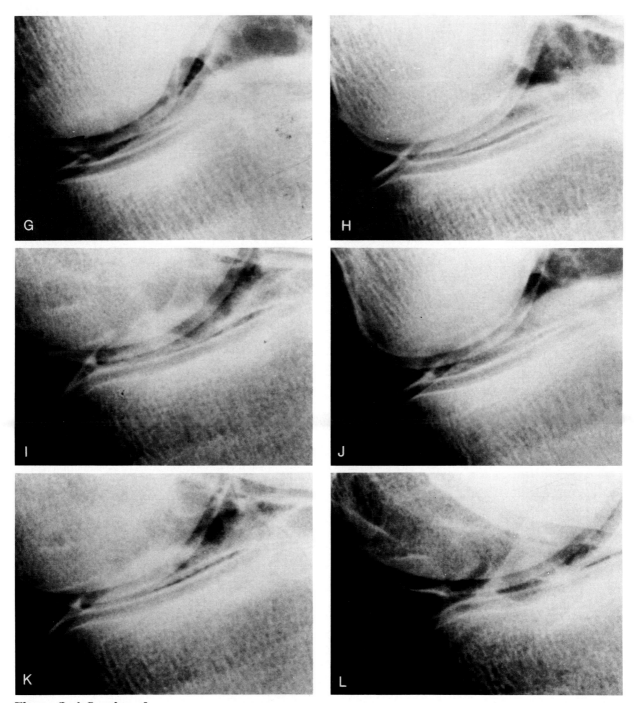

Figure 2–1 *Continued*

tical, horizontal, radial, oblique, or complex (combining several features). The arthrographic appearance of a tear varies depending on location, technique, projection, and the degree of fragment displacement. Vertical concentric tears split the meniscus into central and peripheral portions. When the fragments remain in close contact, contrast material appears as a thin, radiopaque line. With separation, air and positive contrast material can be seen within the tear. Occasionally the central fragment may be com-

pletely displaced within the center of the joint (bucket handle tear), and the remaining meniscus appears as a blunted edge. Parrot beak and vertical radial tears divide the meniscus into anterior and posterior portions and are best seen on tangential views (Figs. 2–2, 2–3).

Horizontal tears can be seen as lines of contrast within the meniscus substance. They split the meniscus into superior and inferior segments (Figs. 2–4, 2–5). Frequently meniscal tears are complex, and

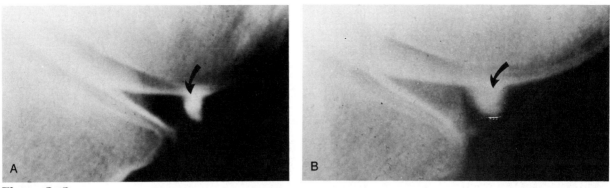

Figure 2–2

A, A vertical tear splits the peripheral posterior horn of the medial meniscus (arrows), a common site for these tears. *B,* Contrast medium can be seen entering the separation between the fragments (arrows).

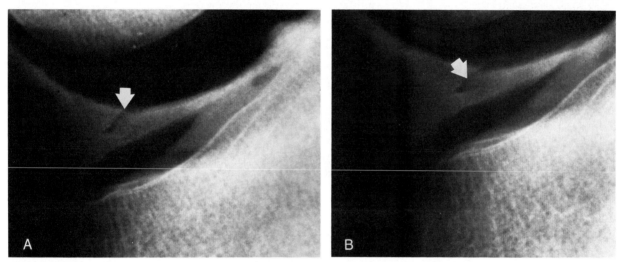

Figure 2–3

A, A vertical (parrot beak) type of tear extending into the anterior horn of the lateral meniscus. *B,* The tear is best seen in this tangential view utilizing double-contrast arthrography.

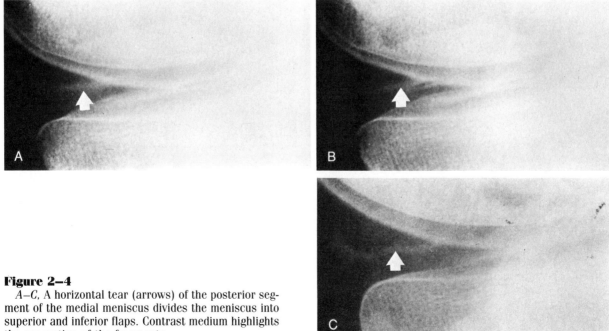

Figure 2–4

A–C, A horizontal tear (arrows) of the posterior segment of the medial meniscus divides the meniscus into superior and inferior flaps. Contrast medium highlights the separation of the fragments.

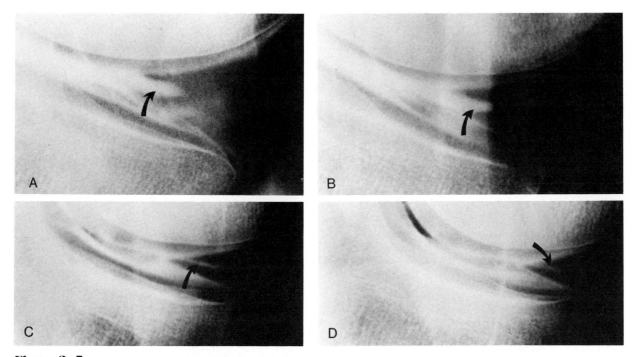

Figure 2–5
A–D, Multiple views of a horizontal tear involving the posterior horn of the lateral meniscus with slight separation of the fragments. This tear can be distinguished from the normal popliteal sleeve, which is anterior and cannot be seen on this view.

multiple linear aberrations may be seen extending throughout the meniscus (Fig. 2–6). Degenerative menisci demonstrate central edge opacification as multiple minute tears allow contrast material to enter.

Meniscal cysts can be demonstrated arthrographically when the associated tear (usually horizontal or oblique) communicates with the cyst, most frequently in the anterior half of the lateral meniscus and less commonly in the posterior half of the medial menis-

cus. The lateral meniscus is uniform in shape in its anteroposterior dimension and is attached to the capsule along its anterior two thirds (Fig. 2–7). The posterior margin is crowded at its periphery by the popliteal tendon, and its bursa normally fills with contrast medium (Fig. 2–7*B,C,D*). This frequently may be misinterpreted as a tear. As a result of its circular shape, the anterior and posterior attachments of the lateral meniscus are deep within the knee and are impossible to evaluate with arthrogra-

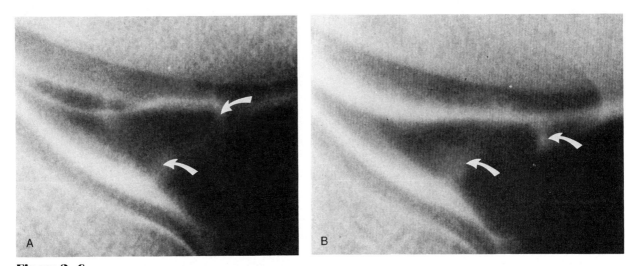

Figure 2–6
A and *B,* Two views of a complex tear of the posterior horn of the medial meniscus with vertical, horizontal and oblique fissures extending throughout.

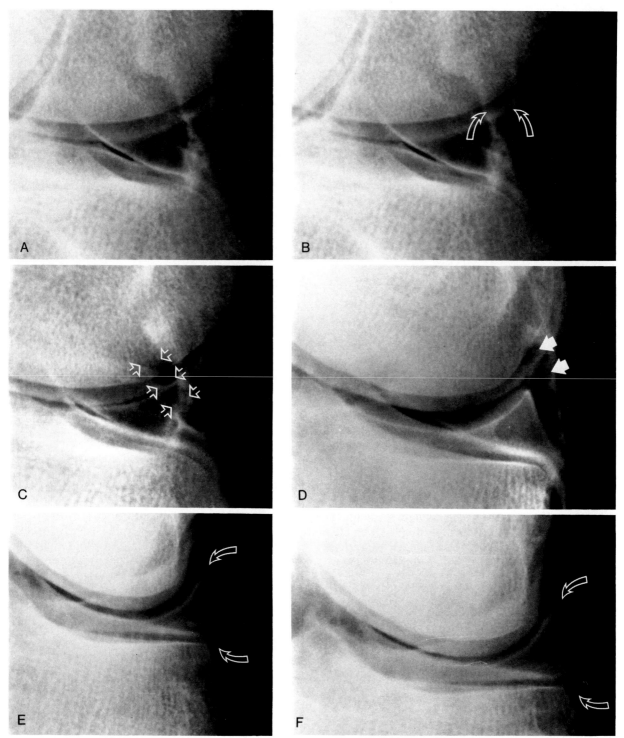

Figure 2–7
See legend on opposite page.

phy. The anterior fat pad is seen quite well overlying the anterior horns of the menisci on lateral projection and is often a cause of a false-positive meniscal reading.[26]

The abnormal shape of a discoid lateral meniscus is easily visualized, but distinction between partial and complete states is difficult (Fig. 2–8). Evaluation

of the posterior horn of the lateral meniscus is particularly unreliable because of the overlying popliteal sleeve that normally fills with contrast material. Peripheral separations are rare in this location, while vertical concentric or longitudinal tears in this region often go undetected.[13,14,25] The accuracy with which meniscal pathology may be demonstrated ranges

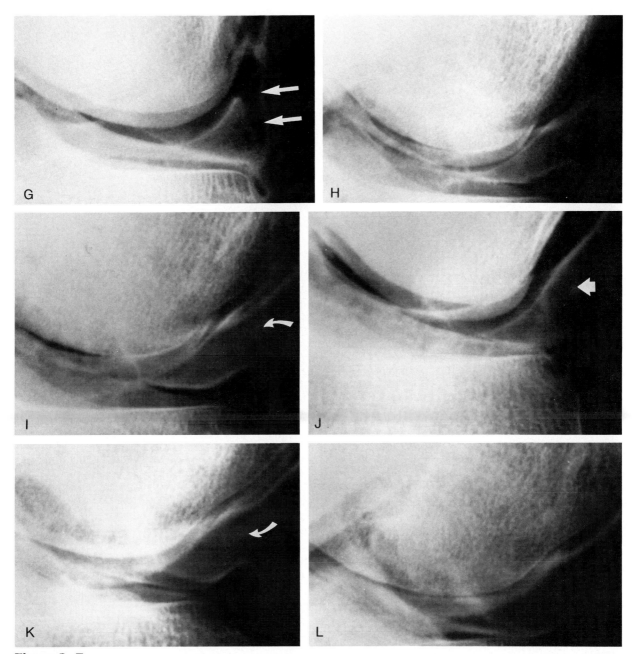

Figure 2–7
Serial views of a normal lateral meniscus viewed from posterior to anterior. The capsular attachments are more lax than the medial mensicus and can be seen filling with contrast medium along the anterior attachment of the meniscus. The small radiodense spots (arrows) represent collections of contrast material within lymphatic channels and should not be confused with a tear (I,J,K). The posterior attachments of the lateral meniscus are complex and have normal defects (arrows) (E,F,G). The popliteus tendon can be seen interrupting the superior capsular attachment crossing the posterior horn (arrows); contrast medium normally fills this bursa (B,C,D). Owing to its more C-shaped contour, the inner border lies deeper within the knee and is more difficult to evaluate with arthrography.

from 68 to 95 percent, depending upon the technique, the location of the tear, and the radiologist's experience. Meniscus tears found at surgery but not seen on arthrography remain a serious concern. These false-negatives most frequently occur in evaluation of the lateral meniscus. False-positive results are rare.

The collateral and cruciate ligaments are extrasynovial, and thus their evaluation by arthrography is indirect.[13,14,42–44] Medial collateral and capsular tears allow leakage of contrast from the joint into the surrounding soft tissues (Fig. 2–9). Small tears may seal over within a few days and are easily missed. The lateral ligaments are separated from the capsule

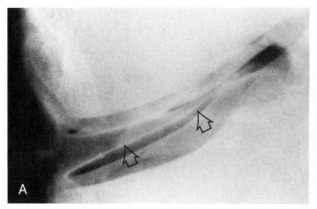

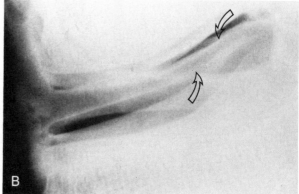

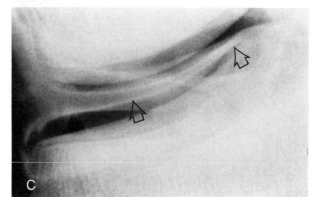

Figure 2–8

A–C, The abnormally broad appearance of a discoid lateral meniscus. The inner apex is seen extending deep within the center of the knee. Tears of the inner margin may be symptomatic but are difficult to diagnose with arthrography.

and thus not seen during arthrography. Evaluation of the cruciate ligaments has been less exacting. The arthrogram reveals the synovia-covered free margins of the normal cruciate ligaments.[1] The intact anterior cruciate ligament is seen as a linear radiopaque band extending from the distal femur to the anterior proximal tibia. The posterior aspect of the posterior cruciate ligament is a contrast band sloping posteriorly and inferiorly from the distal femur to the posterior

margin of the proximal tibia. The ligaments cross and form a triangle of contrast.

Failure to visualize a contrast band in the region of the normal anterior cruciate ligament should be interpreted as an abnormal finding, especially in the presence of a normal posterior cruciate ligament. A wavy, bowed, or irregular contrast margin indicates a torn ligament with intact synovium.[13] Partial tears are almost impossible to diagnose. Isolated posterior

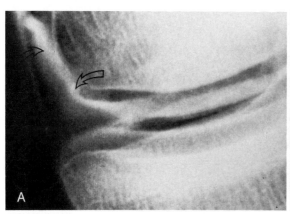

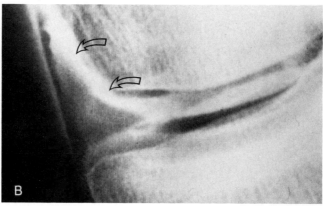

Figure 2–9

A and *B,* Double contrast arthrogram demonstrating extravasation of dye at the meniscocapsular junction at the mid-posterior portion of the medial meniscus, indicating a peripheral separation of the medial meniscus with a tear of the deep medial collateral ligament. The dye appears as a linear streak (arrows) walled off from the surrounding soft tissues by an intact superficial medial collateral ligament.

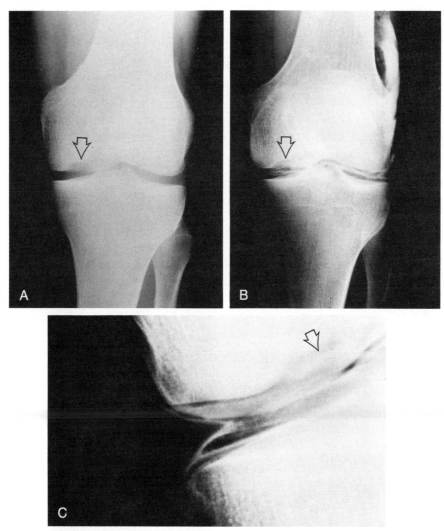

Figure 2–10
     An articular defect of the medial femoral condyle with separation
of the osteochondral fragment. *A*, A plain AP radiograph; *B* and *C* are
of the corresponding arthrogram.

cruciate ligament disruptions may result in the non-visualization of the posterior cruciate ligament with a normal-appearing anterior cruciate ligament. The failure to demonstrate either ligament may occur when both ligaments are damaged, and this failure must not be dismissed as faulty technique.

Arthrographic demonstration of the cruciate ligaments has been considered by many to be unreliable.[13,14,26,39] Often associated hemarthrosis hinders visualization. A few experienced arthrographers report up to 91 percent accuracy, but most workers place their accuracy rate in the 50 to 75 percent range.[14,20,26,39,41,44,59] Few data are available on the accuracy of evaluation of the posterior cruciate ligament by conventional arthrography or postarthrographic CT, although rates as high as 91 percent have been reported.

Osteochondritis dissecans usually can be visualized on plain radiographs as a lucent defect in sub-chondral bone. Arthrography is helpful in determining whether the overlying cartilage is intact or displaced (Fig. 2–10) and whether there is an associated meniscal tear, which is frequently present.[70]

Since the introduction of double-contrast arthrography in 1931, controversy has existed as to whether single- or double-contrast arthrography is the preferred method for diagnosing meniscal injuries. The proponents of single contrast point to its simplicity in both performing the examination and its interpretation.[64] Others point out the preference for single contrast in the evaluation of loose bodies and synovial masses, citing interference by air bubbles with the double-contrast technique. Those who prefer double-contrast arthrography believe it is more accurate and especially valuable in the evaluation of the cruciate ligaments and articular cartilage derangements[44,45,64] (Fig. 2–11).

High-resolution computed tomography (HRCT) has

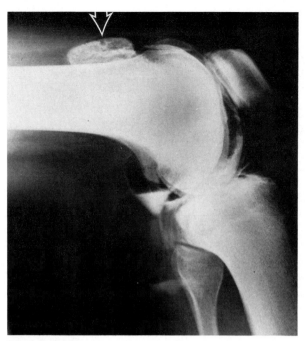

Figure 2–11

A lateral projection of a large loose body (arrow) in the suprapatellar pouch on a double-contrast arthrogram. Air surrounded by contrast medium coats this radiopaque loose body. Air surrounded by contrast alone may be mistaken for a small loose body, and some recommend the use of single-contrast arthrography to identify loose bodies.[64]

been used successfully in the diagnosis of meniscal tears. When compared with arthroscopic findings, accuracy rates as high as 91 percent have been reported[13,14,16] (Figs. 2–12 through 2–15).

The major advantages of HRCT as compared with arthroscopy are: (1) it is noninvasive, requiring no injection of contrast media; (2) the examination is not hindered by the presence of effusion or hemarthrosis; (3) the posterior horn of the lateral meniscus is better visualized, avoiding confusion with the overlying popliteus tendon; (4) the anatomic detail of the type and location is more precisely evaluated; and (5) the study may be performed without special preparation, usually within 20 to 30 minutes.[16] The disadvantages include (1) the inability to detect nondisplaced meniscal tears; (2) lack of visualization of the cruciate ligaments; (3) difficulty in positioning the patient with an acute knee injury; and (4) the cost of a HRCT examination, which is about twice that of conventional arthrography.

HRCT has been combined with conventional double-contrast arthrography to offer more precise detail of the menisci, cruciate ligaments, and articular cartilage.[16] Advantages include (1) exact delineation of the region of the posterior horns of the menisci, differentiating peripheral separation from lax meniscocapsular attachment; (2) visualization of the articular cartilage, especially in the patellofemoral

compartment; and (3) imaging of the intra-articular ligaments. The disadvantages of HRCT combined with arthrography are (1) the invasiveness of the procedure; (2) exposure to ionizing radiation; (3) difficulty encountered in the presence of acute hemarthrosis; (4) difficulty with the patient with a locked knee or other acute injury, as with conventional arthrography and plain HRCT positioning; and (5) time consuming and costly (about 500 dollars) for HRCT combined with arthrography (Figs. 2–12 through 2–15).

Although the advantages of arthrography (alone or combined with CT) have been outlined here, its usefulness and reliability in light of the advent and availability of MRI are limited at best. As MRI technology improves and scan times as well as cost decline, we expect that MRI will replace arthrography as the imaging mode of choice for internal derangements of the knee. MRI is a new, noninvasive diagnostic tool that has already shown promise in the diagnosis of musculoskeletal pathology and has numerous advantages over conventional imaging techniques.

The first reports of magnetic resonance imaging of normal knee anatomy were published in 1983,[36,37,50,51] and shortly thereafter images of normal and abnormal menisci and cruciate and collateral ligaments were available. In 1984, development of the solenoid surface coil for the knee dramatically improved the signal-to-noise ratio and played a key role in improving spatial resolution.[33] This then allowed depiction of a wide range of disorders, including meniscal tears, ligament injuries, synovial dis-

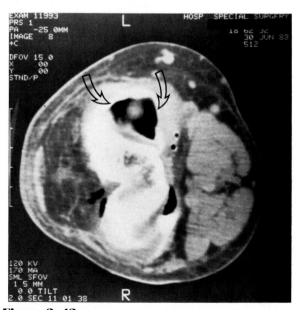

Figure 2–12

A high-resolution CT arthrogram demonstrating a normal medial meniscus. Contrast material coats the sharp, clear inner border of the meniscus while air is seen in the center of the medial joint compartment.

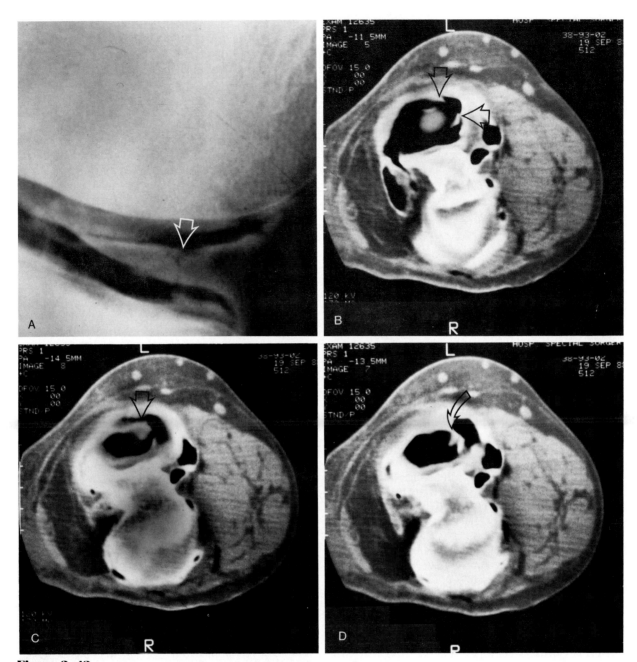

Figure 2–13

A, A double-contrast arthrogram demonstrating a vertical tear of the posterior horn of the medial meniscus (arrow). *B–D,* Corresponding CT arthrogram views of this tear show it to be radial in nature, with fragmentation and displacement of the inner flap into the joint (arrows).

orders, osteochondritis dissecans, bone marrow abnormalities, and soft tissue and bony tumors.

Unlike arthrography, MRI allows direct multiplanar imaging without the need for manipulation, and the presence of an effusion does not detract from imaging quality. Furthermore, its extreme sensitivity in detecting pathologic conditions makes MRI an ideal addition to the arthroscopists' preoperative armamentarium, pinpointing the site of pathology and possibly altering the approach to treatment.

FUNDAMENTALS OF IMAGE FORMATION

The basis for magnetic resonance imaging is the response of protons to an external magnetic field. Protons exist in nature (as hydrogen atoms in tissues), spinning about an axis like a toy top. At equilibrium, all protons are spinning in different directions with a resultant magnetic vector of zero. When

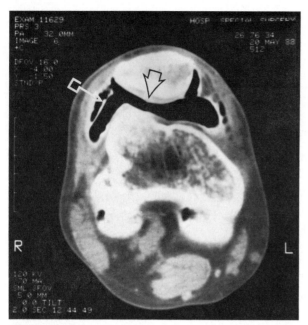

Figure 2–14
This HRCT double-contrast arthrogram illustrates a small medial plica (thin arrow) as well as a small defect in the articular surface of the patella (broad arrow).

protons are subjected to an external magnetic field, they wobble or precess in a particular orientation proportional to the strength of that magnetic field, thus creating a net magnetic vector.

During magnetic resonance imaging, the protons are subjected to radiowaves and are excited to a higher energy level. After the radiofrequency pulse is turned off, the protons return to their previous energy state and emit their own radiowaves in a process known as relaxation. These radiowaves are detected by a receiving coil and are converted into images by computers. The excitation-relaxation cycle must be repeated many times before a sufficient number of signals are acquired to generate an image.

Relaxation time includes both the loss of energy to neighboring molecules (T_1) and return to randomness among adjacent protons (T_2).[23,29,37,38,51] These two processes are independent of each other and are tissue specific. The time between radiofrequency pulses is defined as repetition time (TR), and the time between each administered pulse and sampling of the returning relaxation signal is known as the echo time (TE).[23,29,37,38] TR and TE are measured in milliseconds and can be varied independently by the operator, therefore creating an infinitely possible number of image sequences. Depending on the pulse parameters selected, images may reflect a T_1-weighted or T_2-weighted relaxation image.

T_1-weighted images have a short TE (<30 milliseconds) and short TR (<800 milliseconds), whereas T_2-weighted images have a relatively long TE (>60 milliseconds) and TR (>1500). Imaging sequences have

been developed to clarify specific anatomic areas within the knee, but, in general, T_1-weighted images are used to show basic anatomic structures, while T_2-weighted images are useful to define further a given structure and to allow for better contrast from the surrounding tissues.[17]

Within the most-used range of T_1- and T_2-weighted images about the knee, the relative signal intensity of most structures remains constant. In order of decreasing brightness, they are fat, medullary bone, articular cartilage, muscles, ligaments, tendons, menisci, and cortical bone. MRI has gained much appeal in its recently demonstrated ability to visualize the semilunar cartilages. Owing to the dearth of free H^+ ions within fibrocartilage, the normal meniscus appears as a homogeneously black structure with well-defined borders. The C-shaped menisci have characteristic images in both the coronal and sagittal planes (Figs. 2–16, 2–17), with the medial meniscus demonstrating a larger anterior horn and the lateral meniscus displaying a more equal anterior and posterior horn dimension.

The relationship of the menisci to the tibia must be

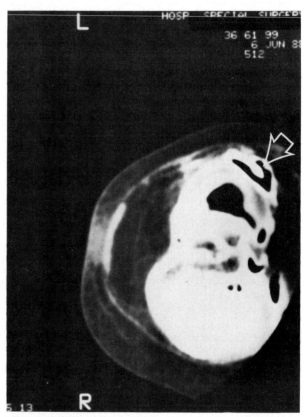

Figure 2–15
A normal-appearing lateral meniscus on an HRCT arthrogram. Note its more circular shape as compared with the medial meniscus, making its inner margin deep within the knee and difficult to visualize on plain arthrography. The arrow points to the popliteal sleeve where air and positive contrast are seen surrounding the popliteal tendon.

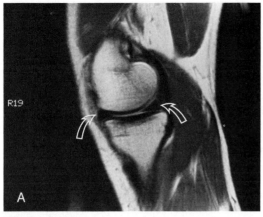
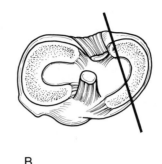
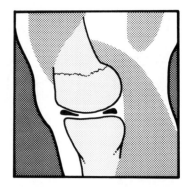

Figure 2–16

A, A normal-appearing medial meniscus on a medial parasagittal view demonstrating the smooth-contoured borders and uniform density of both the anterior and posterior horns. *B,* A schematic illustration showing the section cut of *A.*

evaluated. Normally the peripheral edge of the posterior horn of the medial meniscus extends to within 3 millimeters of the tibial articular cartilage; if this relationship is distorted, one must examine for the possibility of peripheral separation. In addition, the presence of high-intensity signal between the normally tightly bound medial meniscus and deep medial collateral ligament and capsule should alert one to the possibility of peripheral separation as well. Because of increased mobility, the lateral meniscus maintains a less consistent relationship with the tibial plateau, and interference by the popliteal hiatus makes the diagnosis of peripheral separation difficult; however, the fascicular attachments of the lateral meniscus to the capsule can be demonstrated on T_2-weighted sagittal images.

MRI Evaluation of Meniscal Tears

Meniscal tears may be classified by morphology, location, and grade. Location and morphologic description are similar to those described earlier with arthrography, but grading is unique to MRI.

The normal internal substance of knee menisci produces no signal on either T_1- or T_2-weighted images. Meniscal tears and degenerative changes within the meniscus produce signal intensity on T_1- and T_2-weighted images. According to Reicher and Crues, the intrameniscal signal on T_1-weighted images is thought to be secondary to degenerative changes exposing surfaces of macromolecules (within the meniscus) that adsorb water and increase local spin density.[37,49,50] Others have suggested that

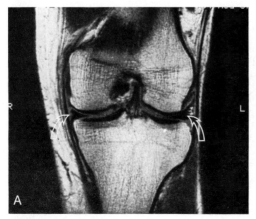
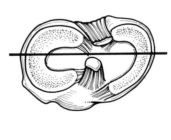
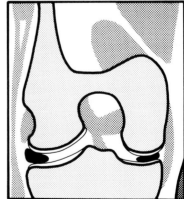

Figure 2–17

A and *B,* Normal-appearing anatomy and schematic of a T1-weighted coronal image of both medial and lateral menisci. Note the clarity and definition of the midportion of both menisci. The entire course of the medial collateral ligament is well seen from its origin to its insertion as a dark, well-defined homogeneous band. The joint capsule next to the medial collateral ligament appears as a bright signal. Contrast this image with Figures 2–29 and 2–30, in which medial collateral ligament is disrupted.

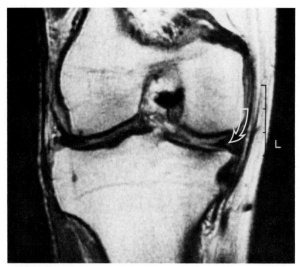

Figure 2–18
T1-weighted coronal section of a parrot beak type of tear at the junction of the body and posterior horn of the medial meniscus. A bright signal can be seen extending to the articular surface, making this a Grade III tear.

the cause of high-intensity signal within the meniscus on T_2-weighted images is the presence of synovial fluid within the tear.[37,63] Stoller and others have correlated the MRI signal present within menisci to histopathologic changes, but this is beyond the discussion of this chapter.

We have adapted a grading system from the work of Crues and Reicher: Grade 0 is a normal, homogeneous black meniscus; a Grade I abnormality shows one or several punctate bright signal densities well within the body of the meniscus; a Grade II tear is a linear signal change through the central portion of the meniscus without extension to an articular surface; a Grade III tear is a linear signal that extends into either the superior or inferior articular margin of the meniscus; and a Grade IV tear is characterized by gross distortion of the meniscal shape.[17]

While Grade III and IV tears are easily visualized at arthroscopy, Grade II tears are often found to extend to the surface when the meniscus is probed.[17,35,37] Reicher points out that intrasubstance tears on MRI not visualized on arthroscopy may be symptomatic, especially in the peripheral one third of the meniscus, and are frequently a cause of false-positive magnetic resonance readings. Although the accuracy of MRI in detecting meniscal abnormalities depends upon the experience of the examiner, accuracy has exceeded 90 percent in recent reports.[47,57,63] Most workers agree that magnetic resonance imaging is the most sensitive test in the evaluation of meniscal tears, and Reicher and associates found the negative predictive value of MRI to be nearly 100 percent[49,50] (Figs. 2–18 through 2–21).

Anterior Cruciate Ligament

The anterior cruciate ligament (ACL) arises from the medial aspect of the lateral femoral condyle and extends anteromedially to insert into the tibial spine. The anterior cruciate ligament is 4 centimeters long and 1 centimeter wide; it consists of two main fiber bundles—the larger anterior medial band and smaller posterolateral band—and lies within the knee in an extrasynovial compartment.

The clinical diagnosis of a torn ACL is especially difficult in the acute setting, and although various clinical tests have been described to aid in making this diagnosis, radiographs alone are of no aid except when a bony avulsion is present. Early reports of evaluation by arthrography revealed a 50 to 75 percent accuracy range. Subsequent attempts to improve diagnoses with and without the addition of CT have yielded somewhat better results, yet the test is invasive, difficult to perform, and hindered often by the presence of a large effusion.[8,13,39,41]

Using MRI, the status of the anterior cruciate ligament is best assessed with the knee in full extension and in 20 degrees of external rotation. Multiple coronal and sagittal images in both T_1- and T_2-weighted imaging sequences are performed.

The normal anterior cruciate ligament appears as a homogeneous dark band extending in continuity through the long axis of the ligament from origin to insertion (Fig. 2–22). The MRI appearance of a torn anterior cruciate ligament depends on the age and location of the lesion and the degree of disruption. A complete acute tear is seen on both T_1- and T_2-weighted images as a bright signal intensity within

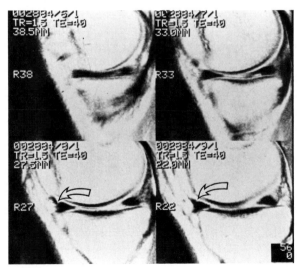

Figure 2–19
Four parasagittal sections of a Grade III meniscal tear involving the medial meniscus. A bright signal can be seen within the normally dark meniscus, blunting the anterior horn.

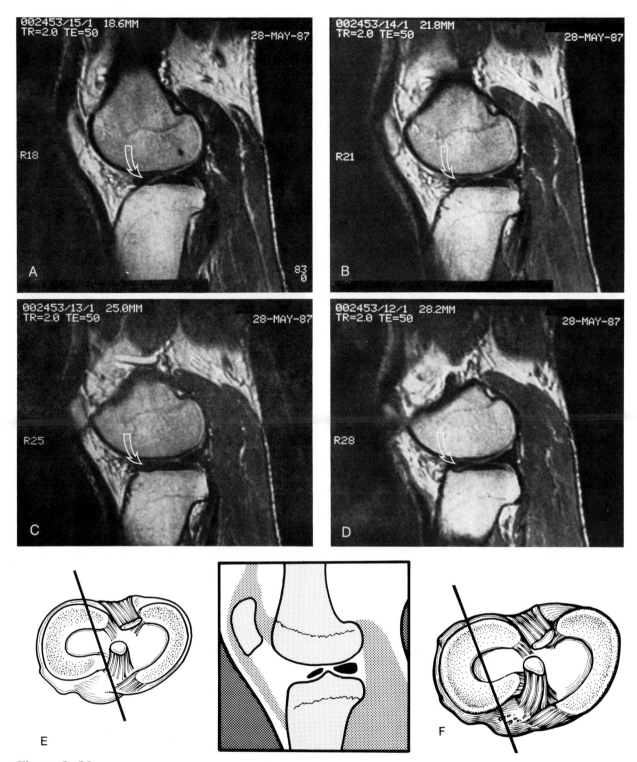

Figure 2–20

Multiple T2-weighted sagittal images and schematics of a complex radial tear of the anterior horn of the medial meniscus. A bright signal is seen within the midsubstance of the meniscus extending to the periphery, making this a Grade III tear. *E*, A schematic drawing corresponding to the level of the cut in image *A; F* corresponds to image *D*.

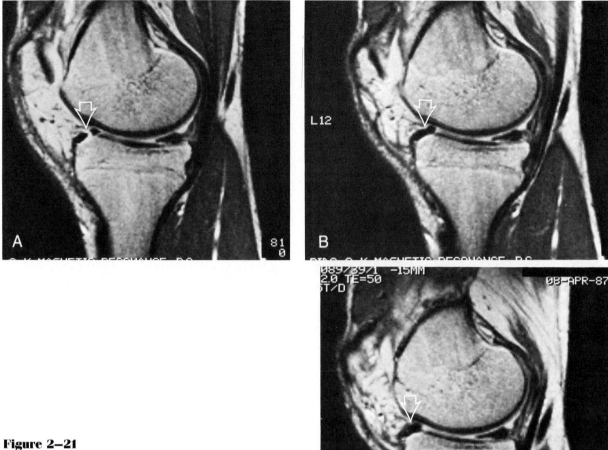

Figure 2–21

Multiple sagittal sections demonstrating a bucket handle tear of the medial meniscus (arrows). Bright signal within the normally dark meniscus indicates the presence of synovial fluid within the substance of the meniscus. Gross distortion of the anterior horn makes this a Grade IV type of tear.

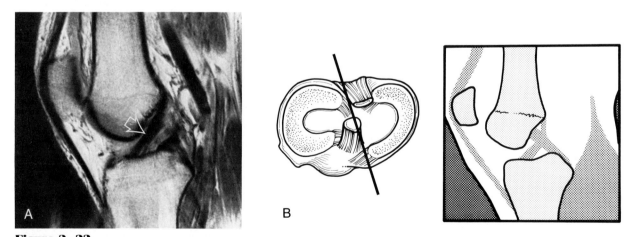

Figure 2–22

A and *B,* A normal-appearing anterior cruciate ligament and schematic on midsagittal section. A dark, homogeneous density can be traced throughout the normal course of the anterior cruciate ligament, indicating an intact ligament. This section is cut in about 20 degrees of external rotation to view the entire anterior cruciate ligament on one image.

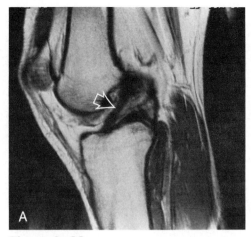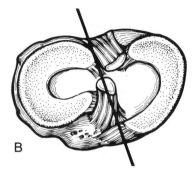

Figure 2–23

An MRI and schematic of a midsubstance tear of the anterior cruciate ligament, identified by interruption of the homogeneous dark signal by an area of brightness within its middle third.

the ligament substance. T_2-weighted sagittal images may show a wavy, irregular anterior margin, indicating a complete tear (Fig. 2–23). Complete chronic tears may be seen as a small remnant of tissue in the area where the anterior cruciate ligament is normally found, often obscured by fat and scar tissue within the intercondylar notch on sagittal images (Fig. 2–24). We have not found coronal imaging to be very helpful in assessing the integrity of the cruciate ligaments.

Clinically significant partial anterior cruciate ligament tears are less reliably detected on magnetic resonance imaging. Criteria for the establishment of partial tears have not been rigidly established, but many parameters are under investigation, including the ratio of maximum signal intensity of anterior cruciate ligament to posterior cruciate ligament, the scope of the anterior cruciate ligament on T_2-weighted sagittal imaging, and the ratio of maximum to minimum width of the anterior cruciate ligament on both T_1 and T_2 sagittal images. The MRI diagnosis of a partial ACL disruption is quite difficult, but, with further improvements in equipment and in imaging techniques, we will be able to make this diagnosis more accurately in the years to come[17] (Fig. 2–25).

The posterior cruciate ligament (PCL) takes origin from the lateral aspect of the medial femoral condyle and fans out in a posterolateral fashion, inserting into the intercondylar region of the tibia.

The posterior cruciate ligament is shorter, thicker and wider than the anterior cruciate ligament. With the knee in slight external rotation, it is seen on a single sagittal image in 95 percent of patients. Because of its size and location, the posterior cruciate ligament is easier to image than the anterior cruciate ligament[17] (Fig. 2–26).

Acute and chronic posterior cruciate ligament disruptions appear as areas of increased signal intensity within the normally dark image on T_1- and T_2-weighted views. The ligament may be broader, suggesting loss of integrity. In acute tears, hemorrhage and edema appear as bright foci on T_2-weighted sagittal views. In chronic tears, fibrous scar tissue replaces the normal substance of the posterior cruciate ligament and may yield little or no increased signal intensity, or alternately may appear as a homogeneous band of increased signal intensity running throughout the entire ligament. As in the anterior cruciate ligament, partial tears are difficult to diagnose. Loss of signal from underlying subchondral bone suggests avulsion of overlying ligament and is often helpful when the ligament is disrupted but re-

Figure 2–24

T2-weighted midsagittal section of a chronic anterior cruciate ligament–deficient knee. The normally dark band seen in this view is replaced by fat and scar tissue, giving the ill-defined, distorted appearance in the region of the intercondylar notch.

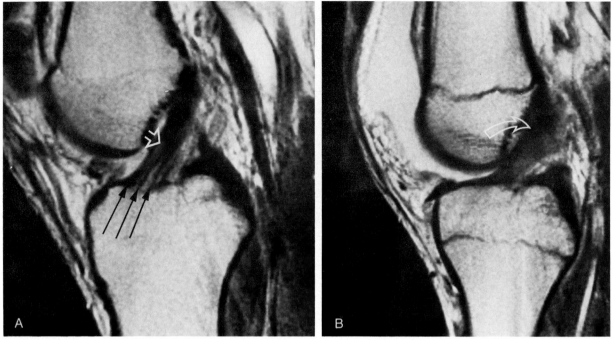

Figure 2–25
Two examples of partial anterior cruciate ligament disruptions on T2-weighted sagittal images. *A* demonstrates three distinct fiber bundles (triple arrows) attaching to the tibia with loss of their definition in midsubstance where the ligament was found torn (arrow). *B* illustrates an area of increased signal in midsubstance, the site of partial disruption in this acute knee injury.

mains closely applied to tibia or femur[36] (Figs. 2–27, 2–28).

The medial collateral ligament arises from the medial femoral epicondyle and inserts onto the medial aspect of the tibia approximately 5 to 7 centimeters below the joint line. It is composed of the superficial medial collateral ligament, which extends the entire course, and the deep medial collateral ligament, which is the thickened medial capsule attaching to the middle one third of the meniscus. The two

layers are separated by an interligamentous bursa that allows for motion between the two.

The superficial medial collateral ligament appears as a thin, straight dark band from the medial femoral condyle to the proximal tibia on T_1- and T_2-weighted coronal images. Frequently the interligamentous bursa and surrounding fat are seen superimposed, and their bright signal should not be mistaken for a meniscocapsular separation.

A complete tear is seen as a loss in continuity of

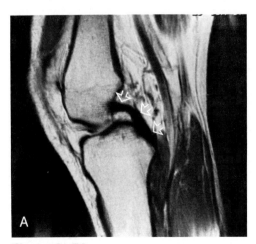

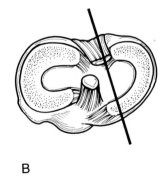

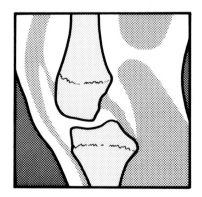

Figure 2–26
The normal appearance of the posterior cruciate ligament and schematic on sagittal view. A dark, homogeneous signal can be traced from femoral to tibial attachment.

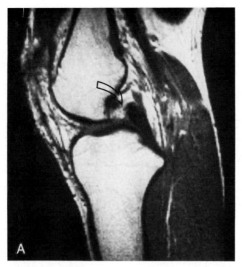
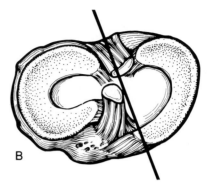

Figure 2—27
A chronic tear of the posterior cruciate ligament and schematic, as evidenced by disruption of the homogeneous dark band running from the posterolateral aspect of the medial femoral condyle to the posterior aspect of the tibia on a T2-weighted sagittal image.

the dark band, with a bright signal intensity in the precise area of disruption on T_2-weighted images. Frequently in acute tears surrounding edema and hemorrhage displace the surrounding fat, resulting in a decrease in signal on T_1-weighted images and an increase in T_2-weighted images. Chronic tears may manifest as a thickened, buckled, and homogeneously ill-defined low signal band in the region of the medial collateral ligament (Figs. 2–29, 2–30).

The complex anatomy of the lateral side of the knee

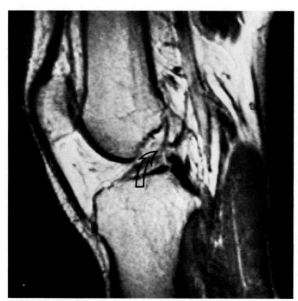

Figure 2—28
A chronic tear of the posterior cruciate ligament from its origin on the femur. A dark band can be traced from the tibia but is interrupted at the posterior region of the joint. The anterior cruciate ligament was seen intact in this patient in a more lateral parasagittal view.

makes MRI an ideal imaging mode. The fibular collateral ligament originates from the lateral femoral epicondyle just posterosuperior to the origin of the popliteus tendon and courses posterior and inferior to insert with the biceps tendon onto the fibular head. The tendon of the popliteus courses deep to the fibular collateral ligament, perforates the posterior horn of the lateral meniscus, and inserts onto the posterior tibia. The fibular collateral ligament, iliotibial band, and popliteus are all extra-articular and make the diagnosis of disruption by arthrography impossible.[13,26]

On MRI, the normal lateral ligaments of the knee produce no signal and appear as homogeneous dark straight bands. On both T_1- and T_2-weighted images the fibular collateral ligament is recognized by its complete absence or by disruption of the straight homogeneous dark band. The normal iliotibial band is usually well visualized as well on coronal images, coursing distally from the lateral thigh, surrounded by bright signal from subcutaneous fat, and it can be followed to its insertion into Gerdy's tubercle.[36] Similarly, a disruption of the iliotibial band appears as a bright signal within the normally dark band or as nonvisualization of the entire band.

OSTEONECROSIS

Osteonecrosis results from lack of or diminished blood supply to bone and is not uncommon about the knee.[42,65] Ischemic necrosis begins within the fatty marrow of subchondral bone; the epiphyseal ends of long bones are affected most, because arterial supply and venous outflow are limited. The causes of osteonecrosis are varied and include a host of disorders, such as hemoglobinopathies, alcohol abuse, steroids,

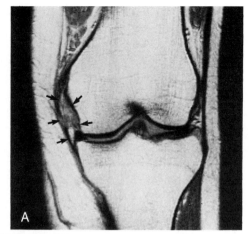
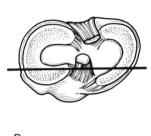
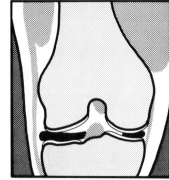

Figure 2—29
A coronal T1-weighted image and schematic of a chronic tear of the medial collateral ligament off the femur. Notice the markedly thickened grayish appearance of the ligament abutting the femur and lack of definition throughout its length. Compare this image with Figure 2–17A, which exemplifies a normal medial collateral ligament as well as normal menisci.

Gaucher's disease, caisson disease, collagen vascular diseases, and others.[5,37,56,65]

Infarcts have been classified by Reicher and others into four zones: central necrosis, surrounding ischemia, hyperemia, and normal bone.[37,65] Initially when cell death occurs, no roentgenographic changes are present, and in fact, bone scan reveals an area of decreased uptake. On MRI, however, T_1-weighted images normally revealing "alive" medullary bone would be decreased as a result of infarction. Edema associated with acute infarction would result in increased signal intensity on T_2-weighted imaging. As the reparative process ensues, there is a continued loss of signal on T_1-weighted views while T_2-weighted

images may be mixed as areas of edema continue. Previous methods for diagnosing osteonecrosis have included plain radiograph, tomography, and bone scan. It is well known that plain radiographs are insensitive until the advanced stage of collapse has occurred. Little has been written about MRI in detecting osteonecrosis about the knee, but early reports suggest that MRI is a more sensitive technique[5,37,48,56,65] and is far superior in detecting the extent of disease, as well as having the ability to distinguish between acute and chronic infarctions.[64]

Osteochondritis dissecans is an area of subchondral bone that undergoes avascular necrosis, accompanied by changes in the overlying cartilage. The

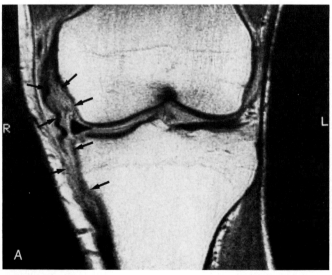
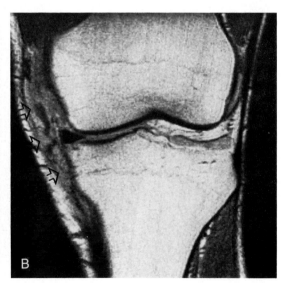

Figure 2—30
Sequential T1-weighted coronal views from anterior to posterior of an acutely torn medial collateral ligament. *A,* Note the thickened, wavy appearance of the ligament throughout its course (solid black arrows) and lack of definition at its site of origin and insertion. *B,* Note the thickening and brightness of the subcutaneous tissues, indicating extra-articular hemorrhage and edema (open black arrows).

exact etiology of osteochondritis dissecans is unclear, but several theories have been proposed, including direct and indirect trauma, abnormal ossification within the epiphysis, and vascular insufficiency secondary to emboli of blood elements and fat.[5,37] In the knee, osteochondritis occurs within the medial femoral condyle 85 percent of the time, classically involving the lateral portion near the attachment of the posterior cruciate ligament. The remaining 15 percent usually occur in the inferocentral or anterior portion of the lateral femoral condyle.[70] Treatment depends on the age of the patient, the size and location of the lesion, and whether the fragment is detached. Although standard radiographs may reveal changes in the subchondral bone or radiopaque displaced fragments, they are unable to assess the overlying cartilage.[37] Arthrography, HRCT, and technetium bone scans have been used to evaluate the extent of bony disease and to determine whether the fragment of bone and cartilage is detached (see Fig. 2–10).

MRI has proved to be the most sensitive test available in diagnosing avascular necrosis of the femoral head in children as well as in adults.[37,65] Early reports and our own experience regarding the use of MRI in osteochondritis dissecans of the knee show great promise in the ability of MRI to detect early changes, the extent of involvement, and the status of the overlying cartilage.[36]

On T_1-weighted images, the subchondral bone yields lower signal intensity than the surrounding normal medullary bone. T_2-weighted imaging, in which synovial fluid appears bright, is helpful in determining whether the fragment of bone and overlying cartilage is detached (Fig. 2–31). MRI is also helpful in identifying concomitant lesions or other conditions considered in the differential diagnosis of osteochondritis dissecans, such as a meniscal tear or loose body. Although these conditions all may be detected with the combined use of plain technetium bone scan, and arthrography with and without CT, MRI has the distinct advantages of being extremely sensitive and yielding this information from a single, noninvasive test.

A large proportion of bone tumors occur around the knee, but these tumors are relatively uncommon in the entire scope of disorders presenting as knee pain, effusion, and loss of motion. Benign and malignant tumors about the knee include osteosarcomas, chondrosarcomas, synovial sarcomas, fibrosarcomas, malignant fibrohistiocytomas, granulocytic sarcomas, giant cell tumors, pigmented villonodular synovitis (PVNS), osteochondromas, enchondromas, nonossifying fibromas, chondroblastomas, and osteoid osteomas. Diseases affecting the bone marrow, such as multiple myeloma, occur about the knee as well. While CT is the study of choice for evaluating cortical bone, MRI has proved quite valuable and more sensitive in delineating the extent of disease and its relationship to bone and surrounding struc-

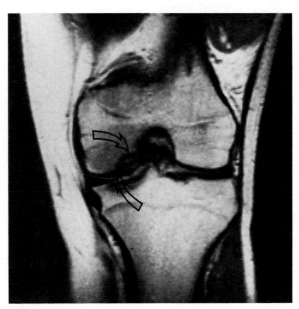

Figure 2–31

An area of osteochondritis dissecans of the medial femoral condyle on a T1-weighted midcoronal section. The overlying cartilage appears disrupted and the lesion is seen extending into subchondral bone (arrows).

tures. Manipulating TR values using a spin echo pulse sequence allows for contrasting signals and differential imaging. In the case of osteosarcoma, for example, short TR values reveal a weak tumor signal similar to that of muscle, whereas with longer TR values the tumor signal increases dramatically, resembling fat in brightness.[37,52] In such a manner it could be determined whether a tumor is expanding from the medullary cavity outward or from the surrounding soft tissue structures invading bone. Fifty percent of all giant cell tumors occur about the knee, evenly distributed between the distal femur and the proximal tibia. While plain x-rays reveal an obvious subchondral lucency, the extent of medullary involvement is impressive on MRI (Fig. 2–32).

PVNS is often a difficult clinical diagnosis to determine when it affects the knee joint. Clinically, patients may present with a knee effusion (up to 75 percent of cases), loss of motion, and joint line tenderness. Plain radiographs most commonly reveal a joint effusion; cystic erosions are more frequently seen in the hip. The differential diagnosis includes synovial sarcoma, rheumatoid arthritis, and synovial hemangioma. The magnetic resonance imaging characteristics of PVNS are unique. On T_1-weighted imaging the synovium demonstrates intermediate signal intensity; long TR/TE pulse sequences show the synovium-containing areas of increased signal interspersed with areas of decreased signal. Hemosiderin deposition is thought to account for areas of decreased signal. The increased signal results from fluid and inflamed synovium, which can be seen proliferating and ballooning from the joint[61] (Figs. 2–33, 2–34).

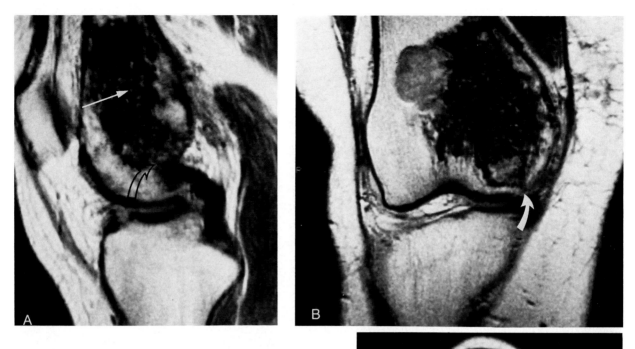

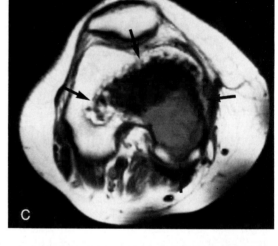

Figure 2–32
Coronal, sagittal, and transverse sections of a giant cell tumor of the medial femoral condyle. *A*, The sagittal section (T2-weighted) shows the septations (solid arrow) within the tumor and its close proximity to the posterior cruciate ligament (open arrow). *B*, On coronal view (T1-weighted), the tumor can be seen extending to the articular surface (arrow) with overlying intact articular cartilage. *C*, The transverse section illustrates the extent of the tumor and its relationship to the anterior and posterior cortices of the femur as well as to the patella (arrows).

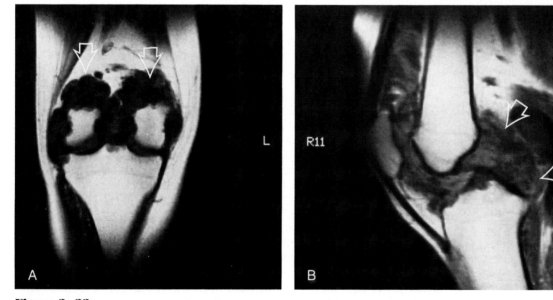

Figure 2–33
Coronal (*A*) and sagittal (*B*) images of a knee with diffuse pigmented villonodular synovitis (PVNS). Proliferating synovium is seen expanding the suprapatellar bursa and posterior regions of the knee.

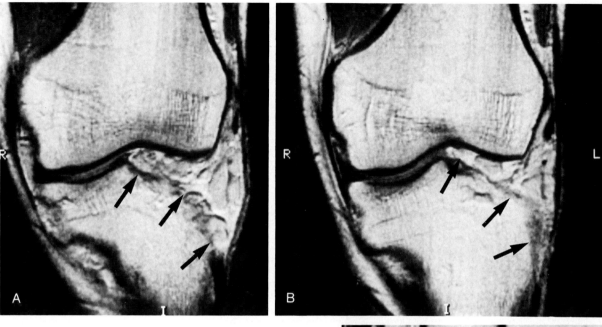

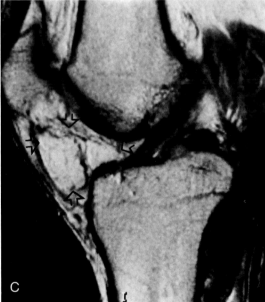

Figure 2–34

A case of localized PVNS involving the medial capsular structures of the knee. *A* and *B*, Mid to anterior coronal sections (TR 0.5/TE 30) illustrating a bright mass encroaching upon the medial joint (arrows). *C*, A T2-weighted sagittal image showing the same mass extending anteriorly to the area of the anterior cruciate ligament attachment to the tibia (arrows).

References

1. Aichroth P: Osteochondritis dissecans of the knee. J Bone Joint Surg 53:440–446, 1971.
2. Aisen AM, Martel W, Braunstein EM, McMillan KI, Phillips WA, Kling TF: MRI and CT evaluation of primary bone and soft tissue tumors. Am J Radiol 146:749–756, 1987.
3. Burgow DW: Arthrographic findings in meniscal cysts. Radiology 101:579–581, 1971.
4. Casscells SW: Arthroscopy of the knee joint; A review of 150 cases. J Bone Joint Surg 53A:287, 1971.
5. Crenshaw AH: Campbell's Operative Orthopaedics. St. Louis, CV Mosby, 1984.
6. Daffner RH, Lupetin AR, Dash N, Deeb TL, Sefczek RJ, Schapiro RL: MRI in the detection of malignant infiltration of bone marrow. Am J Roentgenol 146:353–358, 1986.
7. Dalinka MK, Garofola J: The infrapatellar synovial fold: A cause for confusion in the elevation of the anterior cruciate ligament. Am J Roentgenol 127:589–591, 1976.
8. DeHaven KE: Diagnosis of acute knee injuries with hemarthrosis. Am J Sports Med 8:9–14, 1980.
9. DeHaven KE, Collins HR: Diagnosis of internal derangement of the knee: The role of arthroscopy. J Bone Joint Surg 57:802, 1975.

10. Ehman RL: MR imaging with surface coils. Radiology 157:549–550, 1985.
11. Evarts CM: Surgery of the Musculoskeletal System. New York, Churchill-Livingstone, 1983.
12. Fisher MR, Barker B, Amparo BG, Brandt R, Brant-Zawadzki M, Hrick B, Higgins CB: MR imaging using specialized coils. Radiology 157:443–447, 1985.
13. Freiberger RH, Kaye JJ: Arthrography. New York, Appleton-Century-Crofts, 1979.
14. Freiberger RH, Killoran PJ, Cardona G: Arthrography of the knee by double contrast method. Am J Roentgenol 97:736–747, 1966.
15. Gallimore GW Jr, Harms SE: Knee injuries: High-resolution MR imaging. Radiology 160:457–461, 1986.
16. Ghelman B: Meniscal tears of the knee: Evaluation by high-resolution CT combined with arthrography. Radiology 157:23–27, 1985.
17. Glashow JL, Katz R, Schneider M, Scott WN: Double-blind assessment of the value of MRI for anterior cruciate and meniscal lesions. J Bone Joint Surg 71A(1):113–119, 1989.
18. Hartzman S, Reicher MA, Bassett LW, Duckwiler GR, Mandelbaum B, Gold RH: Magnetic resonance of the knee joint. Clinical update II: Chronic disorders. Radiology 162:553–559, 1987.
19. Insall JN: Surgery of the Knee. New York. Churchill-Livingstone, 1984.
20. Ireland J, Trickey EL, Stoken OJ: Arthroscopy and arthrography of the knee: A critical review. J Bone Joint Surg 62B:3–6, 1980.
21. Jackson RW, Abe I: The role of arthroscopy in the management of disorders of the knee; An analysis of 200 consecutive examinations. J Bone Joint Surg 54B:310, 1972.
22. Jackson RW, DeHaven KE: Arthroscopy of the knee. Clin Orthop Relat Res 107:87–92, 1975.
23. Jacobsen HG: Fundamentals of magnetic resonance imaging. JAMA 258(23):3417–3423, 1985.
24. Johnson LL: Impact of diagnostic arthroscopy on the clinical judgement of an experienced arthroscopist. Clin Orthop Relat Res 167:75–83, 1982.
25. Johnson LL: Diagnostic arthroscopy in clinical practice. *In* Diagnostic and Surgical Arthroscopy: The Knee and Other Joints. 2nd ed. St. Louis, CV Mosby, 1981, pp 69–96.
26. Kaye JJ, Freiberger RH: Arthrography of the knee. Clin Orthop Relat Res 107:73–80, 1975.
27. Kennedy JC, Weinberg HW, Wilson AS: The anatomy and function of the anterior cruciate ligament. J Bone Joint Surg 56:223–235, 1974.
28. Kleinberg S: Pulmonary embolus following oxygen injection of the knee. JAMA 89:172, 1972.
29. Kramer DM: Basic principles of magnetic resonance imaging. Radiol Clin North Am 22(4): Dec 1984.
30. Lee JK, Yao L, Phelps CT, Wirth CR, Czajka J, Lozman J: Anterior cruciate ligament tears: MR imaging compared with arthroscopy and clinical tests. Radiology 166:861–864, 1988.
31. Li DKB, Adams ME, McConkey JP: Magnetic resonance imaging of the ligaments and menisci of the knee. Radiol Clin North Am 24:209–227, 1986.
32. Kindbloom K: Arthrography of the knee: Roentgenographic and anatomical study. Acta Radiol (Suppl) 74:1948.
33. Lufkin RB, Votruva T, Reicher M, Bassett L, Smith SO, Hanafer WN: Solenoid surface coils in magnetic resonance imaging. Radiology 146:409–412, 1986.
34. Manco LG, Kavanaugh JH, Lozman J, Coleman ND, Bilfield BS, Fay JJ: Diagnosis of meniscal tears using high-resolution computed tomography. J Bone Joint Surg 69A:498–502, 1987.
35. Manco LG, Lozman J, Coleman ND, Kavanaugh JH, Bilfield BS, Dougherty J: Non-invasive evaluation of knee meniscal tears: Preliminary comparison of MR imaging and CT. Radiology 163:727–730, 1987.
36. Mandelbaum BR, Finerman GAM, Reicher MA, Hartzman S, Bassett LW, Gold RH, Rauschning W, Dorey F: Magnetic resonance imaging as a tool for evaluation of traumatic knee injuries. Am J Sports Med 14:361–370, 1986.
37. Mink JH, Reicher MA, Crues JV III: Magnetic Resonance Imaging of the Knee. New York, Raven Press, 1987.
38. Moon KL Jr, Genant HK, Helms CA, Chafetz NI, Crooke LE, Kaufman L: Musculoskeletal applications of nuclear magnetic resonance. Radiology 147:161–171, 1983.
39. Nicholas JA, Freiberger RH, Killoran PJ: Double-contrast arthrography of the knee. Its value in the management of 225 knee derangements. J Bone Joint Surg 52A:203, 1970.
40. Passariello R, Trecco F, dePaulis F, Masciocchi C, Bonanni G, Zobel BB: Meniscal lesions of the knee joint: CT diagnosis. Radiology 157:29–34, 1985.
41. Pavlov H, Freiberger RH: An easy method to demonstrate the cruciate ligaments by double contrast arthrography. Radiology 126:817–818, 1978.
42. Pavlov H, Hirshy JC, Torg JS: Computed tomography of the cruciate ligaments. Radiology 132:389–393, 1979.
43. Pavlov H, Schneider R: Extrameniscal abnormality as diagnosed by knee arthrography. Radiol Clin North Am, 19:287–304, 1981.
44. Pavlov H, Torg JS: Double contrast arthrographic evaluation of the anterior cruciate ligament. Radiology 126:661-665, 1978.
45. Pavlov H, Warren RF, Sherman MF, Cayen PD: The accuracy of double-contrast arthrographic evaluation of the anterior cruciate ligaments. J Bone Joint Surg 65:175–183, 1983.
46. Pollack MS, Dalinka MK, Kressel HY: MRI in the evaluation of osteonecrosis of the knee. Proceedings of the Fifth Annual Meeting of the Society of Magnetic Resonance in Medicine. Montreal, 1986.
47. Polly DW, Callaghan JJ, Sikes RA, McCabe JW, McMahon K, Savory CG: The accuracy of selective magnetic resonance imaging compared with findings of arthroscopy of the knee. J

Bone Joint Surg 70:199–202, 1988.

48. Rao VM, Fichman M, Mitchell DG, Steiner RM, Ballas SK, Axel L: Painful sickle cell crisis: Bone marrow patterns observed with MR imaging. Radiology 161:211–215, 1986.
49. Reicher MA, Hartzman S, Duckwiler GR, Bassett LW, Anderson LJ, Gold RH: Meniscal injuries: Detection using MR imaging. Radiology 159:753–757, 1986.
50. Reicher MA, Bassett LW, Gold RH: High resolution MRI of the knee joint: Pathologic correlations. Am J Roentgenol 145:903–909, 1985.
51. Reicher MA, Rauschning W, Gold RH, Bassett LW, Lufkin RB, Glen A Jr: High resolution MRI of the knee joint: Normal anatomy. Am J Roentgenol 145:895–902, 1985.
52. Reis ND, Ben-Arien Y: Localization of a small tumor in the leg by magnetic resonance imaging. J Bone Joint Surg 68:929–931, 1986.
53. Resnick D, Goergen TG, Kaye JJ, Ghelman B, Woody PR: Discoid medial meniscus. Radiology 121:575–576, 1976.
54. Resnick D, Niwayama G: Diagnosis of Bone and Joint Disorders. Philadelphia, WB Saunders, 1981.
55. Rockwood CA, Green CP: Fractures. Philadelphia, JB Lippincott, 1984.
56. Sartoris DJ, Brozinsky S, Resnick D: MRI's role in assessing musculoskeletal disorders. J Musculoskel Med Dec:12–26, 1987.
57. Savoy CG, Polly DW, Sikes RA, Callaghan J, McCabe JM, McMahon K: A prospective comparison study of magnetic resonance imaging and arthroscopy of the knee: Proceedings of the International Society of the Knee. Am J Sports Med 15(4):389, 1987.
58. Scott JA, Rosenthal DI, Brady TJ: The evaluation of musculoskeletal disease with magnetic resonance imaging. Radiol Clin North Am 22(4):Dec 1984.
59. Selesnick FH, Noble HB, Bachman DL, Steinberg FL: Internal derangement of the knee: Diagnosis by arthrography, arthroscopy and arthrotomy. Clin Orthop Relat Res 198:26–30, 1985.
60. Silva I Jr, Silver DM: Tears of the meniscus as revealed by magnetic resonance imaging. J Bone Joint Surg 70:199–202, 1988.
61. Soundry M, Lanir A, Angel D, Roffman M, Kaplan N, Mendes DG: Anatomy of the normal knee as seen by magnetic resonance imaging. J Bone Joint Surg 68B:117–120, 1986.
62. Spritzer E, Dalinka MK, Kressel H: Magnetic resonance imaging of pigmented villonodular synovitis: A report of two cases. Skel Radiol 16:316–319, 1987.
63. Stoller DW, Martin C, Crues JV III, Kaplan L, Mink JH: Meniscal tears: Pathologic correlation with MR imaging. Radiology 163:731–735, 1987.
64. Tegtmeyer CJ, McCue FC III, Higgins SM, Ball DW: Arthrography of the knee: A comparative study of the accuracy of single- and double-contrast techniques. Radiology 132:37–41, 1979.
65. Thickman D, Axel L, Kressel HY, Steinberg M, Chen H, Velchick M, Dalinka M: Magnetic resonance imaging of avascular necrosis of the femoral head. Skel Radiol 15:133–140, 1986.
66. Thijin CJP: Accuracy of double-contrast arthrography and arthroscopy of the knee joint. Skel Radiol 8:187–192, 1982.
67. Turner DA, Prodomos CC, Petasnick JP, Clark JW: Acute injury of the ligaments of the knee: Magnetic resonance evaluation. Radiology 154:717–722, 1983.
68. Tyrrell RL, Gluckert K, Pathria M, Modil MT: Fast three-dimensional MR imaging of the knee: Comparison with arthroscopy. Radiology 166:865–872, 1988.
69. Wang JB, Marshall JL: Acute ligamentous injuries of the knee. Single contrast arthrography—a diagnostic aid. Trauma 15:431–440, 1975.
70. Wershba M, Dalinka MK, Coren GS, Cotler J: Double contrast knee arthrography in the evaluation of osteochondritis dissecans. Clin Orthop Relat Res 107:81–86, 1975.
71. Wojtys E, Wilson M, Buckwalter K, Braunstein E, Martell W: Magnetic resonance imaging of knee hyaline cartilage and intraarticular pathology. Am J Sports Med 15(5):455–463, 1987.
72. Zimmer WV, Berquist TH, McCleod RA, Sim FH, Pritchard DJ, Shives TE, Wold LE, May GR: Bone tumors: Magnetic resonance imaging vs. computed tomography. Radiology 155:709–718, 1984.

3

Nigel E. Sharrock
H. Keith Pinchot
Anesthetic Considerations in Arthroscopy

Arthroscopic knee surgery is now one of the most commonly performed surgical procedures, and no doubt, with surgical advances, it will be more widely available in years to come. A major advantage is the minimal surgical trauma to the knee joint, which usually enables rapid recovery. For reasons of economics and patient convenience, many of these procedures are now performed on an outpatient basis.

Typically, the patients have been young and fit, but, as experience has accumulated, the elderly and infirm are being considered suitable candidates for ambulatory surgery. At present, between 40 and 50 percent of all surgery in the United States is performed in an outpatient setting. This chapter, therefore, will highlight anesthetic techniques designed to enable early ambulation and discharge from surgical units. Table 3–1 grades anesthetic techniques in various patient conditions.

Table 3–1
Grading of Anesthetic Techniques

	GENERAL	FEMORAL ± SCIATIC	SPINAL	EPIDURAL	LOCAL	LOCAL + SEDATION
Safety in healthy patients	+	+	+	+	++	+
Safety in ASA II and III	0	+	+	+	++	+
Speed to perform	++	00	++	0	+	+
Skill required of anesthetist	++	00	++	0	++	++
Headache risk	++	++	00	00	++	++
Postoperative nausea and vomiting	00	++	+	+	++	+
Rapid discharge	0	+	0	+	++	+
Aspiration risk	00	++	+	+	++	+
Urinary retention	+	++	00	0	++	++
Postoperative disorientation	00	++	++	++	++	++
Backache	+	++	0	0	++	++
Surgical condition	++	+	++	++	00	0
Tourniquet pain	++	0	+	++	00	0

  0 Possible disadvantage
 00 Clear disadvantage
  + Favorable
++ Highly favorable

Factors Influencing Ability to Perform Outpatient Surgery

Size of the Surgical Procedure Longer and more extensive procedures are not suitable for outpatient surgery. For example, ligament augmentation and possibly meniscal repair should be done on an inpatient basis.

Anticipated Postoperative Pain It is not feasible to administer parenteral narcotics on an outpatient basis. If the patient's disposition or prior drug tolerance or the gravity of the surgery suggests that postoperative pain will be considerable, hospital admission may be advisable. Lateral release for patellar realignment, although easily performed, may entail considerable postoperative pain. Admission following ambulatory surgery is frequently due to uncontrolled pain or side effects of analgesics.

Age Ambulatory surgery is performed on elderly patients more frequently nowadays, so age per se is not a limiting factor. However, home support systems and concurrent medical problems may militate against ambulatory surgery.

Patient Condition Traditionally, only healthy candidates were considered for outpatient surgery, but now patients in ASA (American Society of Anesthesiology) categories II and III have been found suitable for minor surgery under appropriate anesthetic techniques.[3]

Preoperative Testing

Urinalysis, blood tests, chest radiographs, and electrocardiograms are generally unnecessary prior to ambulatory surgery as they are not considered cost effective. However, many states or hospitals have minimal standards that have to be adhered to.

Eating or Drinking Preoperatively Liquids are generally cleared from the stomach within 4 hours if the patient is not taking narcotics. Individual units performing surgery in the afternoon may choose to allow a patient to have a liquid breakfast, but, in general, it is preferable to have patients fast after midnight of the day of operation (NPO).

After Discharge

Home Setting It is important that a patient who is discharged to the home following arthroscopic surgery have a responsible companion.

Postoperative Instructions These should be made clear to the patient preoperatively or given in written form, as recall following a general anesthetic or intravenous sedative is variable.

ANESTHETIC OPTIONS

Local anesthesia.
Local anesthesia with sedation.
General anesthesia.
Epidural anesthesia.
Spinal anesthesia.
Femoral nerve block.

Local Anesthesia With or Without Sedation

The advantages of this form of anesthesia include relative safety, minimal medical contraindications, minimal postoperative pain and nausea, and ease of discharge. The disadvantages are mainly surgical and include the inability to leave a tourniquet comfortably inflated for more than 15 to 20 minutes, and the inability to fully manipulate the knee joint into varus or valgus.

Intravenous sedation may be used to obtund some of the patient's discomfort. Typically, midazolam (Versed), in doses of 0.03 mg/kg initially followed by 1- to 2-mg increments, in combination with fentanyl, 25 to 50 μg, or sufentanyl in 2- to 5-μg increments can be used.

Once intravenous sedation is utilized, many of the theoretical advantages of local anesthesia are lost, but on the other hand, it may make the procedure more effective. If intravenous sedation is to be used, electrocardiograms, pulse oximeter, and blood pressure should be monitored and nasal oxygen supplied. Furthermore, an anesthesiologist must be present to monitor the patient and adjust the level of sedation.

Properly sedated, the patient can communicate with the surgeon and watch the procedure on the monitor, but he or she is subject to a more prolonged recovery room stay and perioperative amnesia from midazolam.

TECHNIQUE OF LOCAL ANESTHESIA

The key to an adequate block in the knee joint is to use enough volume of local anesthetic to bathe the synovial membrane and to allow enough time for the local anesthetic to take effect.

A small-gauge (25 or 27) needle is used to anesthetize the skin overlying the portals to be used. The capsule is then anesthetized at these sites, with care taken not to distend the capsule or fat pad into the joint with excessive anesthetic. The joint is distended with 40 to 60 ml of the anesthetic mixture via a larger

(18-gauge) needle inserted through the superior medial portal (usually at the junction of the medial patella and the quadriceps tendon). The anesthetic mixture may contain a combination of drugs, such as 1 percent lidocaine (for more rapid onset) combined with an equal volume of 0.25 percent bupivacaine (Marcaine) for postoperative analgesia. Epinephrine, added to a concentration of 1:300,000 to 1:500,000, tends to decrease bleeding into the joint during the procedure, reduce vascular reuptake of the local anesthetic, and prolong the local anesthetic action.

Femoral With or Without Sciatic Nerve Block

These blocks may be more useful under special circumstances or in clinical situations in which neither spinal, epidural, nor general anesthesia can be used safely.

Significant anesthesia of the knee joint can be obtained using the so-called three-in-one block (femoral, obturator, and lateral femoral cutaneous). This is done by eliciting a paresthesia when performing a femoral nerve block beneath the inguinal ligament and injecting 20 to 30 ml of local anesthetic at the site of a paresthesia. Local anesthetic tracks proximally along the fascial plane in which the femoral nerve runs and anesthetizes the other two components of the lumbar plexus. For complete anesthesia of the knee joint and to provide prolonged relief from tourniquet pain, a sciatic nerve block should also be performed. This requires additional positioning, preparation, and needle insertions, adding to the time, complexity, complications, and patient discomfort. The landmarks taught for the performance of sciatic blocks may be inaccurate, accounting for the low popularity of this block (the nerve appears to be closer to the ischium than the descriptions in anesthetic texts aver). Furthermore, sciatica is a common symptom that subsequently may be ascribed to the nerve block.

For reasons of technical difficulty, multiple injection sites, and significant recovery time plus the fact that there are good alternatives, these blocks are infrequently used for arthroscopic surgery. However, severe pain following arthroscopy, especially lateral release, may be readily controlled by a femoral nerve block alone. Unfortunately, this may prevent early discharge because of quadriceps weakness.

General Anesthesia

PROBLEMS

Relative *medical contraindications* include:
1. Difficult airway management especially in obese patients or heavy, athletic patients.

2. Asthmatic patients or heavy smokers with bronchospasm and irritable airways.
3. Other medical problems, such as ischemic heart disease, diabetes, and hypertension, in which general anesthesia may complicate perioperative management.
4. Gastrointestinal dysfunction—e.g., hiatus hernia with an increased risk of aspiration or persistent nausea and vomiting.

Delayed discharge, to include dizziness, disorientation, nausea, and vomiting. Nausea and vomiting occur in 20 to 25 percent of patients following knee arthroscopy under general anesthesia and may be more common if narcotics are used. Nitrous oxide diffuses into the middle ear, nasal sinuses or stomach, contributing to nausea and vomiting, especially when patients are moved.

Aspiration. The risk of significant aspiration in an ambulatory setting is probably about 1:5000, but it can be a serious complication.

Prophylactic H_2 blockers (ranitidine and cimetidine), *metoclopramide* (Reglan), and *antacids* are probably unnecessary. High-risk patients include those with obesity, diabetes, pregnancy, and gastrointestinal dysfunction, such as hiatus hernia or peptic ulcers. Rapid-sequence induction with intubation or regional anesthesia should be considered in this high-risk group.

Postoperative *muscle pains* from succinylcholine may be a problem.

Minor Disadvantages
Many patients like to watch the television, enjoy the sense of participation, or fear lack of control. Others have a fear of general anesthesia.

Advantages
Excellent operative condition.
Speed of induction.
Relatively well accepted by patients, although this may be changing with increased patient sophistication.
Excellent track record of safety in skilled hands.

RECOMMENDATIONS

1. Thorough preoperative assessment by the anesthesiologist.
2. Avoid general anesthesia, if a history of airway problems, severe medical conditions, or postoperative nausea and vomiting is obtained.
3. Utilize perioperative antiemetics, e.g., droperidol with or without metoclopramide.
4. Careful airway management to minimize air entry into the stomach.
5. Intraoperative local anesthesia to the knee joint with 0.25 percent bupivacaine to minimize postoperative pain and the need for narcotics.

6. Avoid succinylcholine; use vecuronium or atracurium if intubation is necessary.

INDUCTION AGENTS

It is preferable to use agents with a short duration of action and minimal side effects. Sodium thiopental is the most widely used agent. Alternatives include:

1. Methohexital, which may have a slightly quicker recovery time.
2. Propofol, which has a smooth induction and gives a "clearer head" postoperatively. This may become the agent of choice following Food and Drug Administration approval.
3. Midazolam—initially recommended doses may have been excessive; smaller doses, 0.05 to 0.1 mg/kg, followed by a mask inhalation anesthetic, are quite satisfactory.
4. Alfentanyl, which is an ultrashort-acting narcotic. It may necessitate muscle relaxants plus intubation.

MAINTENANCE AGENTS

Combinations of nitrous oxide, with or without enflurane, isoflurane, and halothane, are all used and differ little in emergence, discharge patterns, or postoperative clarity. Intraoperative narcotics may result in rapid emergence but more postoperative nausea and vomiting.

MUSCLE RELAXANTS

Generally, muscle relaxants are needed only if intubation is performed. Short-acting succinylcholine should be used only if a difficult intubation or a short procedure is contemplated. Intermediate-acting nondepolarizing agents (vecuronium and atracurium) are associated with fewer postoperative body aches, last 20 to 40 minutes following an intubating dose, and should be the agent of choice if an intubation is planned.

POSTOPERATIVE PAIN

Generally, it is preferable to prevent postoperative pain by intraoperative infiltration with 0.25 percent bupivacaine, 30 to 50 ml.

Intravenous narcotics in smaller doses (e.g., 25 μg of fentanyl) are generally preferable to the intramuscular route. It is preferable to prevent nausea and vomiting by the use of small doses of droperidol, e.g., 0.625 to 1.25 mg intravenously, but excessive doses may result in dizziness on standing, thus delaying discharge.

Spinal Anesthesia

Lidocaine, bupivacaine, and tetracaine are commonly used. Tetracaine and bupivacaine will provide at least 3 hours of anesthesia but it may take 6 to 7 hours before a patient can ambulate. This limits their use in ambulatory surgery. Lidocaine, on the other hand, may last 45 to 90 minutes per single dose, which may be insufficient if the surgery is more prolonged than expected.

Unfortunately, spinal anesthesia is a single-shot technique, making it less flexible than epidural or general anesthesia.

Advantages

1. Most anesthesiologists are skilled at spinal anesthesia.
2. It is relatively quick and simple to perform.
3. There is reliable, quick onset of anesthesia, with complete anesthesia and muscle paralysis.
4. The patient can be awake to watch the procedure on the monitor.
5. Physiologic changes in circulation are readily treated with a vasopressor having both α and β effects, e.g., ephedrine, epinephrine, or dopamine.
6. It avoids airway difficulties.

Disadvantages

1. *Headaches.* Headache following lumbar puncture is particularly difficult to manage on an outpatient basis and may not become apparent for 2 to 4 days postoperatively.
2. *Dural punctures.* Headache rates vary widely in studies, but they seem related to needle size (less common with small 26-gauge needles), sex (more common in women), age (less common in the elderly), and the angle of needle entry (if the cutting edge of the needle pierces the dura at an acute angle and parallel to the direction of the spine, headaches are said to be less common). Early ambulation may or may not affect headache rates. Postoperative follow-up of the patient is necessary so that treatment (e.g., an epidural blood patch) can be implemented.
3. *Hypotension.* This is readily treated with intravenous fluid and/or ephedrine, IV and/or IM.
4. *Bradycardias and/or Asystole.* This may follow spinal anesthesia if no chronotropic catecholamines are given. This complication can be avoided by the use of an epinephrine infusion, 2 to 4 μg/minute, or ephedrine intramuscularly, 25 to 50 mg. Intravenous injections of ephedrin, 5 to 10 mg, or epinephrine, 4 to 8 μg, can be used to treat bradycardia or hypotension.
5. *Total Spinals.* Unexpectedly high levels may occur, particularly if large doses of hyperbaric local

anesthetic are used, or when the patient coughs or is placed in the head-down position.

6. *Management.* All patients with spinal anesthesia should have nasal oxygen and close monitoring of pulse oximetry, electrocardiogram, and blood pressure. Constant surveillance and monitoring by the anesthetist are mandatory.

7. *Backache.* This may follow spinal anesthesia and may be related to the midline approach or the difficulty with the technique. Prior backache or sciatica is not a contraindication to spinal or epidural anesthesia.

8. *Urinary retention* is common with long-acting agents like bupivacaine or tetracaine.

Epidural Anesthesia

Many of the issues pertaining to spinal apply to epidural anesthesia.

Avoid bupivacaine or long-acting agents for ambulatory surgery.

Chloroprocaine may be used, but it requires insertion of and reliance on the function of an epidural catheter and has been associated with postoperation back pain.

Lidocaine, 1.5 and 2 percent plain, has a duration of 60 to 90 minutes. Lidocaine, 2 percent with 1:300,000 epinephrine injected at L3–L4, is recommended in doses of 20 to 30 ml, depending on age. This provides between 2 and 3 hours of excellent surgical anesthesia and discharge within 2 to 3 hours of arrival in the recovery room.

It is important to inject at the L3–L4 or L4–L5 interspace to achieve maximal anesthetic effect. Added epinephrine with or without bicarbonate, 1 to 2 mEq in 30 ml, provides more rapid onset with more intense motor blockade. The epinephrine also reduces circulating local anesthetic levels, maintains cardiac output, and may reduce the likelihood of circulatory collapse.

The excellent anesthesia, reliable duration, and ease of discharge make this an excellent approach. Epidural catheters may be inserted as a back-up should the surgery be prolonged or additional local anesthesia needed (especially in the young athletic patient with presumably larger nerve roots).

Attempts to finesse the duration of anesthesia in order to discharge patients 30 minutes sooner seem foolhardy if the safety and quality of anesthesia suffer.

Advantages

1. Complete surgical anesthesia with good motor paralysis.

2. The patient is able to watch the procedure on the screen.

3. Outcome studies suggest that the discharge time is shorter following epidural than general anesthesia.

4. Nausea, vomiting, and postoperative dizziness are less frequent.

5. Management of coexisting medical problems seems easier.

6. It circumvents airway and aspiration difficulties.

7. High patient satisfaction is noted.

8. The surgeon can relate to the patient better perioperatively.

9. It may be safer than general anesthesia, but any risk difference must be extremely small.

10. A major advantage of an epidural over a spinal anesthetic is that if no dural puncture occurs the patient can be told that a headache will not occur. This simplifies follow-up. With spinal anesthesia, a headache may occur regardless of skill and technique.

11. An epidural catheter enables the anesthesia to be maintained for longer procedures.

Disadvantages

Many anesthesiologists are not experienced at giving epidural anesthesia, so the success rate is lower and the interval between cases can become considerable.

Headache following dural puncture is considerable. Our practice is to admit a patient if a #17 dural puncture has occurred and do an epidural blood patch the following day if the patient has a headache. We also keep the patients in bed for 24 hours following an epidural blood patch. If dural puncture rates exceed 2 to 3 percent in a particular institution, it is preferable to avoid epidural anesthesia for routine cases. Epidural anesthesia should be used only in an ambulatory setting if the anesthesiologists are skilled at performing them. Teaching epidural anesthesia to residents in an ambulatory setting may be inadvisable.

Hypotension Hypotension, asystole, and total spinal anesthesia may occur as with spinal anesthesia. In addition, intravascular injections of local anesthesia (especially via a catheter) can cause seizures and circulatory collapse. Intraoperative monitoring and vigilance are identical to those for spinal or general anesthesia.

Urinary Retention This is related to the use of long-acting agents such as bupivacaine, and excessive fluid administration. Our experience with 2 percent lidocaine with epinephrine 1:300,000 is that urinary retention has not been a problem resulting in unexpected admission. Urinary retention may also follow spinal and general anesthesia.

Summary

Arthroscopic surgery is usually performed under general anesthesia. Current general anesthetic medications and techniques have definite difficulties and limitations. In the future, improved anesthetic agents with fewer side effects may make general anesthesia more suitable.

Regional anesthesia in competent hands offers a suitable alternative and may become more commonly used owing to consumer pressure, as has occurred in obstetric practice. However, the lack of skill in performing regional anesthesia and postoperative side effects (headache) may impair its expanded use in the outpatient setting.

We foresee improvements and changes in this area over the next 10 years that will make arthroscopic surgery even more appealing for the patient and orthopedist.

References

1. Cousins MJ, Bridenbaugh PO (eds): Neural Blockade in Clinical Anesthesia and Management of Pain. 2nd ed. Philadelphia, JB Lippincott, 1988.
2. Doze VA, Shafer A, White PF: Nausea and vomiting after outpatient anesthesia: Effectiveness of droperidol alone and in combination with metoclopramide. Anesth Analg 66:S41, 1987.
3. Meridy HW: Criteria for selection of ambulatory surgical patients and guidelines for anesthetic management; A retrospective study of 1553 cases. Anesth Analg 61: 921, 1982.
4. Wetchler BV (ed). Anesthesia for Ambulatory Surgery. Philadelphia, JB Lippincott, 1985.
5. White PF: Outpatient anesthesia. In Miller RD (ed): Anesthesia. New York, Churchill-Livingstone, 1987, p 1895–1919.

Andrew G. Franks, Jr.
Synovial Fluid Characteristics

In the patient with undiagnosed articular disease of the knee, examination of the synovial fluid is essential. This analysis of synovial fluid (synovianalysis) is also an integral part of the arthroscopic evaluation of the knee, along with direct visualization and synovial biopsy. It is generally more clinically useful than synovial biopsy, with the exception of the granulomatous diseases and amyloid; and, when combined with the clinical examination and general laboratory data, synovianalysis facilitates early diagnosis by rapidly distinguishing between noninflammatory and inflammatory disorders.

Synovianalysis may be performed prior to or concurrently with arthroscopy, depending upon the clinical setting. Thus, when acute arthritis occurs without a history of trauma, and bacterial infection or crystal-induced arthritis is suspected, synovianalysis performed immediately with a 19-gauge needle (arthrocentesis) may guide initial therapy. Alternatively, in those patients with more indolent disease in whom ancillary studies, including radiographs, blood cultures, and blood chemistry determinations, are unrevealing, synovianalysis may be performed at the time of arthroscopy. Small effusions are best analyzed prior to arthroscopy, in order to avoid bleeding caused by the introduction of the arthroscope.

Two circumstances require careful exclusion prior to synovianalysis, whether by arthrocentesis or arthroscopy, in order to avoid septic contamination of a sterile joint. Patients with septicemia or with cutaneous or soft tissue infection mimicking an acute arthritis should not be subjected to arthrocentesis or arthroscopy, since direct introduction of the offending organisms into the joint space may occur.

NORMAL SYNOVIAL FLUID

The normal knee joint contains up to 4 ml of synovial fluid with fewer than 200 white cells per cubic millimeter. In general, small lymphocytes and monocytes predominate, with few, if any, polymorphonuclear cells. This fluid is not simply an ultrafiltrate of plasma as is that of serous cavities, because the synovial lining cells (synoviocytes) produce hyaluronate (mucin), a heavy, asymmetrically branched glycosaminoglycan that significantly alters viscosity as well as composition by diminishing water content and interfering with the permeability of large molecules such as fibrinogen, other clotting factors, and globulins. Therefore, normal synovial fluid is of scant volume with few white cells, is highly viscous, does not clot, is transparent, and is colorless or pale yellow (Table 4–1). These features are the basis upon which correct interpretation of synovianalysis of the abnormal knee joint depends.

Abnormal Synovial Fluid

Diseases that affect the knee may change the normal characteristics of the synovial fluid in a number of ways, allowing distinctions to be made. Grossly, increased volume, decreased viscosity, ability to clot, diminished clarity, and change in color all contribute to the interpretation of synovianalysis. Microscopic analysis for the number and type of cells, as well as the presence or absence of crystals, is equally important. The addition of bacteriologic, chemical, and immunologic tests further enhances the ability to discriminate between the vast number of disorders that

Table 4–1
Normal Synovial Fluid

Volume (knee)	Up to 4 ml
Viscosity (string or mucin clot)	High
Color	Colorless/pale yellow
Clarity	Transparent
Total WBC/mm^3	Less than 200
Differential WBC	
Polys (%)	25% or less
Lymphs (%)	25% or less
Monos (%)	50% or more
Crystals	None
Protein	2.5 gm/dl or less
Glucose	90% of blood
Culture	Negative

may affect the knee. However, the total white cell count and the identification of bacteria or crystals are considered the most important factors in most diagnostic and therapeutic decisions.

Initial descriptions of abnormal joint fluid were simply divided into those that were noninflammatory and those that were inflammatory. The usefulness of this division was eventually increased by the separation of those fluids that were septic, and subsequently of those that were hemorrhagic. Therefore, at the present time, four clinically useful groups of abnormal synovial fluid have been defined (Table 4–2). Distinction among these groups is based upon synovial fluid volume, viscosity (hyaluronate), clarity, color, cellularity (amount and type), and culture. Further subdivision, particularly within inflammatory, noninfectious (Group II) synovial fluid, has recently been suggested.

TECHNIQUE OF SYNOVIANALYSIS

Inadequate or improper technique in performing synovianalysis has been responsible for misinterpretation, sometimes diminishing the importance of its place in the assessment of joint pathology. It is often more informative than synovial biopsy alone. Unfortunately, there are more pitfalls in its collection and preparation than are found in other body fluids, and many clinical and hospital laboratories are not thoroughly familiar with the preferred techniques. Therefore, it becomes the responsibility of the physician who performs synovianalysis to become adept in this area, either performing the tests personally or documenting the correct handling of specimens sent to the laboratory. Although a complete review of specific technique is beyond the scope of this chapter, some general guidelines are suggested. The reader is referred to detailed descriptions on this subject in the bibliography.

When profuse amounts of extraneous blood are caused by introduction of the needle or arthroscope, the validity of synovianalysis is questionable. However, when smaller numbers of red blood cells may interfere with white cell counts, lysing the red blood cells may be helpful (discussed later). Once synovial fluid is obtained, approximately 10 to 15 ml are sufficient for complete synovianalysis, although basic studies such as cell count and culture can be obtained with smaller amounts.

The fluid obtained in a sterile syringe should be gently shaken, any needle is removed from the syringe, and then the fluid is immediately separated, as follows:

1. *Sterile tube with sodium heparin*
   (Green-topped tubes in many laboratories, if sterile)
   3 to 5 ml for stains and cultures, including aer-

obic, anaerobic, tubercular and fungal vials, and direct inoculation on chocolate agar for gonococci. Use the same media as for blood cultures. Do not use transport media.
Gram and special stains are best performed on a centrifuged aliquot.

2. *Sterile tube with sodium heparin or EDTA*
   (Green- or purple-topped tubes in many laboratories)
   2 to 3 ml for cell count, differential, cytology, and crystals.

3. *Two clean tubes without anticoagulant*
   (Plain red-topped tubes in many laboratories)
   1 to 2 ml for color, viscosity (string or mucin clot), inclusions, crystals (option from anticoagulated).
   1 to 2 ml for total protein, rheumatoid factor, complement, etc.

4. *Clean tube with preservative, e.g., oxalate*
   (Gray-topped tube in many laboratories)
   1 ml for glucose.

Volume

The total volume aspirated may help determine the severity of the disease process, although it is generally not helpful in distinguishing between the various groups of abnormal fluids. Low volume does not rule out significant pathology; rather, the volume of synovial fluid removed on several subsequent synovianalyses is sometimes helpful in determining response to treatment, such as in septic arthritis. Generally more than 4 ml obtained from the knee is considered abnormal.

Viscosity

Reduced viscosity results from either the degradation of hyaluronate caused by inflammation, or the rapid accumulation of fluid after trauma, which dilutes hyaluronate concentration. Direct measurement of viscosity or hyaluronate is not usually performed; instead, indirect assessment is based upon two relatively simple procedures: string test and mucin clot.

1. When a drop of normal synovial fluid is held between the thumb and index finger, a "string" effect will be noted as the fingers are slowly separated. If viscosity is reduced, separation of the fingers occurs without any bridge of synovial fluid between them. An alternate method is to express fluid one drop at a time from a syringe with the needle removed. Normal synovial fluid droplets form a long "string" suggesting honey, whereas low-viscosity fluid appears like water droplets with short tails.

Table 4–2
Characteristics of Abnormal Synovial Fluid

GROUP I, NONINFLAMMATORY

Volume (knee)	Often > 4 ml
Viscosity (string or mucin clot)	High
Color	Straw-colored to yellow
Clarity	Transparent
Total WBC/mm^3	200 to 3000
Differential WBC	
Polys (%)	25% or less
Lymphs (%)	25% or less
Monos (%)	50% or more
Crystals	None
Protein	Usually normal
Glucose	90% of blood
Culture	Negative

Partial list of associated conditions:
    Trauma
    Internal derangement
    Osteoarthritis
    Aseptic necrosis
    Osteochondritis dissecans
    Osteochondromatosis
    Polymyalgia rheumatica
    Amyloidosis
    Early or resolving inflammation
    Acquired immunodeficiency syndrome

GROUP II, INFLAMMATORY

Volume (knee)	Often > 4 ml
Viscosity (string or mucin clot)	Low
Color	Yellow to white
Clarity	Translucent
Total WBC/mm^3	2000 to 75,000
Differential WBC	
Polys (%)	>50%
Lymphs (%)	25% or less
Monos (%)	25% or less*
Crystals	May be present
Protein	>3.0 gm/dl
Glucose	75% of blood or lower
Culture	Negative for bacteria

Partial list of associated conditions:
  a) Often highly inflammatory:
    Rheumatoid arthritis
    Crystal arthritis
    Reiter's syndrome
    Acute rheumatic fever
    Lyme disease
  b) Often mildly inflammatory
    Psoriatic arthritis
    Bowel-related arthritis

    Juvenile arthritis
    Ankylosing spondylitis
    Connective tissue disease
    Viral arthritis (including parvovirus)*
    Tubercular or fungal arthritis*

GROUP III, SEPTIC

Volume (knee)	Usually > 4 ml
Viscosity (string or mucin clot)	Low
Color	Variable
Clarity	Opaque
Total WBC/mm^3	Usually > 100,000
Differential WBC	
Polys (%)	>75%
Lymphs (%)	10% or less
Monos (%)	10% or less
Crystals	None
Protein	>3.0 gm/dl
Glucose	50% of blood or lower
Culture	Positive for bacteria, overlaps with Group II for tubercular and fungal

Partial list of associated conditions:
    Bacterial infections
    Tubercular or fungal arthritis (rarely)

GROUP IV, HEMORRHAGIC

Volume (knee)	Usually > 4 ml
Viscosity (string or mucin clot)	Variable
Color	Pink to bloody
Clarity	Variable
Total WBC/mm^3	Variable
Differential WBC	
Polys (%)	Variable
Lymphs (%)	Variable
Monos (%)	Variable
Crystals	None
Protein	Variable
Glucose	Variable
Culture	Negative

Partial list of associated conditions:
    Trauma (exclude fracture)
    Hemorrhagic diatheses:
      Thrombocytopenia
      Anticoagulant therapy
      Hemophilia
      Sickle cell disease
      Malignancy
    Neuroarthropathy (Charcot joint)
    Joint prostheses
    Tumor:
      Pigmented villonodular synovitis
      Synovial hemangioma

*monocytosis may predominate

2. The mucin clot test also correlates with the amount of hyaluronate present and therefore reflects viscosity. When one part of normal synovial fluid is added to four parts of 2 per cent acetic acid and shaken, a firm button of clotted hyaluronate–protein complex forms at the bottom of the tube after standing for 5 minutes. With degraded hyaluronate from inflammation, no button forms, and the synovial fluid may contain friable shreds of clotted material.

The string test and mucin clot are generally interchangeable in the interpretation of synovial fluid viscosity, with most clinicians performing the former because of its simplicity.

Clarity

The clarity of normal synovial fluid can be reduced by any particulate matter, most commonly increased cellularity, but also by crystals, inclusion bodies, and lipids. The method for detecting loss of clarity generally involves placing black text on a white background, such as newsprint, behind a test tube containing synovial fluid. If the text can be read through the fluid in a bright light, its clarity is normal (transparent).

Color

Normal synovial fluid is colorless or pale yellow (straw-colored). When blood is found that is not caused by the procedure, it generally does not form clots and is distributed evenly throughout the fluid. Inflammatory fluid may appear as a deep yellow. Pus may be found, but its appearance may be mimicked by large numbers of crystals or inflammatory debris.

Cell Counts

A grossly bloody fluid may be caused by introduction of the needle or arthroscope and is usually evident during the procedure, since the blood obtained may be unevenly distributed, often clots, and may decrease as the procedure continues. A hematocrit reading from an anticoagulated tube should be obtained on all bloody effusions to determine whether it is blood per se, since only moderate amounts of red cells may simulate the appearance of whole blood. If red cells are actually present in the synovial fluid from the disease process, they are usually evenly distributed, do not clot, and remain consistent throughout the procedure. Furthermore, since the intra-articular breakdown of these disease-related red cells releases heme, a centrifuged specimen produces xanthochromia.

Considered one of the most important aspects of synovianalysis, the total and differential white cell count may be inaccurate if precautions are not observed. It is important that synovial fluid be promptly placed in appropriate anticoagulant and that no clumps of cells are found after gently shaking the tube. If clots remain, this should alert one that the total white count may be falsely low. Even if this is correctly done, differences may occur depending on whether manual or automated counting methods are employed. Manual counts are considered most accurate but have one pitfall: if acetic acid is inadvertently used as the diluent, synovial protein clots will entrap white cells and falsely lower the total count. Therefore, it is imperative that normal saline be used as the diluent. If the effusion is bloody, hypotonic (0.3 per cent) saline should be used to lyse the red cells, after a hematocrit determination is performed. Automated counters are not recommended, because of the large number of technical artifacts that may occur.

Crystals

The presence or absence of crystals in synovial fluid is as essential in the evaluation of disorders of the knee as the total cell count and differential, particularly since crystal-induced arthritis may produce inflammation with very high white counts overlapping those of septic arthritis. As with the cell count, precautions must be observed in order to obtain an accurate result. Considerable variation in correctly identifying crystals has been documented in clinical and hospital laboratories, and it is strongly recommended that the clinician personally perform the analysis to ensure accuracy, just as the hematologist does with the bone marrow examination.

Collection of the specimen into appropriate tubes is essential for success. As noted earlier, anticoagulated tubes may be used, but only with sodium heparin or EDTA. If lithium heparin or calcium oxalate are inadvertently used, crystalline artifacts will be produced and cause totally inaccurate results. Although nonanticoagulated specimens may also be used, inaccuracies may be caused by white cell clumps, obscuring the identification of crystals. An additional pitfall is the presence of corticosteroid crystals, which may be present for weeks after their instillation into the joint cavity.

Once collected into a tube containing sodium heparin or EDTA, a "wet mount" should be prepared as soon as possible. This requires placing a drop of synovial fluid on a slide free of dust or scratches, placing a clean coverslip over the drop, and sealing it on all four sides with clear nail polish. Sealing the coverslip avoids the streaming of cells as well as the de novo precipitation of crystals caused by dehydration of the specimen.

Assuming the correct collection of the specimen and preparation of the wet mount, the identification of crystals requires the use of a compensated polarized light microscope with a rotating stage. All clinicians who perform synovianalysis should have access to this equipment and be familiar with its use. Without it, significant joint pathology will be surely missed.

At the present time, four types of pathologic crystals may be identified: monosodium urate monohydrate (MSUM) in gout, calcium pyrophosphate dihydrate (CPPD) in pseudogout, calcium oxalate (CO) in chronic dialysis arthropathy, and hydroxyapatite (HA) in rotator cuff (Milwaukee shoulder) syndrome and erosive osteoarthritis.

The purpose of the compensated polarized light is twofold: it provides a black background that causes the crystalline material, which is most frequently found intracellularly, to stand out from the cells and other particulate material, allowing an estimation of size and shape; and it provides two optical characteristics of crystals, extinction and elongation (birefringence), which further aids in differentiating the specific type of crystal seen. The reader is referred to the bibliography for detailed discussions on identification of crystals.

Microbiology

The swift identification of septic arthritis of the knee depends upon analysis of the synovial fluid similar to those techniques used on the blood. As noted earlier, in patients in whom septicemia or soft tissue infection is suspected, synovianalysis should be deferred until ancillary data are obtained, to avoid contaminating a sterile joint.

Once fluid is collected in a sterile tube, aliquots should be placed into both aerobic and anaerobic blood agar vials, including tubercular and fungal media, and an additional aliquot should be immediately inoculated onto chocolate agar if gonococcal disease is suspected. Gram stain for bacteria and special stains for mycobacteria and fungi are best performed on a concentrated (centrifuged) aliquot.

Chemistry and Serology

The total protein of normal synovial fluid is usually about 2 gm/dl, or approximately 25 per cent that of the blood. If greater than 2.5 gm/dl, it is abnormal, with higher levels reflecting the degree of inflammation present.

Although fasting specimens are most accurate, normal synovial fluid glucose is about 90 per cent that of simultaneous blood. With inflammation, the levels of synovial fluid glucose diminish, the lowest levels generally occurring in septic arthritis.

Rheumatoid factor may be found in synovial fluid even in those patients with negative serum levels. Presumably, this is due to production by the synovial cells themselves, and may occur as a nonspecific reaction to many kinds of inflammation. It should not be used as an indicator of rheumatoid arthritis.

Many other components such as ANA, DNA, complement, globulins, cryoprecipitates, enzymes, and so on may be found in synovial fluid but are of little clinical value at present; they are mainly of research interest.

CLASSIFICATION GROUPS OF ABNORMAL SYNOVIAL FLUID

GROUP I (NONINFLAMMATORY)

These include the noninflammatory synovial fluids typically found in trauma (including internal derangement) and osteoarthritis. Rapid accumulation of a high volume of fluid after trauma may dilute the concentration of hyaluronate and reduce the viscosity, thereby causing an abnormal string test or mucin clot. Generally, the white cell counts are low (an average of 1000 per cubic millimeter) and rarely exceed 3000 cells per cubic millimeter. Grossly bloody synovial fluid (see Group IV) may occur after an injury without fracture, although careful exclusion should be performed. Reaccumulation of grossly bloody fluid should suggest other Group IV disorders. If osteoarthritis is suspected clinically but synovianalysis suggests otherwise, evaluation for superimposed crystal arthritis, particularly pseudogout (see Group II) or infection (see Group III) should be pursued. Advanced osteoarthritis may produce cartilage fragments and other debris. Worn or damaged prostheses may produce metallic, polymethylmethacrylate, or polyethylene fragments that can sometimes be confused with crystals. Immunodeficiency syndromes, including AIDS, may be associated with arthritis, with the synovial fluid being noninflammatory in the few reported cases.

GROUP II (INFLAMMATORY)

Because of the large number of inflammatory disorders included within this broad category, it is useful to divide those that are mildly inflammatory from those that are moderately or severely inflammatory. For mildly inflammatory fluid, this distinction is usually based upon the total and differential white cell count, which ranges between 1000 and 5000 per cubic millimeter, less than 30 per cent being polymorphonuclear. Although there is much overlap within Group II, disorders such as psoriatic and bowel-related arthritis, lupus, juvenile arthritis, and seronegative arthritis may demonstrate only mild inflammation. Many viral diseases may be associated with joint effusions that produce mild inflammation, generally with large numbers of mononuclear cells. Recent outbreaks of parvovirus infection in adults (after exposure to children with erythema infectiosum caused by the same agent) have been associated with arthritis with mild inflammatory fluid and a predominance of monocytes. Moderate-to-severe inflammatory fluid is typically found in rheumatoid arthritis and crystal-induced arthritis, with counts generally ranging from 10,000 to 50,000 per cubic millimeter, more than 50 per cent being polymorphonuclear. Acute rheumatic fever and Reiter's syndrome may also cause high cell counts. Rarely, counts approaching 100,000 cells per cubic millimeter may be found, but infection should be diligently excluded. Lyme arthritis has recently been shown to have varying white cell counts with a range from 5000 to above 300,000 per cubic millimeter. Cultures from the synovial fluid have not grown the spirochete. Tubercular and fungal infections may have low white cell counts and appear as Group II fluid. Also, sarcoma and other malignancies may be found within Group II fluid and can be identified by standard cytologic analysis.

GROUP III (SEPTIC)

Joint fluid, unlike serum, diminishes the normal phagocytic function of cells and allows uninhibited growth of microbial organisms. Infection, therefore, must be excluded in any patient with an unexplained arthritis, as well as in those patients with other arthritic diseases whose joint remains disparately inflamed. Acute bacterial infection, particularly with *Staphylococcus aureus,* produces very high white counts, typically 100,000 or more per cubic millimeter, with polymorphonuclear cells comprising at least 90 percent. However, lower white counts are not unusual, particularly in patients treated with antibiotics for any reason, prior to synovianalysis. Opportunistic organisms or tubercular or fungal infections may also produce lower white counts, with varying amounts of mononuclear and polymorphonuclear cells, and overlap with Group II fluids. Gonococcal arthritis may be a difficult diagnosis to establish unless the fluid is plated immediately onto chocolate agar. Disseminated gonococcal infection with arthritis may present with white cell counts below 20,000 per cubic millimeter.

GROUP IV (HEMORRHAGIC)

As little as a 10 per cent admixture of red cells may make a joint fluid look like whole blood, but when the fluid is determined to be truly hemorrhagic (Group IV), a number of disorders should be considered. If trauma has occurred, fracture should be excluded. Hemorrhagic diatheses, including hemophilia, sickle cell anemia, and thrombocytopenia, in addition to anticoagulant therapy, must be eliminated. Neuroarthropathy (Charcot's joint) may also produce a hemorrhagic fluid. Pigmented villonodular synovitis and synovial hemangioma must be eliminated. In addition, worn or damaged prostheses may cause bleeding within the joint.

Conclusion

In summary, synovianalysis is a critical component in the evaluation of knee joint pathology and rapidly allows the clinician to make specific diagnostic and therapeutic decisions. The routine use of synovianalysis can reveal clues to new developments in established disease, such as the superimposition of pseudogout on osteoarthritis, or infection in a rheumatoid knee. If, however, synovianalysis is to remain a valuable tool, it is essential that it be precisely performed.

Bibliography

1. Cohen AS, Brandt KD, Krey PR: Synovial fluid. *In* Laboratory Diagnostic Procedures in Rheumatic Disease. 2nd ed. Boston, Little, Brown, 1975, pp 1–62.
2. Culp RW, Eichenfield AH, Davidson RS, Drummond DS, Christofersen MR, Goldsmith DP: Lyme arthritis in children; An orthopedic perspective. J Bone Joint Surg 69:96–111, 1987.
3. Gatter RA: A Practical Handbook of Joint Fluid Analysis. Philadelphia, Lea and Febiger, 1984, pp 1–105.
4. Goldenberg DL, Reed JI: Medical progress—Bacterial arthritis. N Engl J Med 312:764–771, 1985.
5. Hasselbacher P: Variation in synovial fluid analysis by hospital laboratories. Arthritis and Rheum 30:637–642, 1987.
6. McCarthy DJ Jr: Synovial fluid. *In* Arthritis and Allied Conditions. 10th ed. Philadelphia, Lea and Febiger, 1985, pp 54–75.
7. Ropes MW, Bauer W: Synovial Fluid Change in Joint Disease. Cambridge, MA, Harvard University Press, 1953, pp 1–150 (the classic).
8. Schumacher HR: Synovial fluid analysis. *In* Kelley WN, Harris ED, Ruddy, S, Sledge C (eds): Textbook of Rheumatology. Philadelphia, WB Saunders, 1981, pp 568–579.
9. Semble EL, Agudelo CA, Pegram SP: Human parvovirus B19 arthropathy in two adults after contact with childhood erythema infectiosum. Am J Med 83(3):560–562, 1987.

5

Robert M. Wilson
Peter Fowler
Arthroscopic Anatomy

ANATOMY

When viewed through an arthroscope, the anatomy of the knee may seem very different from what is expected. The lens and water medium lead to distortion of shapes and sizes, and the angle of the lens may further change the orientation. Even normal tissue may appear unusual, and frank pathology may be missed. Without a clear understanding of the anatomy, the difficulty and time required for successful knee arthroscopy may be greatly increased.

The knee is a hinged synovial joint providing flexion and extension. Once partially flexed it also rotates, which allows rapid direction changes. The knee has little inherent stability when only its osseous structures are considered. It depends on the ligaments, the menisci, and the dynamic action of its muscles all working in concert to provide stability, especially in flexion. The joint consists of two major articulations, the femoral tibial joint and the patellofemoral joint. It is conveniently thought of as having three major compartments—lateral, medial, and patellofemoral. Each compartment has its own personality and often its own particular pathology.

Femoral Condyles

The distal articular end of the femur is composed of the two femoral condyles (Fig. 5–1). They are separated by the intercondylar notch. The lateral femoral condyle is wider in the anteroposterior (AP) and transverse planes and has an increased curvature; the medial projects further distally to allow for the normal genu valgum. The condyles are convex in their articulation with the tibia, and the area of articulation changes as the knee goes from full extension to full flexion.

Tibial Plateau

The tibial plateaus are essentially flat, although the lateral has a slight convexity. They slope posteriorly 10 degrees relative to the shaft of the tibia. The lateral articular surface extends farther posteriorly than the medial surface. This allows the lateral meniscus room to move with knee flexion. The medial meniscus does not enjoy this advantage. Between the tibial plateaus are the tibial spines, small projections that help provide static stability to transverse (sideways) motion. Nothing attaches to the tibial spines themselves. Just anterior to them, in the anterior intercondyloid fossa, the anterior horn of the medial meniscus, the anterior cruciate ligament, and then the anterior horn of the lateral meniscus are attached, in that order, going from anterior to posterior. The relatively poor contact area between the convex femoral condyle and the flat tibial surface is improved dramatically by the presence of the menisci.

Menisci

The menisci are semilunar spacers composed of firm fibrocartilage. They help increase the contact area, dissipate peak stresses, and provide increased stability and joint lubrication. They are avascular in the majority of their intra-articular portion but contain blood vessels and nerves in the peripheral one third. They attach to the tibia and femur by meniscotibial (coronary) and meniscofemoral ligament thickenings of the fibrous capsule (Fig. 5–2). The menisci are triangular in cross section, tapering centrally to a thin edge (the loss of this tapered edge may be one of the first clues to the presence of a meniscal tear). The collagen fibers are specifically arranged within the meniscus, with the outer fibers running

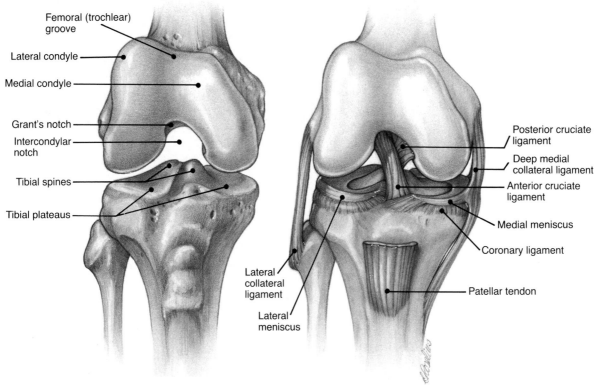

Figure 5–1
    Anterior view of the flexed knee. Note:
(1) lateral femoral condyle higher than medial;
(2) the two components of the anterior cruciate ligament (ACL) (anteromedial and posterolateral);
(3) posterior cruciate ligament (PCL) passing behind the ACL;
(4) deep medial collateral ligament (MCL) in contact with the medial meniscus.

circumferentially, to resist compressive displacement and longitudinal loading. It is important to avoid cutting into this outer one third peripheral portion when performing a partial meniscectomy. Most meniscal tears start out as a circumferential separation in line with these fibers and then progress inward to form either bucket handle or flap tears. The meniscus is a white, firm, rubbery structure. With age, the meniscus slowly discolors and loses its elasticity and recoil. The fringe will degenerate, losing its normal tapered edge (see Fig. 5–22*G*). In older menisci, horizontal cleavage tears are often seen.

The medial meniscus is less mobile than the lateral meniscus, partially because the deep fibers of the medial collateral ligament attach directly onto the midportion of the meniscus. This decreased mobility may help explain why the medial meniscus is injured more often than the lateral meniscus.

The lateral meniscus is thicker, wider, more circular, and more mobile than the medial meniscus (Fig. 5–3). It covers up to two thirds of the articular surface of the tibia and occasionally is seen as a discoid meniscus covering the entire surface. The anterior horn attaches posterior to the anterior cruciate liga-

ment (ACL) in the intercondylar fossa of the tibia. The posterior horn, which is more firmly attached, often has meniscal femoral ligaments going up to the medial femoral condyle. Specifically, the ligament of Wrisberg runs posterior to the posterior cruciate ligament (PCL) and the ligament of Humphrey anterior to the PCL (Figs. 5–3 and 5–4). In the posterior lateral attachment of the lateral meniscus is a 1-cm hiatus for the passage of the popliteus tendon (Fig. 5–4; see also Fig. 5–23). This area, the popliteal recess, is a common site for loose bodies to collect.

The popliteus muscle arises from the posterior medial surface of the tibia above the soleal line. It forms a strong, cordlike tendon sloping upward and lateral, approximately 2.5 cm long. This tendon passes beneath the arcuate ligament, entering the joint through an aperture in the lateral capsule to become invested with synovium. It passes through the hiatus in the attachment of the lateral meniscus and inserts onto the lateral condyle of the femur just anterior to the lateral collateral ligament. A portion of the tendon attaches directly to the lateral meniscus to assist in pulling it posterior with knee flexion (Fig. 5–4). It is the only muscle capable of rotating

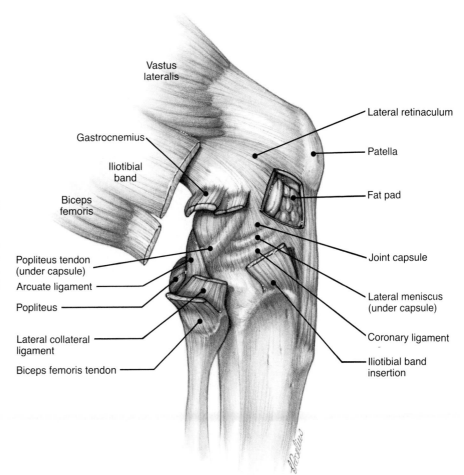

Figure 5-2
Lateral view of the flexed knee. Note:
(1) the coronary ligament;
(2) the popliteus tendon passing through a hiatus in the lateral meniscus to insert anterior to the lateral collateral ligament.

the leg on the extended knee. Its principal function is to unlock the knee from full extension, reversing the so-called "screw home mechanism." It is also a component of the posterolateral support of the knee, providing stability along with the arcuate ligament, biceps tendon, and lateral collateral ligament.

Intercondylar Notch

Between the condyles is the intercondylar notch. This is a cavelike area housing the cruciate ligaments. The notch must be wide enough not to impinge on the cruciates. In individuals with congeni-

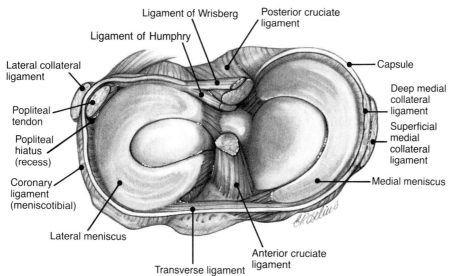

Figure 5-3
Superior view of the tibial plateau with the meniscus preserved. Note:
(1) the thicker, more circular, lateral meniscus;
(2) the popliteal hiatus;
(3) the C-shaped medial meniscus anchored to the deep collateral ligament.

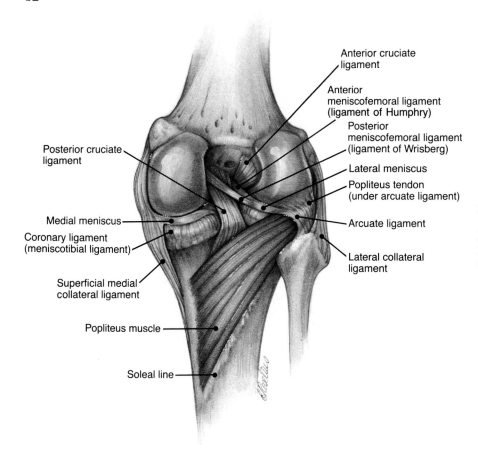

Posterior cruciate
ligament

Medial meniscus

Coronary ligament
(meniscotibial ligament)

Superficial medial
collateral ligament

Popliteus muscle

Soleal line

Anterior cruciate
ligament

Anterior
meniscofemoral ligament
(ligament of Humphry)

Posterior
meniscofemoral ligament
(ligament of Wrisberg)

Lateral meniscus

Popliteus tendon
(under arcuate ligament)

Arcuate ligament

Lateral collateral
ligament

Figure 5–4
Posterior view of the knee.
Note the popliteus tendon passing upward through the lateral
meniscus.

tally narrow notches, anterior cruciate ligament ruptures may be more common. The notch extends farther anteriorly to provide clearance for the anterior cruciate ligament in full extension. This extension is called Grant's notch (see Fig. 5–1). In individuals with chronic cruciate insufficiency, the entire notch may be narrowed by osteophyte formation. These impinging osteophytes must be removed at the time of cruciate reconstruction.

Anterior Cruciate Ligament

The anterior cruciate ligament (ACL) is the most frequent ligament reconstructed after sports injuries. It is often injured in a noncontact pivoting deceleration injury, in which case it may be an isolated injury, or following severe valgus or varus stress after the collateral ligaments are injured. Occasionally, with hyperextension, both the ACL and posterior cruciate ligament (PCL) may be ruptured.

The ACL is approximately 4 cm long by 11 mm wide. It arises from the anterior tibia between the anterior horns of the medial and lateral menisci: it remains intra-articular to insert on the lateral femoral condyle posteriorly. It is responsible for guiding the tibia during flexion and extension and assisting in proper rollback of the femoral condyle. Without a

properly functioning ACL the tibia is able to sublux forward. This improper excursion during knee motion may cause meniscal damage and increased articular cartilage destruction, especially in the medial compartment.

The ligament spirals as it passes through the joint, forming two major functional components. The portion arising more anteromedially from the tibia twists over the more posterolateral component and inserts farther posteriorly on the femur (see Fig. 5–1B). Because of this more anterior origin and posterior femoral insertion, these fibers tighten with knee flexion. The shorter posterolateral component comprises the bulk of the ligament and tightens with knee extension. The two portions acting together provide stability throughout the range of motion in the normal knee. If just the posterolateral fibers are ruptured, one may see an unstable knee with a positive Lachman sign and pivot shift test but there may be a negative drawer sign as the anteromedial fibers remain to resist anterior displacement in flexion. In acute ACL repairs, a better anatomic repair is possible if separate sutures are placed in each portion, with the anteromedial portion pulled more posteriorly in an over-the-top fashion, while the posterolateral sutures are secured to the lateral femoral condyle slightly more anteriorly through drill holes. Both portions of the ACL and PCL are tightened with internal tibial rotation.

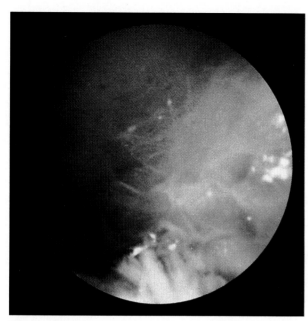

Figure 5–5
Crystal synovitis. Note particles of calcium pyrophosphate imbedded within the synovium.

Posterior Cruciate Ligament

The posterior cruciate ligament (PCL) is the strongest ligament in the knee. It arises extra-articularly from the posterior surface of the tibia. It becomes invested in synovium and has a broad insertion on the anterior portion of the medial femoral condyle. It is tightened in full flexion and with internal rotation. It is a very important stabilizer of the knee, providing the main restraint to posterior tibial displacement. It is also crucial in guiding the rotation of the knee to produce the "screw home mechanism." Without a PCL, the normal center of axis of rotation at the joint shifts from the midportion of the medial compartment to a more lateral position in the center of the joint. This abnormal motion leads to greatly increased peak stresses. This may help explain the occasional disastrous consequence of PCL insufficiency: early severe degeneration of the articular cartilage of the medial compartment.

Unlike chronic ACL insufficiency which often presents with the chief complaint of episodic instability and giving way, chronic PCL instability usually presents with a history of chronic pain. (There may be a feeling of almost daily instability, especially when descending stairs, but this is usually not the chief complaint.) The chronic pain is associated with the degeneration of the articular surface, which may happen many years after the initial injury.

The common mechanisms of PCL injury include hyperflexion (in which it may be an isolated injury); hyperextension (in which the ACL may also be injured); a direct violent posterior displacement (a so-called dashboard injury); or after a severe valgus or varus force after complete tearing of the collateral structures.

After an acute isolated PCL injury the patient may not have the tense hemarthrosis seen in ACL tears, since the bleeding portion of the PCL tends to be extrasynovial and therefore the swelling remains outside the knee joint.

Synovium

The knee joint is completely lined with synovium, which is a tough, waterproof layer containing numerous cells capable of producing the synovial fluid necessary for normal knee lubrication and cartilage nutrition. The synovium invests the ACL, PCL, and popliteus tendons. Its border goes right up to the beginning of the meniscus and the edge of the articular cartilage. It extends superiorly into the suprapatellar pouch almost 3 inches above the patella. In a normal young patient the synovium is flat, glistening, thin, and almost transparent. It is richly innervated and very vascular. Synovial disorders can be best evaluated arthroscopically. They include pigmented villonodular synovitis (PVNS), crystal synovitis (chondrocalcinosis) (Fig. 5–5), synovial chondrometaplasia, proliferative synovitis of rheumatoid arthritis, or the chronically irritated synovium seen with degenerative joint disease (Fig. 5–6). The arthroscope is used to perform directed biopsies (which are especially important in localized PVNS), and for

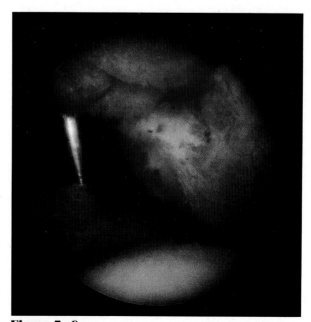

Figure 5–6
Chronic synovitis in a 54 year old patient with degenerative joint disease.

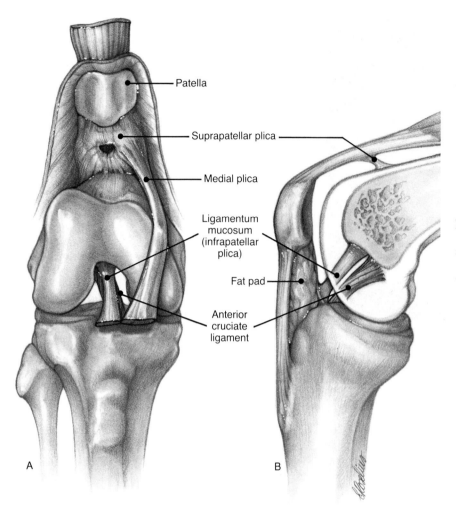

A

B

Figure 5–7
A, Anterior view of the knee showing the suprapatellar and medial plicae. *B,* Lateral view of the knee and ligamentum mucosum.

irrigation and partial debridement in chondrocalcinosis or in total synovectomy (which is the procedure of choice for PVNS).

Plicae

Plicae are synovial shelves within the knee joint. The fetal knee is divided into compartments by septa that recede before birth except for small remnants called plicae. In some individuals these embryonic synovial septa persist into adult life, often as firm fibrous bands. The suprapatellar plica may persist as a wall across the suprapatellar pouch completely separating it from the rest of the knee joint. The medial plica is the one most often implicated as a pathologic condition. It extends from the suprapatellar pouch parallel to the medial gutter, ending at the ligamentum mucosum (Fig. 5–7). In flexion it will cross the medial femoral condyle. With repeated trauma it may thicken (Fig. 5–8), leading to medial jointline pain with symptoms of snapping, instability, and occasionally even a block to extension. These may

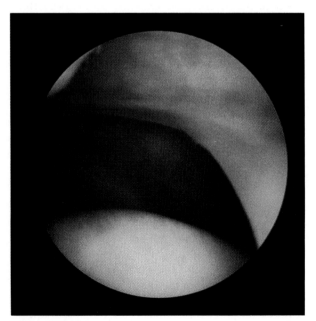

Figure 5–8
Mildly thickened medial plica.

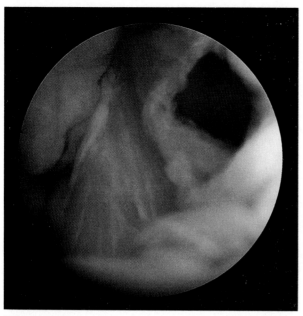

Figure 5–9
Ligamentum mucosum. In this patient the thin ligamentum mucosum divided the knee except for the oval foramen visible on the right.

mimic the symptoms of a torn medial meniscus. The most successful treatment has been by arthroscopic division and partial excision.

The final portion of this embryologic septum is the ligamentum mucosum (the infrapatellar plica). This normally is a synovial band of tissue extending from the femur at the top of the intercondylar notch inserting onto the fat pad (Fig. 5–7B). When first viewed arthroscopically this may be confused with the anterior cruciate ligament. The two can be rapidly differentiated by probing and by proper visualization. Occasionally the ligamentum muscosum persists as a larger, fanlike synovial wall separating the medial and lateral compartments, making it more difficult to pass the arthroscope or instruments from one compartment into the other (Fig. 5–9).

Patella

The patella is a large sesamoid bone within the quadriceps tendon. It functions biomechanically to increase the efficacy of the quadriceps muscle and also to physically protect the articular surface of the femoral condyle. It is composed of two major facets—the medial and the lateral, which are separated by a central keel (Fig. 5–10). There is also a smaller odd

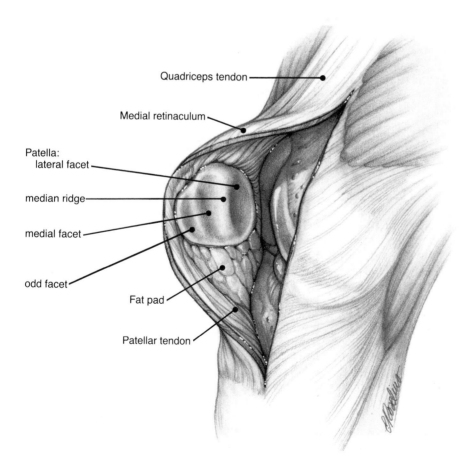

Quadriceps tendon
Medial retinaculum
Patella:
    lateral facet
median ridge
medial facet
odd facet
Fat pad
Patellar tendon

Figure 5–10
Lateral view of the everted patella following medial arthrotomy.

medial facet at the far medial side that comes into contact with the femur only with full flexion. The medial facet is usually smaller and more convex than the lateral facet. An unfused superolateral ossification center is present in the bipartite patella. This may be misdiagnosed on radiographs as a patellar fracture but can usually be differentiated by its superolateral position, rounded scalloped edge, and sclerotic lines. It very occasionally becomes symptomatic after trauma and may require excision.

The femur has a sulcus, or trochlear groove, in which the patella tracks during its excursion from full extension to flexion. Normally the lateral lip (the anterolateral femoral condyle) is wider and higher than the medial. If hypoplastic, this shallow sulcus may contribute to a subluxating patella. Another anatomic cause of recurrent subluxation is patella alta (or high-riding patella).

Patients may complain of anterior knee pain without evidence of instability, the so-called patellofemoral syndrome. Classically, this is most symptomatic during activities that involve the dynamic compression of the patella, such as climbing stairs or squatting, or with unrelieved static compression, such as prolonged sitting (the so-called "movie sign"). Abnormal tracking may contribute to this syndrome, with findings of malalignment, including lateral deviation of the patellar tendon (abnormal Q angle), squinting patella with lateral tracking, increased femoral anteversion, hindfoot hyperpronation, and abnormal muscle development or insertion (such as a hypoplastic vastus medialis). Excessive lateral facet pressure syndrome may be seen with contracture and fibrosis of the lateral retinaculum. Many of these conditions are at least partially ameliorated by performing an arthroscopic lateral release. More severe cases may require proximal or distal realignment procedures or tibial tubercle elevation.

Cartilage

All articular bone surfaces are covered by hyaline cartilage (articular cartilage). This is composed of chondrocytes embedded in an abundant matrix composed of glycosaminoglycans and collagen fibers (primarily type II). This matrix has an organized arrangement of collagen fibers, with the outer zones having horizontally aligned fibers to resist shear stress and maintain structural integrity; in the deeper zones, the fibers become more vertically aligned to resist compression. Glycosaminoglycans are extremely hydrophilic, attracting and holding water molecules. This provides the firmness and maintains the shock absorption of cartilage by placing the collagen fibers under tension within the matrix.

In young individuals, cartilage is a white, firm, smooth, glistening surface. With age or degeneration it becomes softer and less able to efficiently reduce

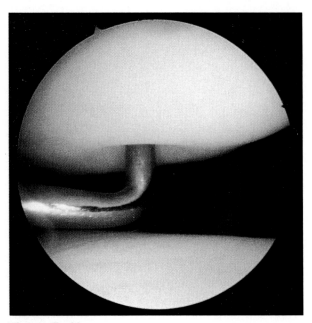

Figure 5–11
  Grade I chondromalacia. A normal-appearing patella until probing revealed softening.

the peak stress to the underlying bone. Microscopically, there is basal degeneration with rupture of the collagen fibers, and they lose their ordered arrangement. The composition of the glycosaminoglycans changes, with a decrease in their water-holding ability, leading to a loss of turgor. The cartilage surface becomes softer, with small areas of bulging and blister formation. The color becomes yellowish and the normal slippery translucent surface changes to a dull, slightly colored one. Fissuring, blister rupture, and surface degeneration with a "crabmeat" appearance and fragmentation occur. Finally there is the full-thickness loss of cartilage with exposed subchondral bone. This continuum of degeneration is often divided into stages for arthroscopic classification. Grade I is the mild softening, blister formation, and slight irregularity (Figs. 5–11 and 5–12); Grade II includes fissuring, fibrillation, and the crabmeat appearance (Figs. 5–13 and 5–14); and Grade III is exposed subchondral bone with severe degeneration (Figs. 5–15 and 5–16).

Normal cartilage, once damaged, has little intrinsic ability for repair; however, following a full-thickness lesion to the subchondral bone there is access to undifferentiated fibroblasts from the vascular system. If stimulated, these may produce a fibrocartilage (scar cartilage) capable of filling in some defects. The cartilage produced is weaker, less organized, and less able to resist compressive or shear stress, but it is better than articulating with raw bone.

Stimulation of these fibroblasts by debridement down to bleeding bone is the principle of "abrasion" arthroplasty (Fig. 5–17).

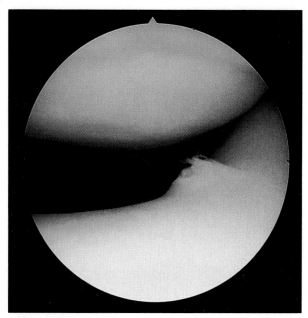

Figure 5–12
Grade I chondromalacia. Femoral groove with a small blister lesion.

PUNCTURE SITES

The proper selection of portal sites may be the key to successful arthroscopy. We will describe primary and auxiliary portals. The primary (or routine) portals are used in most arthroscopies and are often the

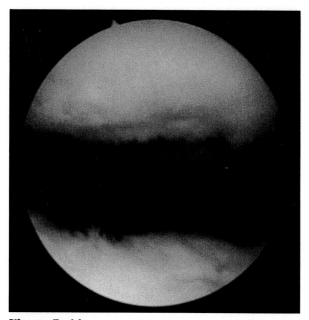

Figure 5–14
Grade II chondromalacia. Both patellar and femoral surfaces show fissuring and a "crabmeat" appearance.

only ones needed, but to be truly successful as an arthroscopist it is important to be thoroughly familiar and comfortable with all the sites (Figs. 5–18 and 5–19). Occasionally only one of the auxiliary portals will provide the proper positioning of the scope or surgical instrument necessary to successfully complete an arthroscopic procedure.

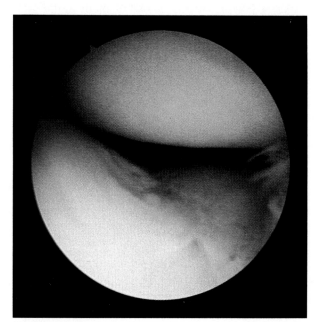

Figure 5–13
Grade II chondromalacia. Femoral groove with mild cartilage fissuring and fibrillation.

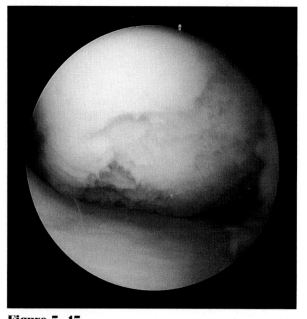

Figure 5–15
Grade III chondromalacia. Medial femoral condyle with full-thickness loss of articular cartilage.

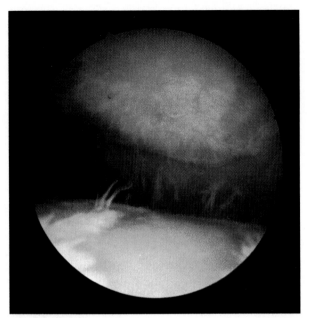

Figure 5–16
Grade III chondromalacia. Patellofemoral joint with full-thickness cartilage loss. Note reactive synovium.

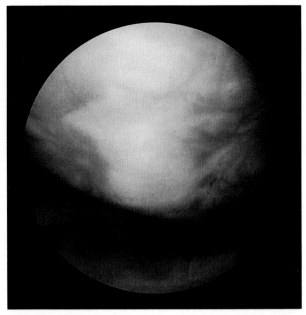

Figure 5–17
Fibrocartilage. A medial femoral condyle 8 months following abrasion chondroplasty for Grade III chondromalacia.

Primary Portals

SUPEROMEDIAL

This is usually the first portal made. It is used to insert the inflow cannula into the knee joint and distend the knee. (Some prefer a superolateral portal for this, possibly to avoid injury to the vastus medialis muscle, which would prolong rehabilitation, but we have rarely observed any prolonged tenderness or fibrosis.) The superomedial insertion places the in-

flow (or outflow) cannula into the suprapatellar pouch (or medial gutter) away from the actual compartments. The muscle bulk of the vastus medialis provides a good watertight seal, decreasing fluid leakage. The medial placement of the cannula positions it out of the way of the commonly used lateral post or leg holder. The superomedial position is also the best for viewing patellar tracking.

The puncture site is 2 fingerbreadths above the superior pole of the patella and medially in line with the medial patellar border (Fig. 5–19A). We use a

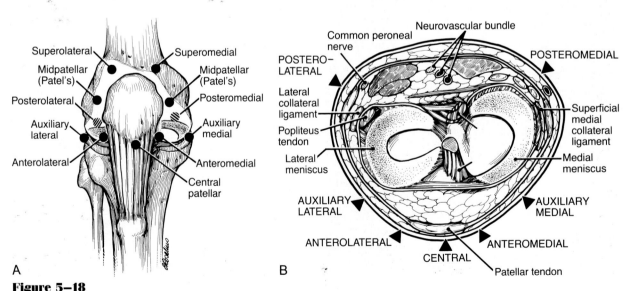

Figure 5–18
A, Anterior view of the knee, showing various portals used in knee arthroscopy. *B*, Transverse section of the knee, showing various arthroscopy portals.

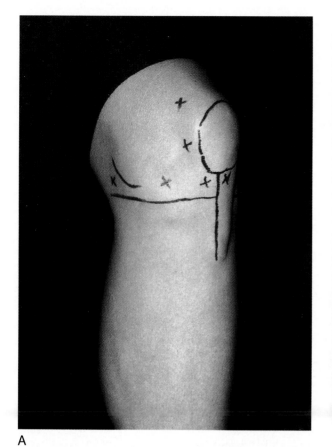

A

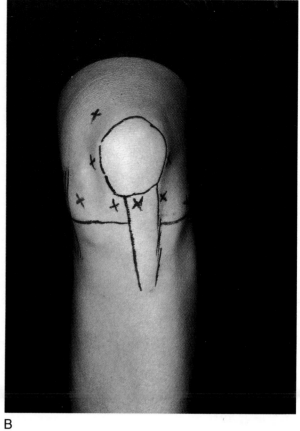

B

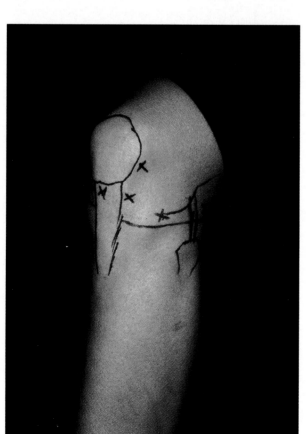

C

Figure 5–19

The knee marked for proper portal placement. *A*, Medial; *B*, anterior; *C*, lateral. (Photographs courtesy of Jayne Papac.)

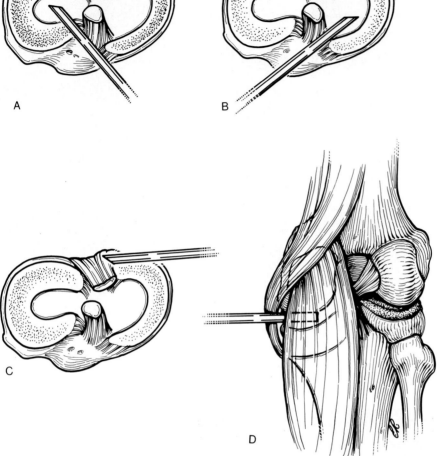

Figure 5–20
   A, Anteromedial portal, with arthroscope in lateral compartment. *B,* Anterolateral portal, with arthroscope in medial compartment. *C,* Posteromedial portal. *D,* Posterior view of the knee with arthroscope in the posteromedial portal.

number 15 scalpel directed posteriorly with the knee flexed, and then the knee is extended and the blade is angled distally and laterally and pierces the capsule. The inflow cannula with the blunt obturator is then inserted into the suprapatellar pouch, first underneath the patella and then angled superiorly out of the way of the patellofemoral articulation. It is important not to make the puncture site too far posteriorly where large circumflex vessels could be injured.

SUPEROLATERAL

   This portal is less frequently used. The fibers of the vastus lateralis in this area are thin and tough, which often leads to fluid leakage and loss of joint distention.

ANTEROMEDIAL

   The anteromedial (Fig. 5–20A) and the anterolateral (Fig. 5–20B) are the two routine working portals of arthroscopy. Generally each portal provides optimal visualization of the ipsilateral compartment. We prefer to start with the anteromedial as our initial portal for scope insertion. The knee is flexed and a point is chosen 1 fingerbreadth above the anterior joint line (to be above the medial meniscus) and at the medial edge of the patellar tendon. (Some prefer that the incision be made 1 cm medial to the patellar edge, feeling that the insertion will then avoid the fat pad.) We have found that the more central location aids significantly in visualization of the medial compartment and provides room for a second medial auxiliary portal. The number 15 knife blade is placed at the selected location and directed into the intercondylar notch area, with the cutting blade turned away from the patellar tendon (see Figs. 5–18B and 5–19B). The skin and capsule are pierced with a single straight puncture, after which an arthroscopic sheath with a blunt obturator can be inserted through the synovium and into the knee.

Advantages
   The anteromedial portal is more central than the anterolateral portal, providing better overall visualization of both the medial and lateral compartments.

Disadvantages

Femoral osteophytes may hinder scope placement from this portal into the patellofemoral joint. It occasionally is difficult to visualize the posterior horn of the medial meniscus from this portal.

ANTEROLATERAL

This is the primary portal for many arthroscopic surgeons due to its good visualization of the medial compartment (Fig. 5–20*B*). It is made by flexing the knee to 60 degrees and palpating the tibial joint surface. A stab incision is made 1 fingerbreadth superior to the palpable tibial plateau and at the lateral edge of the patellar tendon (see Fig. 5–19*B*). The knife is directed into the intercondylar notch.

Advantages

This is the best anterior portal for viewing the patellofemoral joint or a medial synovial plica and for searching for loose bodies in the lateral gutter. If the arthroscope is placed into the anteromedial portal, this then is the primary insertion for the probe or surgical instruments.

Disadvantages

The patellar tendon is lateral to the midline and hence the lateral portal is placed farther away from the center of the joint than the medial portal. This may cause difficulty viewing the posterior horn of the lateral meniscus. The more superficial location of the lateral meniscus at this site, as compared with the medial meniscus, may make manipulation of the arthroscope slightly more difficult.

MEDIAL AUXILIARY

With the arthroscope in the anteromedial portal, it is often very helpful to have a second medial portal. This can be made approximately 1 inch medial to the routine anteromedial portal to allow the use of two instruments (see Figs. 5–18*B* and 5–19*A*). One instrument is brought in through this medial auxiliary portal and the second instrument through the standard anterolateral portal. This two-instrument technique is useful so that traction can be applied while cutting. Also, the more posterior location of the medial auxiliary portal places it behind the convexity of the femoral condyle and allows a more direct line to the posterior horn of the medial meniscus.

The portal is made immediately above the medial meniscus approximately 1 inch from the anteromedial portal. A spinal needle can be inserted first to check the position and confirm that there is a straight passage to the area of pathology. The number 15 blade should be placed parallel to the meniscus and the portal made with a single insertion. A similar portal can be made on the lateral side if needed.

MIDPATELLAR (PATEL'S)

This is a slightly superior portal used for arthroscope placement. It is made 5 mm from the patellar edge in the midportion of the patella (see Figs. 5–18*A* and 5–19). It allows the arthroscope to be placed in the anterior portion of the desired compartment and then, by rotating the arthroscope backward, a clear view of the contralateral meniscus is possible. Instruments may be placed through the anteromedial or anterolateral portals for surgical procedures while the arthroscope remains anterior and "out of the way."

CENTRAL

This portal is placed directly through the patellar tendon just distal to the tip of the patella (above the fat pad). It is located at the center of the joint, *not* at the center of the patellar tendon (see Fig. 5–18). The skin incision may be made horizontally if desired, but the stab incision through the tendon must be performed with the blade turned 90 degrees vertically so it is parallel to the fibers of the tendon. This portal has been popularized by Gillquist in Europe (it is sometimes called the "Swedish portal"). It allows good visualization of both compartments. It also is useful in the three-portal technique of arthroscopic surgery in which the grasping and cutting instruments are then placed through anteromedial and anterolateral portals.

Disadvantages

In violating the patellar tendon there is the possibility of causing a mild, prolonged postoperative tendinitis. Also, the prominent fat pad may increase the soft tissue impingement, interfering with arthroscope motion and intra-articular placement. We feel that the centrally placed anteromedial portal is almost a "central" portal and has its advantages without requiring violation of the patellar tendon. The patellar tendon portal should not be used routinely.

POSTEROMEDIAL (Fig. 5–20*C, D*)

This portal allows direct observation or instrument passage into the posteromedial compartment. It is useful for fully evaluating the posterior cruciate ligament (Fig. 5–21), removal of loose bodies, exploration of Baker's cysts, or dealing occasionally with posterior horn tears of the medial meniscus. The skin incision is made with the knee flexed. A point is chosen 1 inch above the palpable posterior tibial plateau and posterior to the medial collateral ligament. This should be in a soft spot that is overlying the posterior oblique ligament. By first placing the arthroscope in the anterolateral portal and through the intercondylar notch, it is possible to view the posteromedial compartment. The light of the arthroscope will then transilluminate outside the joint and assist in placing

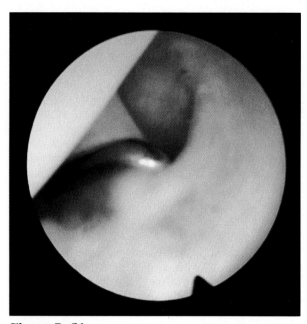

Figure 5—21
Posterior cruciate ligament, viewed through a postero-medial portal with a probe on the ligament.

the skin incision. The position can be confirmed with a spinal needle that is inserted and then seen intra-articularly. A Number 15 blade is inserted in the same spot and directed parallel to the needle. The knife is used to pierce the skin and capsule. A cannula with a blunt obturator can then be inserted to pierce the synovium. The most common mistake is placing the skin incision too far anterior. Just prior to piercing the capsule the knee can be momentarily distended by having an assistant squeeze on the saline bags. If necessary, a second accessory portal can be made 1 cm superior for instrument insertion.

POSTEROLATERAL

This portal is seldom used. Occasionally it is needed for removal of a loose body, to evaluate more fully the posterior horn of the lateral meniscus, or to explore the popliteus tendon. A skin incision is made with the knee flexed. A point is chosen at the insertion of a line drawn along the inferior border of the iliotibial band and a line along the posterior border of the fibula. This is a soft spot immediately behind the lateral collateral ligament (which can be palpated with the knee in a figure four position) and above the biceps tendon. There is more soft tissue here than on the posteromedial side, and maximal joint distention is necessary. A large spinal needle placed in this spot and directed just posterior to the femoral condyle (see Fig. 5–19C) will enter the joint with a palpable pop and clear saline should return. A knife is used to make the portal, after which a cannula with a blunt obturator is inserted into the joint.

COMPARTMENTS

In arthroscopy, one should consider the knee as containing three main compartments: the lateral, the medial, and the patellofemoral. Also, an assessment of the intercondylar notch, suprapatellar pouch, medial and lateral gutters, and posteromedial and posterolateral recesses is usually required. Each compartment has its own particular anatomy and often its own pathology. It is important to evaluate each area systematically and fully. This should be done methodically, following a set pattern of examination each time to avoid overlooking any pathology. We prefer to begin the arthroscopic surgery by placing the inflow cannula into the superomedial portal and distending the knee with saline. The anteromedial portal is then made, and the arthroscopic sheath with the blunt obturator is placed into the knee. It is directed slightly superiorly and into the intercondylar notch. There is often a palpable "pop" as it pierces the synovium. The knee is now placed in a figure four position by flexing, internally rotating, and abducting the hip and flexing the knee. The arthroscopic sheath can be placed in front of the anterior cruciate ligament and into the lateral compartment. The obturator is now removed and the arthroscope inserted. The first compartment visualized is the lateral one.

Lateral Compartment

With the arthroscope in the anterior portion of the compartment and angled posteriorly, the posterior horn of the lateral meniscus is visualized (Fig. 5–22B). This is wider, thicker, and more firmly attached than the anterior horn. By rotating the arthroscope the entire meniscus can be evaluated. It should have a fine, tapered edge throughout its length. Any suspicious area should be probed. The probe is usually inserted through the anterolateral portal. The probe is used to lift the meniscus gently to inspect its undersurface, to probe gently the meniscal synovial junction, and to hook the posterior horn and pull it forward, noting its excursion. The popliteal hiatus is visualized (Fig. 5–23) and should not be mistaken as a tear. This is a common area for small loose bodies to collect. The lateral meniscus is more mobile than the medial meniscus and can be drawn farther into the joint with a probe. It is extremely rare though, for the meniscus to be so "hypermobile" as to cause symptoms. The lateral meniscus has an O shape, with its anterior and posterior horns brought much closer together, and it is wider, covering a larger portion of the tibial surface than the medial surface.

Articular cartilage of the femur and tibia is inspected by taking the knee through a range of motion from extension to full flexion. The entire femoral cartilage will then pass in front of the arthroscope.

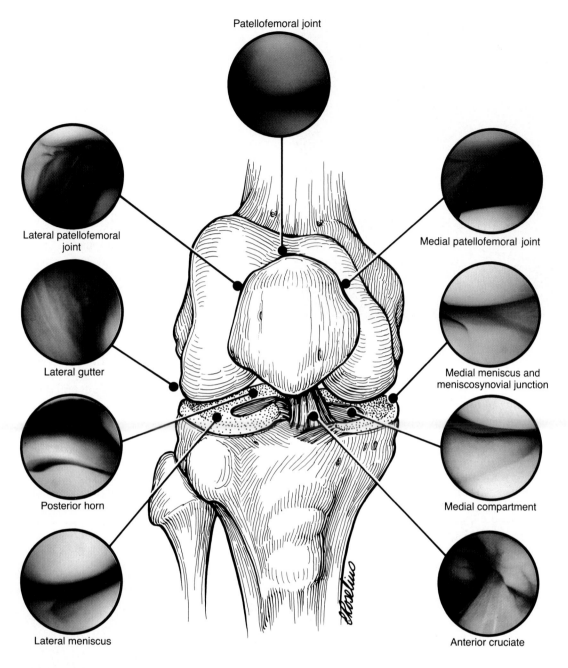

Figure 5—22
Anterior view of the knee showing each section as it appears with arthroscopy.

(If a meniscal tear extending into the anterior horn has been identified, this area often can be better visualized by placing the arthroscope through a mid-patellar [Patel's] portal.)

The anterior horn of the meniscus is followed around to enter the intercondylar notch. The knee is then placed in 70 to 90 degrees of flexion and the intercondylar notch inspected.

Intercondylar Notch

The intercondylar notch is best viewed through the anteromedial portal. We continue with the routine arthroscopy by slightly elevating the arthroscope superiorly and rotating the lens downward for a full panoramic view of the notch. The arthroscope should be withdrawn far enough to visualize both walls of

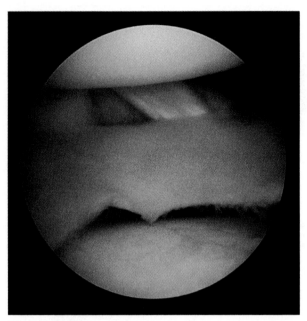

Figure 5–23
Lateral meniscus, with popliteal tendon passing through its hiatus.

the notch. The anterior cruciate ligament should be seen clearly arising from the lateral femoral condyle and then inserting onto the tibia (Fig. 5–24; see also Fig. 5–22*I*). Frequently a large blood vessel is noted on the surface of the ligament. Occasionally the synovial covering is very thick; in cases of suspected injury this may need to be partially stripped or cleared by carefully inserting the probe and pulling down parallel to the fibers of the ACL. Only then can an actual disruption of the ACL fibers be noted.

The smaller, more superior, and unsubstantial structure, the ligamentum mucosum, is often present and should not be confused with the ACL (see Figs. 5–7 and 5–9). It does not arise from the lateral femoral condyle but from the superior portion of the notch. When probed it does not have the firm longitudinal fibers that the ACL possesses.

Partially hidden behind the ACL will be the posterior cruciate ligament. This is covered by an even thicker synovium, and the ligament must be carefully probed to determine its integrity. Both its anterior portion inserting on the medial femoral condyle and the more posterior portion in the posterior medial recess can be evaluated. The arthroscope can now be directed along the wall of the medial femoral condyle and straight posterior. The small opening between the ACL and the posterior horn of the medial meniscus is seen; aiming for this area and rotating the arthroscope allows it to pass along the tibial spine and into the posteromedial recess. The arthroscope is then slowly withdrawn as it is angled medially. The posterior horn of the medial meniscus will come into view. By rotating the arthroscope laterally, the posterior cruciate ligament with its synovial covering is

visible. The posteromedial compartment is a common site for loose bodies to collect.

If further evaluation or surgery in the posteromedial compartment is required, a posteromedial portal can be made. This will allow even better visualization of the posterior cruciate ligament, and a probe can then be passed from the anterolateral portal posteriorly to apply traction on the ligament while it is viewed with the arthroscope placed in the posteromedial portal (see Fig. 5–21). This is also the best way to remove loose bodies from the compartment. A Baker's cyst may be explored from this portal.

To continue the routine arthroscopy, the knee is then partially extended to approximately 30 degrees of flexion and a valgus force is applied while the arthroscope is inserted into the medial compartment.

Medial Compartment

The medial compartment is best visualized from the anterolateral portal (see Fig. 5–20*B*) (although in routine diagnostic arthroscopy, if the arthroscope is still in the anteromedial portal this is usually adequate) (Fig. 5–25). With the knee positioned as noted, the arthroscope is directed into the far medial side of the compartment, with the lens angled posteriorly to bring the posterior horn of the medial meniscus into view. In very tight knees this may require some trial manipulation to assess whether slightly more flexion or extension is best. Also, external rotation of the tibia and valgus stress open up the compartment. The posterior horn of the medial meniscus is farther posterior than that of the lateral meniscus. The probe is usually necessary to assess its integrity.

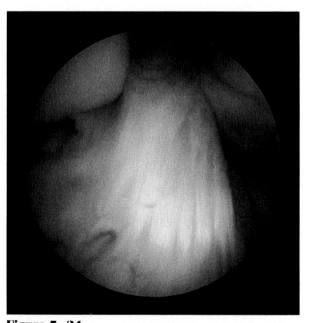

Figure 5–24
Normal anterior cruciate ligament.

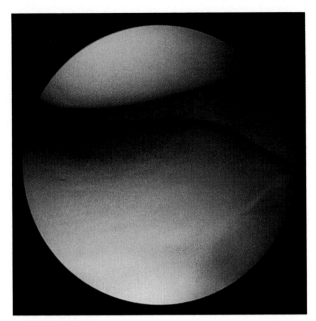

Figure 5–25
Medial compartment with normal meniscus.

The probe is placed through an anterior portal and is used to gently lift up the leading edge of the meniscus to visualize the ventral surface and inspect for tears. The probe is then used to hook gently along the meniscal synovial junction, evaluating for longitudinal separations, and the leading edge is carefully probed for any small flap tears. In a very tight knee, an auxiliary medial portal will allow the probe a more direct path to the posterior horn of the medial meniscus. Occasionally it is desirable to switch arthroscope portals to inspect the compartment fully. Again, a midpatellar (Patel's) portal will allow excellent evaluation of the anterior horn.

The cartilage surfaces should be carefully inspected and probed, and the knee is again taken through a full range of motion.

The medial gutter is inspected by releasing the valgus stresses and slightly flexing the knee. The condition of the synovium is noted and loose bodies are sought. The knee is now extended and the arthroscope rotated superiorly over the top of the medial gutter and inserted into the suprapatellar pouch.

Patellofemoral Joint (Suprapatellar Pouch)

An easy way to view the patellofemoral joint is with the arthroscope through the anterolateral portal with the knee extended. This gives a direct route to the undersurface of the patella. If patellar debridement is necessary, it may be done using a midpatellar (Patel's) portal, or else the shaver is inserted in the

anterolateral site and the arthroscope remains in the anteromedial portal.

With the arthroscope inserted all the way into the suprapatellar pouch, this area is carefully checked by rotating the lens and then directing the arthroscope back and forth. The synovium is carefully inspected. This is another common area for loose bodies to collect. At the end of the suprapatellar pouch is the beginning of the medial synovial plica as it courses down along the medial gutter (see Fig. 5–7). This can be checked for any thickening or fibrosis, and by slowly flexing the knee, any impingement across the femoral condyle (see Fig. 5–8) can be noted.

Slowly withdrawing the arthroscope and rotating the lens superiorly and centrally brings the patella into view (see Fig. 5–22D, E, F). By manipulating the patella externally, it can be fully visualized. With the arthroscope placed medially and the lens rotated back into the joint, the far medial (odd) facet can be seen. This often has an area of asymptomatic chondromalacia (this area only makes contact with a fully flexed knee). The medial and lateral facets are probed and inspected for chondromalacia. The arthroscope can then be rotated downward to evaluate the femoral groove. With the arthroscope anterior and distal to the patella and the lens rotated back toward the suprapatellar pouch, the knee is slowly flexed. In this position the patella will be seen to slowly settle down and make contact with the femoral groove. The full articulation of the patellofemoral joint can be visualized as the knee is further flexed (see Fig. 5–22E). Patellar tracking is noted.

Normally the lateral facet of the patella first makes contact with the femur at 30 degrees of flexion. The medial facet contact should occur at 45 degrees of flexion, at which time the patella should be centered in the femoral groove.

The patellar overhang can be best appreciated by placing the arthroscope into the lateral gutter through the anterolateral portal and visualizing the patella by rotating the lens superiorly (see Fig. 5–22D). The knee is then slowly flexed and the amount of lateral overhang noted. (Often the fat pad may cover the lens, obscuring the view. This can be corrected by rapidly inserting the arthroscope farther into the knee and then very slowly withdrawing it; the fat pad will then be partially pulled out of the way.) An even better view of the patellar tracking can be obtained from the superomedial portal by switching the inflow cannula and the arthroscope.

Lateral Femoral Gutter

Finally, the lateral femoral gutter can be inspected. The arthroscope should be in the anterolateral portal, and it is brought down from the patellofemoral joint with the knee only slightly flexed and mild valgus stress applied. The gutter is inspected for

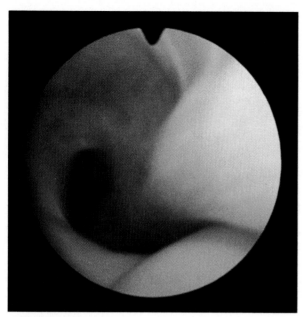

Figure 5–26
Popliteal tendon sheath.

loose bodies and the synovial condition noted. The popliteal tendon sheath can be seen posteriorly by rotating the scope downward (Fig. 5–26). This area is carefully observed for loose bodies while intermittent compression is applied from outside.

Posterolateral Compartment

Further evaluation of this compartment is rarely necessary. Occasionally, small loose bodies may lodge here. These may be detected through the intercondylar notch with an approach similar to that for the posteromedial recess. Better visualization and any removal may require a posterolateral portal to be made. The synovial junction, the posterior horn of the lateral meniscus, and the posterior portion of the lateral femoral condyle also may be inspected from this portal.

References

1. Brantigan OC, Boshell AF: The mechanics of the ligaments and menisci of the knee joint. J Bone Joint Surg 23:44, 1941.
2. Crenshaw AH: Campbell's Operative Orthopaedics. 7th ed. St. Louis, CV Mosby, 1987.
3. Girgis FG, Marshall JL, Al Monajem ARS: The cruciate ligaments of the knee joint. Clin Orthop 105:216, 1975.
4. Hardaker WT, Whipple TL, Bassett FH: Diagnosis and treatment of a plica syndrome of the knee. J Bone Joint Surg 62(A):221, 1980.
5. Herzmark MH: The evolution of the knee joint. J Bone Joint Surg 20(A):77, 1938.
6. Hughston JC: The posterior cruciate ligament in knee joint stability. J Bone Joint Surg 51(A):1045, 1969.
7. Insall JN: Surgery of the Knee. New York, Churchill-Livingstone, 1984.
8. Johnson L: Arthroscopic Surgery. St. Louis, CV Mosby, 1986.
9. Kaplan EB: Some aspects of functional anatomy of the human knee joint. Clin Orthop 23:18, 1962.
10. Last RJ: Some anatomical details of the knee joint. J Bone Joint Surg 30(B):683, 1948.
11. Last RJ: The popliteus muscle and the lateral meniscus. J Bone Joint Surg 32(B):93, 1950.
12. Last RJ: Anatomy, Regional and Applied. 6th ed. Edinburgh, Churchill-Livingstone, 1978.
13. Mann RA, Hagy, JL: The popliteus muscle. J Bone Joint Surg 59:924, 1977.
14. Parisen S: Arthroscopic Surgery. New York, McGraw-Hill, 1988.
15. Seebacher JR, Inglis AE, Marshall JL, et al: The structure of the posterolateral aspect of the knee. J Bone Joint Surg 64:536, 1982.

6

Thomas D. Rosenberg
Patricia A. Kolowich

Arthroscopic Diagnosis and Treatment of Meniscal Disorders

The menisci are important structural and functional components of the knee. Sutton (1897) incorrectly suggested that the menisci were developmental remnants of leg muscle origins that arose intra-articularly and were functionless in the knee.[24]

As early as 1936, King documented the healing potential of meniscal tears.[15] He performed meniscal surgery on dogs and concluded there were four functional roles of the meniscus: (1) protection of the articular hyaline cartilage by absorbing shock, (2) increasing joint stability by deepening the tibial articulation for the convex femoral surface, (3) improving congruity and increasing mobility between the articulating surfaces of the femur and tibia by acting as "peripheral, elastic, movable washers," and (4) lubrication (Fig. 6–1). He performed partial and complete meniscectomies and described partial regeneration of fibrocartilage in medial meniscal defects if a synovial rim was present. However, degenerative changes in the articular surfaces developed and were worse with complete medial meniscectomy than with partial meniscectomy.

This information was not extrapolated to humans until 1948 when Fairbank described significant roentgenographic changes in patients with long-term follow-up after meniscectomy.[8] These changes included sclerosis of the tibial plateau, narrowing of the joint space, squaring of the tibial margin, ridging of the femoral condyle in the anteroposterior direction, and flattening of the femoral articular surface, as well as combinations of these findings (Fig. 6–2). These changes were recorded from a retrospective review observing degenerative roentgenogram changes after meniscectomy.

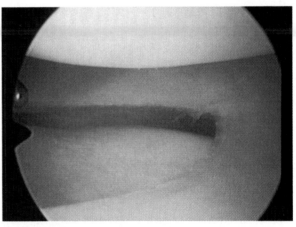

Figure 6–1
A normal lateral meniscus, left knee. The meniscus functions as a load-transmitting tissue between the femur and tibia.

Biomechanical studies eventually showed proof of the functional role of the meniscus and its importance in load distribution. A meniscal contact area was demonstrated by Walker and Erkman with a casting method using self-curing methylmethacrylate.[25] Contact pressures were measured with a miniature pressure transducer and revealed high loads on the posterior and lateral portions of the lateral meniscus and the midmedial portion of the medial meniscus as well as the tibial articular surface near the medial tibial spine. The lateral meniscus appeared to carry most of the load in the lateral compartment while in the medial compartment the load

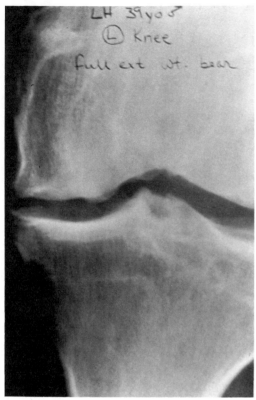

Figure 6–2
Left knee with typical "Fairbank's" changes following meniscectomy.

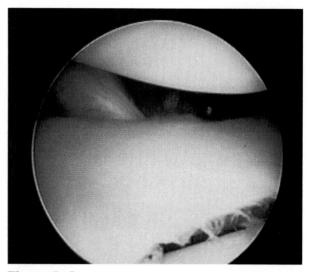

Figure 6–3
The normal separation of the lateral meniscal rim from the capsule at the popliteus hiatus (seen toward the top of the picture) accounts for the increased mobility of the lateral meniscus.

was shared between the meniscus and exposed articular surface. Increasing loads across the knee transferred most of the load through the lateral meniscus in the lateral compartment. The medial compartment shared loads equally between the articular surface and the medial meniscus with increasing loads.

Shrive from Oxford tested human and canine knee joints in an Instron device and calculated mathematically that the menisci carried up to 60 per cent of the total load across the knee joint.[22] Incision of the menisci altered the amount of load transmitted via the meniscus.

Frankel and associates studied the biomechanics of knees with an internal derangement and demonstrated abnormal wear patterns on the articular surface when a torn meniscus was present.[10] A displaced torn meniscus could interfere with the normal "screw home" mechanism of knee extension. Abnormal surface velocities were associated with meniscal tear patterns.

Functional stability on the medial side is related to the attachment of the posterior oblique ligament to the junction of the middle and posterior one third of the meniscus at the meniscal capsular junction. A peripheral tear disrupting this attachment can alter meniscal contact patterns and can contribute to anteromedial rotary instability if the anterior cruciate ligament is also compromised. The lateral meniscus

is normally much more mobile than the medial and consequently contributes less to stability (Fig. 6–3).

Prior to the development of arthroscopy, accepted treatment for meniscal tears consisted of complete or subtotal meniscectomy. With the advancement of arthroscopic surgery and new, finer instrumentation, partial meniscectomy was facilitated and has become the treatment of choice for many meniscal lesions. Degenerative changes can be anticipated in the long term following arthroscopic partial meniscectomy, although to a lesser degree than with total meniscectomy. Therefore, the alternative treatment of meniscal repair, either arthroscopic or open, must be considered in meniscal tear patterns when primary healing can be anticipated. This is especially true of meniscal tears in young patients and when associated with anterior rotary instability of the knee. With arthroscopic or open repair, preliminary studies have revealed that healed menisci approach a normal contact distribution pattern.[3,4]

Treatment of meniscal injuries begins with recognition of tear patterns. A knowledge of functional importance and anatomy is prerequisite. Normal variations such as rippling or buckling of the ridge of the meniscus must be recognized and not mistaken for meniscal pathology (Fig. 6–4). To detect meniscal tears, which often are not obvious to initial inspection, a thorough systematic probing of both superior and inferior aspects of each meniscus must be performed (Fig. 6–5). Tears need to be described relative to the three-dimensional structure of the meniscus: vertical, transverse, horizontal, longitudinal, or oblique (Fig. 6–6). Tears may be complete or incomplete and described as simple, complex, multiple, or degenerative. Incomplete tears generally are visible

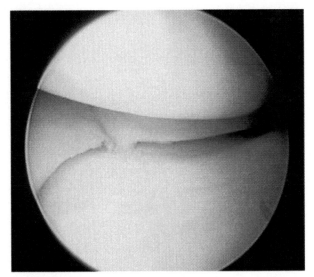

Figure 6–4
Buckling of the free edge of a normal medial meniscus, left knee.

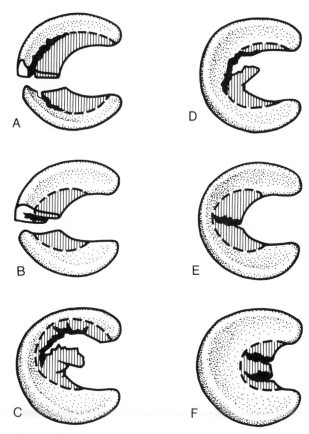

Figure 6–6
Common meniscal tear patterns, with recommended areas of excision shown by dotted lines. *A,* Bucket handle. *B,* Flap tear. *C,* Horizontal cleavage tear. *D,* Radial tear. *E,* Degenerative flap tear. *F,* Double radial tear of a discoid meniscus.

on the superior or inferior surface of the meniscus and frequently are stable tears that may not require excision (Fig. 6–7). Complete tears can also be referred to as a bucket handle tear (vertical, horizontal, longitudinal) (Fig. 6–8), a radial tear (vertical, transverse) (Fig. 6–9), a flap tear (vertical, oblique) (Fig. 6–10), or a horizontal cleavage tear (horizontal, longitudinal) (Fig. 6–11).

EXCISION VERSUS REPAIR

Partial excision of a torn meniscus is superior to complete excision of the meniscus. Some remaining normal meniscal tissue continues to function as a

"shock absorber" in load distribution and is believed to contribute to functional stability (especially in an anterior cruciate ligament–deficient knee). Attention

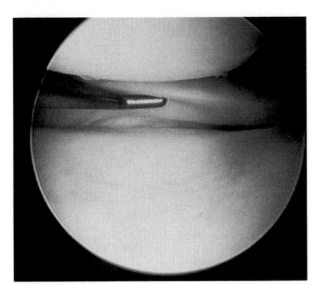

Figure 6–5
Thorough probing of the meniscus is routine.

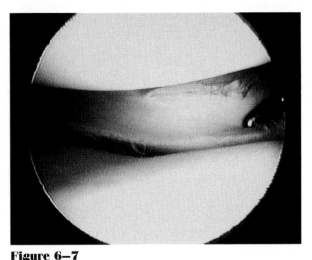

Figure 6–7
An incomplete vertical tear in the posterior horn of the medial meniscus, left knee.

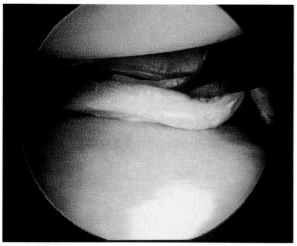

Figure 6–8
A probe is demonstrating a bucket handle tear in the posterior horn of the medial meniscus, right knee.

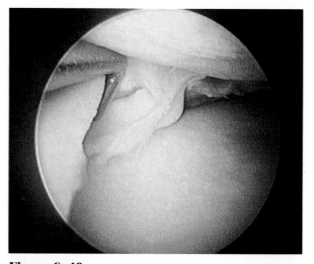

Figure 6–10
A flap tear in the medial meniscus, left knee. Flap tears often occur as a result of oblique tears in the meniscal substance.

to detail in the technique of meniscal excision can facilitate the procedure.

Repair of a torn meniscus retains the entire meniscal structure to provide normal or near-normal stress distribution patterns and functional stability. Patients undergoing meniscal repair in association with an anterior cruciate ligament reconstruction had significantly fewer Fairbank's changes.[8] Work by Arnoczky and Warren[1,2] and Scapinelli[20] demonstrated good vascular supply to the peripheral one third of the meniscus (Fig. 6–12A). A tear in this region, usually longitudinal and vertical, provides the best setting for healing of a repaired meniscus (Fig. 6–12B).

PRINCIPLES OF ARTHROSCOPY

Visualization, or adequate exposure, is paramount in evaluating and treating meniscal tears. A combination of exposure and meticulous technique is necessary to avoid iatrogenic injury to the articular surface of the knee by arthroscopic instruments. Inadequate

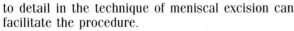

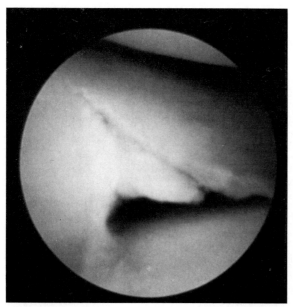

Figure 6–9
Early development of a radial tear in the middle third of the lateral meniscus, right knee.

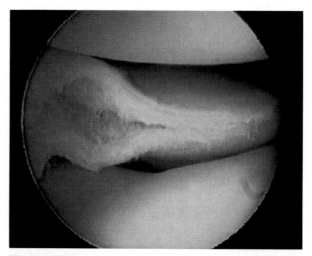

Figure 6–11
A horizontal cleavage tear in the lateral meniscus, right knee. This tear extends peripherally into the body of the meniscus, often through degenerative tissue.

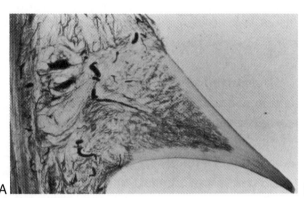

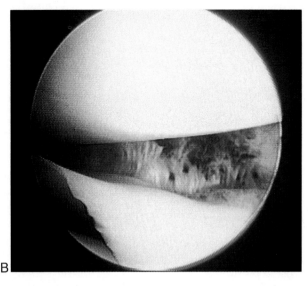

Figure 6–12

A, Cross-section of a meniscus demonstrates the blood supply in the peripheral one third (by Scapinelli). *B*, A longitudinal tear in the vascular peripheral zone of the meniscus is suitable for repair.

exposure, poor portal placement, or lack of attention to detail may exacerbate this potential problem of damage to the articular surface.

Positioning on the operating table can aid exposure. The use of a "well-leg" support for the opposite leg will abduct and flex the hip.[18] This provides adequate access to the medial side of the leg being operated on and supports the well leg, avoiding a strain on the lumbar spine or stretch on the femoral nerve (Fig. 6–13). A low profile leg holder will allow safe

varus and valgus stress to be applied to the knee without interfering with the operative field. When a general anesthetic with muscle paralysis is utilized, the patient offers no resistance to positioning during the operation. An assistant with knowledge of the procedure, anatomy, and inherent risks should position and hold the leg during the procedure to facilitate exposure and minimize risks of damage to the articular surface or collateral ligaments.

Evaluation of the tear includes an estimate of the

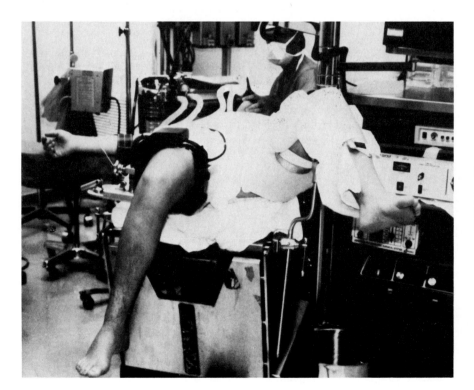

Figure 6–13

The right limb is secured in a leg-holding device; the left leg is carefully positioned in well-leg support.

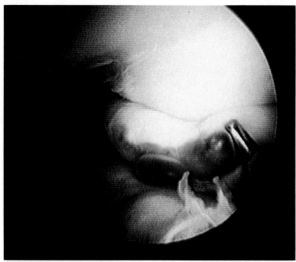

Figure 6–14
Unreducible, swollen, and hemorrhagic displaced bucket handle tear.

size, direction, and location in the meniscus and the presence or absence of degenerative meniscal changes. Once a meniscal tear is determined to be irreparable and unstable, a partial meniscectomy is performed. The goal of partial meniscectomy is to remove all damaged or torn tissue while sculpting a smooth transition zone and sparing as much normal meniscal tissue as possible (see Fig. 6–6).

ARTHROSCOPIC PARTIAL MENISCECTOMY

Bucket Handle Tears (Vertical, Longitudinal)

These tears are more common in younger patients who have significant trauma to the knee. They are frequently associated with tears of the anterior cruciate ligament. Bucket handle tears are three times as prevalent in the medial meniscus compared with the

lateral meniscus. Large tears can displace into the notch, producing symptoms of a "locked knee" or a knee that lacks full extension (Fig. 6–14). Shorter tears, especially in the posterior one half of the meniscus, may be only partially displaceable, rendering them unstable and therefore symptomatic, but not capable of locking the knee (Fig. 6–15). Shorter, complete, stable tears of less than 1 cm or incomplete, stable tears may be left alone. Tears in the peripheral one third may be candidates for meniscal repair. Degenerative or less peripheral tears that are unstable are usually excised by partial meniscectomy.

Performing a partial meniscectomy of a displaced tear is facilitated by reducing the displaced portion with a probe. Application of the appropriate varus or valgus stress will simplify reduction of the displaced meniscal fragment. This maneuver will also enhance visualization of the tear by opening the joint compartment. The posterior attachment is detached first with small straight or curved punch forceps (Fig. 6–16A). A helpful hint is to leave a tissue bridge posteriorly (less than 1 mm) to tether the fragment and prevent it from obscuring visualization of the remaining tear and its anterior extent (Fig. 6–16B). A punch forceps (frequently 30, 45, or 90 degrees) or angled scissors (60 degrees for very anterior tears) is used to transect the anterior tissue bridge (Fig. 6–16C). An arthroscopic grasper is used to grasp the loose anterior portion of the meniscus. The torn portion is removed by a firm pull to avulse the small posterior tether. The remaining meniscal rim is trimmed to a smooth contour, using a combination of the punch forceps and the motorized cutter. Repeat examination of the remaining meniscus is necessary to ensure stability and avoid missing a double or triple longitudinal tear. Shorter longitudinal tears of the posterior horn of the medial meniscus generally propagate. They can be entered with punch forceps and excised as demonstrated in Figure 6–17). The 70-degree arthroscope inserted through the intercondylar notch into the posteromedial compartment may be used to look at the posteromedial meniscal rim to verify its stability.

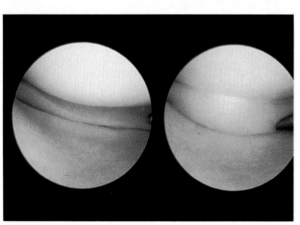

Figure 6–15
Probing of a short posterior horn bucket handle tear in the medial meniscus demonstrates instability.

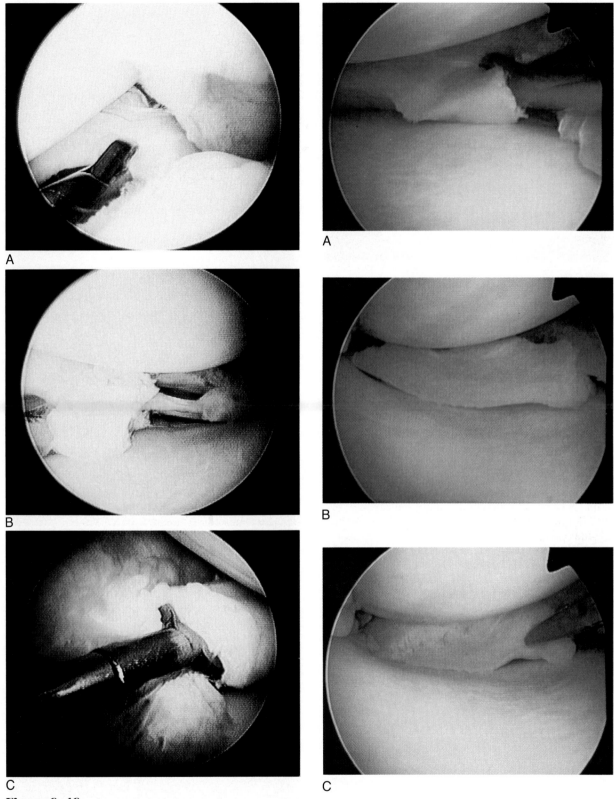

Figure 6–16

A, The posterior attachment of a medial bucket handle tear is divided by means of a small punch forceps. *B,* A small tissue bridge serves to tether a bucket handle fragment. *C,* A 60-degree angle scissors is seen transecting the meniscal fragment at the anterior extent of the tear.

Figure 6–17

A, B, and *C,* Short longitudinal tears of the posterior horn of the medial meniscus generally propagate. They can be entered with punch forceps and excised as demonstrated.

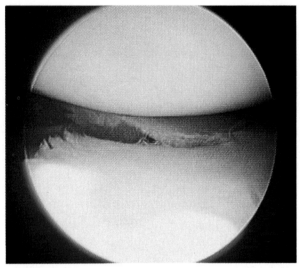

Figure 6—18
A radial tear in the middle third of the lateral meniscus.

Radial Tears (Vertical, Transverse)

Radial tears are most commonly located in the middle one third of the lateral meniscus (Fig. 6–18). Radial tears in the medial compartment usually occur posteromedially and demonstrate degenerative changes (Fig. 6–19). Laterally they may be attributable to excessive valgus stress on the knee. A radial tear of the posterior horn of the lateral meniscus, referred to as a "root tear," is associated with tears of the anterior cruciate ligament. Tears of less than 3 mm may be an incidental finding and usually are not symptomatic. Radial tears greater than 5 mm are usually symptomatic and should be resected. Resection of this tear involves excision of the anterior and posterior edges of the tear only as deep as the apex of the tear. As described previously, the remaining meniscal rim should be smoothed and contoured by use of the motorized cutter and arthroscopic punch forceps. Deep radial tears are often associated with meniscal cyst formation (Fig. 6–20). Treatment of the intra-articular pathology generally will lead to cyst regression. Rarely, open cyst excision is required.

Flap Tears (Vertical, Oblique)

A flap tear is one of the most common meniscal tear patterns. The etiology has been described by several mechanisms, either propagation from a simple radial tear or transection of a bucket handle tear, leaving either an anterior- or posterior-based flap, or two flaps with central transection of the bucket handle (Fig. 6–21). Partial meniscectomy is performed in these tears by sharp division at the base of the

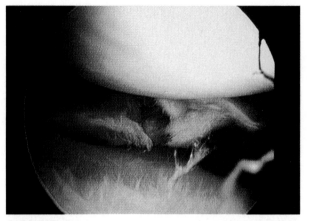

Figure 6—19
A radial tear with degenerative extension.

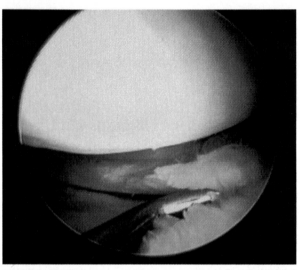

Figure 6—20
A probe is within a deep, long-standing radial tear of the lateral meniscus, which leads to the opening of a meniscal cyst.

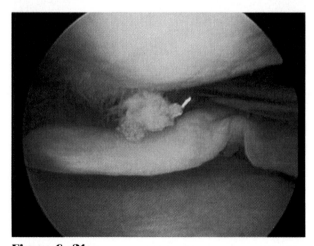

Figure 6—21
A long flap tear that developed after spontaneous posterior transection of a bucket handle tear.

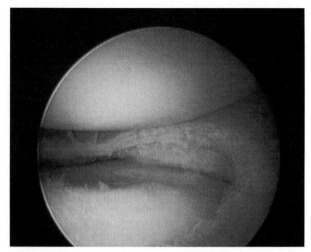

Figure 6–22
Balanced meniscal rim after resection of a flap tear.

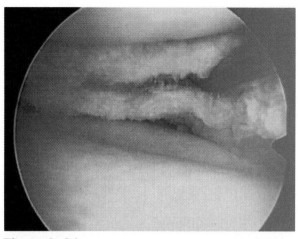

Figure 6–24
Probing demonstrates stability of the remaining leaflets after initial trimming.

tear with punch forceps. The meniscal rim must be contoured as the flap is excised (Fig. 6–22). The remaining meniscus must be stable without a residual tear.

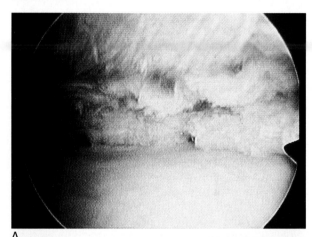

A

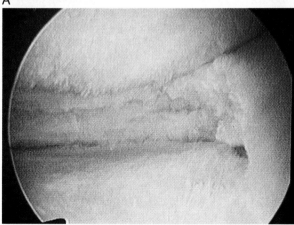

B
Figure 6–23
A, Horizontal cleavage tear before resection and *B*, after resection.

Horizontal Cleavage Tears (Horizontal, Longitudinal)

Horizontal cleavage tears occur most often in association with other meniscal tears, specifically flap tears, degenerative tears, or bucket handle tears. They can occur primarily and occasionally are referred to as "fish-mouth" tears. Horizontal cleavage tears have been described as the most frequently occurring tear pattern (Fig. 6–23*A*). A horizontal tear is the tear pattern most commonly associated with meniscal cysts. Pathologic study of these tears reveals extension to the base of the meniscus. There was a high correlation with tears extending to the base of the meniscus and parameniscal cyst formation, implying a causal relationship.[9] Hypermobile or unstable portions of the superior or inferior leaflets should be excised (Fig. 6–23*B*). It is not necessary to trim the meniscal leaflets completely back to the periphery (Fig. 6–24). A leaflet rim of 3 mm is generally acceptable if the leaflet falls behind the condyle in flexion so that it will not impinge and tear further. Tear excision may be facilitated by using a 15-degree upcurve punch for the superior leaflet and posterior digital pressure along the joint line to better visualize the tear (Fig. 6–25). As stated, earlier meniscal cysts frequently undergo involution after treatment of the intra-articular pathology.

Degenerative and Complex Tears

Chronic tears frequently present as a combination of complete, unstable tears in a variety of tear patterns (Fig. 6–26). The meniscal rim may be edematous. This swollen tissue does not have to be excised. The edema will resolve after the torn portion is resected (Fig. 6–27). The torn portion may be discolored, fibrillated, and edematous (Fig. 6–28). This

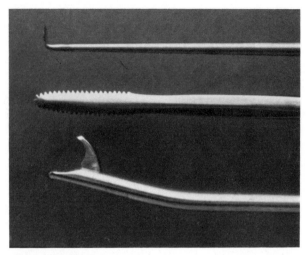

Figure 6–25
Upcurved punch contrasted with straight instruments.

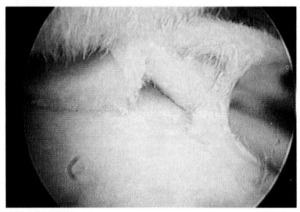

Figure 6–26
Motorized instrumentation is used initially to debride a complex degenerative tear.

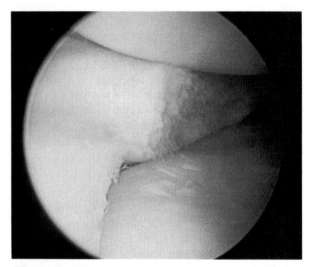

Figure 6–27
Marked edema of the remaining rim following excision of a degenerative tear.

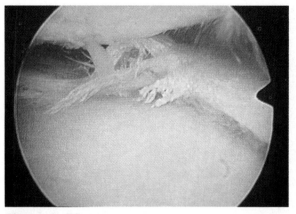

Figure 6–28
A fibrillated degenerative tear of the medial meniscus. Note calcium pyrophosphate crystals.

torn portion needs to be excised. These tears are much more common in the older age group who have associated degenerative changes of the articular surface (Fig. 6–29A,B). Arthroscopic partial meniscectomy is performed, utilizing aforementioned techniques and principles (Fig. 6–30). Frequently, degenerative fibrillated tissue is easily removed with a motorized cutter, allowing better visualization of the tear for more complete tear excision and contouring of the remaining rim.

DISCOID MENISCI

Discoid lateral menisci can tear and become symptomatic. When the peripheral rim is stable, excision of the tear and saucerization of the central discoid portion of the meniscus are performed. The goal is to shape a semilunar meniscus by excision of the central turn portion usually with punch forceps. The remaining tissue is usually thicker than a normal meniscus (Fig. 6–31). Encouraging results have been reported with this procedure.[11,23] Occasionally the discoid meniscus will not have a stable rim; it will possess a deficient posterior attachment or no posterior attachment at all. This is referred to as the Wrisberg ligament type of discoid meniscus and is associated with locking. Peripheral reattachment has been advocated for this type.[17]

Meniscal Repair

Studies by Arnoczky and Warren[1,2] and Scapinelli[20] have demonstrated a vascular supply to the peripheral third of the meniscus (Fig. 6–32). Arnoczky and Warren surgically created meniscal tears in canine menisci, and histologic and gross studies revealed healing by 10 weeks. Cabaud and associates demonstrated meniscal healing in dogs and rhesus monkeys.[6] Transverse incisions in the anterior horn of the medial meniscus contiguous with the synovium and

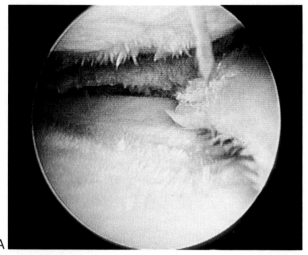 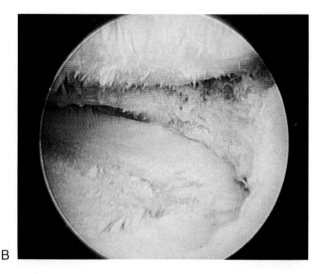

A   B

Figure 6–29

A, A degenerative medial meniscus tear is seen before excision and *B*, after excision. Note degenerative changes of the articular surface as well.

coronary ligament were created. Repairs were performed with a single 3-0 Dexon mattress suture. The limbs were immobilized at 60 degrees for 6 weeks in casts. Inspection 4 months later revealed 38 per cent of the subjects with complete healing and 56 per cent with partial healing; 6 per cent demonstrated failure to heal.

Many subsequent studies have demonstrated meniscal healing in humans.[7,12–14,26] Rosenberg et al reported on 29 meniscal repairs followed by arthroscopy 3 months later to demonstrate healing.[19] Twenty-four of 29 healed completely. Five showed partial healing and four of these five were in anterior cruciate ligament–deficient knees. All tears repaired were peripheral one third, displaceable longitudinal tears. Some studies demonstrated excellent results in up to 98.6 per cent of patients with similar tear patterns.[16]

Henning and colleagues repaired most meniscal tear patterns, not just longitudinal and transverse peripheral tears.[14] In addition to suturing the tear, blood clot is injected into the tear after rasp preparation and suture placement. This must be done in an air or gas medium to avoid blood clot displacement. Their studies demonstrated a 98 per cent stable bond in menisci treated with rasp and suture and a 100 per cent stable bond in those treated with rasp, suture, and blood clot. Healing was evaluated by arthrogram for both medial and lateral menisci. There was a gradual decrease in healing rates for tears of more than 30 mm in length. More recently, research using fibrin clot to aid healing has shown promising results.

As with partial meniscectomy, technique, preparation, and knowledge of anatomy are very important when performing a meniscal repair. The torn meniscal edges should be prepared with a rasp or motorized trimmer to obtain bleeding surfaces. Sutures

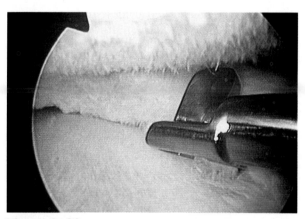

Figure 6–30

A 90-degree rotary punch is used for contouring at the anterior extent of a degenerative tear.

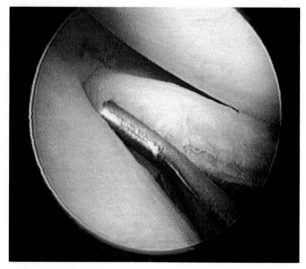

Figure 6–31

A tear is demonstrated through the abnormal central portion of a lateral discoid meniscus, right knee.

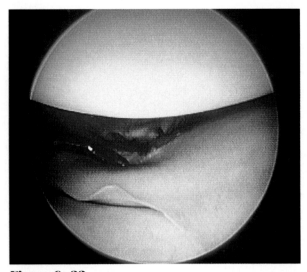

Figure 6–32
A peripheral tear in the vascular zone of the posterior medial meniscus, demonstrating hemorrhage.

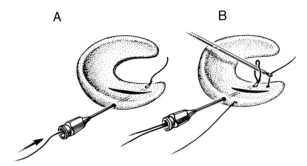

Figure 6–33
"Outside-in" method utilizes straight needles as cannulas for suture-passing devices.

should be meticulously placed for reapproximation of meniscal tissue. Neurovascular structures should not be compromised. Three basic techniques have been described in the literature,[12] although many variations on these techniques exist.

OPEN TECHNIQUE

The open repair was popularized by DeHaven.[7] A longitudinal incision and dissection protects the neurovascular structures. The torn meniscal capsular edge is identified. Sutures are placed through the meniscus and out through the capsule where they are tied. DeHaven's patients have experienced re-tears of their menisci in only 7 of more than 160 cases. This method is extremely effective in very peripheral tears, although it is difficult to reach the far posterior horn. Tears extending into the substance of the meniscus are difficult to identify and repair with this method.

OUTSIDE-IN TECHNIQUE

The outside-in technique was described in 1986 by Morgan and Casscells.[16] This technique was developed in an effort to avoid injury to the peroneal nerve laterally or the sartorial branch of the saphenous nerve medially. An 18-gauge spinal needle is inserted and directed, under arthroscopic visualization, through the capsule and meniscus tear (Fig. 6–33). A 0-gauge absorbable suture is threaded through the spinal needle, retrieved intra-articularly with an arthroscopic grasper, and pulled out the portal. Three knots are tied in the suture and the tail end trimmed. The suture knot is pulled back into the knee until the knot abuts the meniscus, reducing and stabilizing it. This is repeated as many times as necessary. The tails of the sutures are tied to each other

over the capsule with the knee in full extension. Patients are kept in a straight-leg knee immobilizer for 4 weeks but allowed immediate weight-bearing. Based on symptoms and physical examination, 98.6 per cent of patients healed with excellent results. One patient (1.4 per cent) failed to comply with the postoperative immobilization and re-injured his knee 2 months postoperatively while wrestling.

This technique does not require specialized instruments yet allows repair of longitudinal tears. Tears in the extreme posterior zone of either meniscus can be difficult to repair by this technique.

INSIDE-OUT TECHNIQUE

Arthroscopic meniscal repair has been described by many.[5,17,21] Performing meniscal repair via the inside-out technique requires the use of specialized cannulae (Fig. 6–34). Most commonly, curved cannulae are used, which are zone specific depending upon the location of the tear (Fig. 6–35). A longitudinal incision is made on either the posteromedial or posterolateral side for the appropriate site of repair

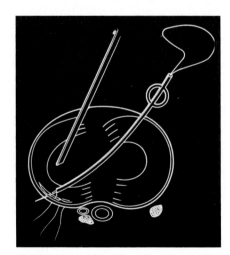

Figure 6–34
A curved cannula is inserted from the contralateral portal while the arthroscope is positioned on the same side as the tear.

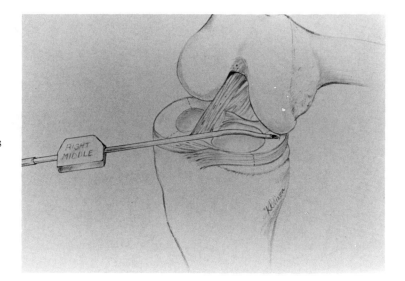

Figure 6–35
  A prebent zone-specific cannula facilitates arthroscopic placement of sutures.

(Fig. 6–36). This protects the neurovascular bundle from the needles and sutures. Under arthroscopic visualization, sutures are placed across the meniscal tear and retrieved through the open wound under direct visualization (Figs. 6–37 and 6–38). When enough sutures have been placed across the tear, the ends are tied over the capsule with the knee in extension. Sutures may be passed from the superior or inferior surface as horizontal or vertical mattress sutures as appropriate for the tear pattern (Fig. 6–39). Absorbable 2-0 gauge suture (PDS) or nonabsorbable 2-0 gauge suture (Ethibond) may be used. This method does require specialized instrumentation. Those proficient in this technique feel that more exact suture placement can be achieved and large intra-articular suture knots are avoided. All longitudinal tears, without regard to location, can be repaired with this method.

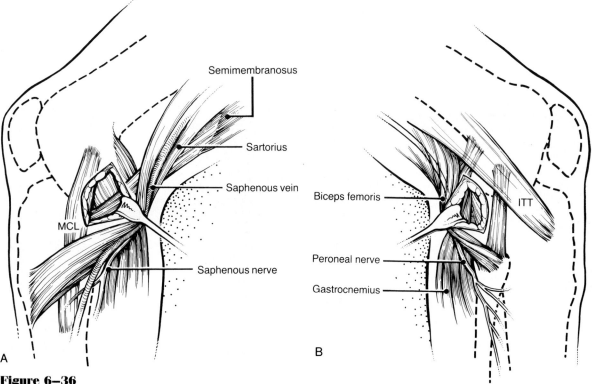

Figure 6–36
  Incisions for retrieval of needles and important neurovascular structures are shown for (A) medial and (B) lateral meniscal repairs.

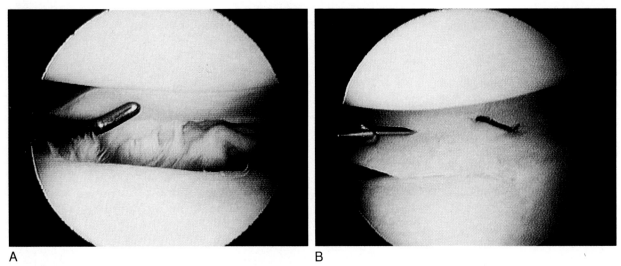

A   B

Figure 6–37
A, A probe is demonstrating a tear in the posterior horn of the lateral meniscus. *B*, Placement of the final suture, using a zone-specific cannula.

Indications

The indications for meniscal repair include longitudinal, peripheral third tears in young patients. Most would advocate repair over partial meniscectomy, particularly for patients under 40 years of age, if the conditions are appropriate. The meniscus should not show significant degenerative changes. There should not be a double or triple longitudinal tear. Ligamentous stability, by virtue of an intact or reconstructed anterior cruciate ligament, is necessary. Longitudinal tears propagating to the middle and anterior portions of the meniscus are often more readily approached by arthroscopic exposure than by an open technique (Fig. 6–40). Animal studies have demonstrated meniscal healing in transverse tears that extend through the meniscal rim. Repairs of this nature have not proved to heal as reproducibly in humans. There is no doubt that a repaired meniscus is superior to partial or complete meniscectomy. When in doubt, repair the meniscus with meticulous technique and careful meniscal bed preparation. If the experience of Henning and associates[14] and others continues to demonstrate successful results, indications for meniscal repair may expand to include more tear patterns.

Contraindications

The contraindications for meniscal repair include knees with ligamentous laxity, specifically anterior

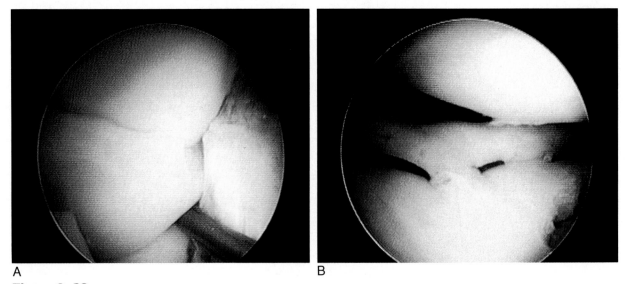

A   B

Figure 6–38
A, Bucket handle tear of the medial meniscus displaced into the intercondylar notch. *B*, The meniscus has been reduced, and horizontal mattress sutures are holding the torn surfaces in close approximation.

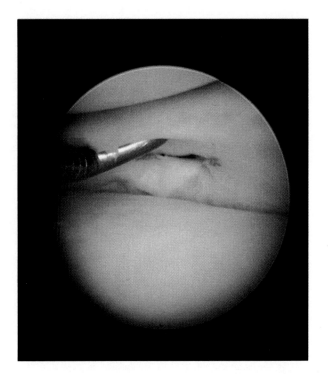

Figure 6–39
　A meniscus repair suture from the interior surface of the meniscus closely approximates the tear.

cruciate ligament tears. The incidence of a successful repair in an unstable knee is markedly decreased. Most surgeons recommend a 4-week period of using crutches with no weight on the operated extremity; however, Morgan and Casscells did allow immediate weight-bearing on the operated leg immobilized in the extended position.[16] A relative contraindication is fraying or degenerative changes at the meniscal tear. Usually, there is poor blood supply to this tissue. Severe articular degenerative changes in an older patient may not warrant the surgery and rehabilitation necessary for meniscal repair. The articular changes have already occurred and will not be prevented by saving the meniscus.

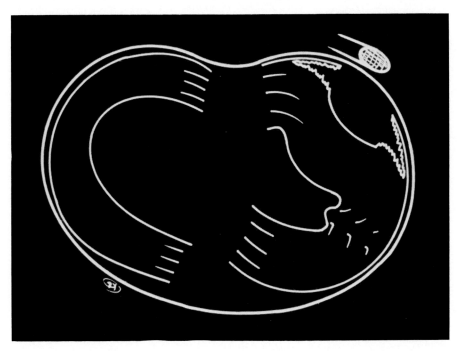

Figure 6–40
　A peripheral longitudinal tear of the lateral meniscus is easier to approach by the arthroscopic technique than by a comparable open method.

References

1. Arnoczky SP, Warren RF: Microvasculature of the human meniscus. Am J Sports Med 10(2):90–95, 1982.
2. Arnoczky SP, Warren RF: The microvasculature of the meniscus and its response to injury: An experimental study in the dog. Am J Sports Med II(3):131–141, 1983.
3. Baratz ME, Fu FH, Mengata R: Meniscal tears: The effect of meniscectomy and of repair on intra-articular contact areas and stress in the knee. Am J Sports Med 14:270–275, 1986.
4. Baratz ME, Rehak DC, Fu FH, Rudert MJ: Peripheral tears of the meniscus: The effect of open versus arthroscopic repair on intraarticular contact stresses in the human knee. Am J Sports Med 16(1):1–6, 1988.
5. Barber FA, Stone RG: Meniscal repair: An arthroscopic technique. J Bone Joint Surg 67-B(1):39–41, 1985.
6. Cabaud HE, Rodkey WG, Fitzwater JE: Medial meniscus repairs: An experimental and morphologic study. Am J Sports Med 9(3):129–134, 1981.
7. DeHaven KE: Meniscus repair in the athlete. Clin Orthop 198:31–35, 1985.
8. Fairbank TJ: Knee joint changes after meniscectomy. J Bone Joint Surg 30-B:664–670, 1948.
9. Ferrer-Roca O, Vilalta C: Meniscal lesions. Part II: Horizontal cleavages and lateral cysts. Clin Orthop 146:301–307, 1980.
10. Frankel VH, Burstein AH, Brooks DB: Biomechanics of internal derangement of the knee. J Bone Joint Surg 53-A:945–962, 1971.
11. Fujikawa K, Iseki F, Mikura Y: Partial resection of the discoid meniscus in a child's knee. J Bone Joint Surg 63-B:391–395, 1981.
12. Graf B, Docter T, Clancy W Jr: Arthroscopic meniscal repair. Clin Sports Med 6(3):525–536, 1987.
13. Hamberg P, Gillquist J, Lysholm J: Suture of new and old peripheral meniscus tears. J Bone Joint Surg 65-A(2):193–197, 1983.
14. Henning CE, Clark JR, Lynch MA, Stallbaumer R, Yearout KM, Vequist SW: Arthroscopic Meniscus Repair with a Posterior Incision. In Bassett FH III (ed): AAOS Instructional Course Lectures. Vol 37, pp 209–221, 1988.
15. King D: The function of semilunar cartilages. J Bone Joint Surg 18:1069–1076, 1936.
16. Morgan CD, Casscells SW: Arthroscopic meniscus repair: A soft approach to the posterior horns. Arthroscopy 2(1):3–12, 1986.
17. Rosenberg TD, Paulos LE, Parker RD, Harner CD, Gurley WD: Discoid lateral meniscus: Case report of arthroscopic attachment of a symptomatic Wrisberg-ligament type. Arthroscopy 3(4):277–282, 1987.
18. Rosenberg TD, Paulos LE, Parker RD, Harner CD, Kolowich PA: The well leg support. Arthroscopy 4(1):41–44, 1988.
19. Rosenberg TD, Scott SM, Coward DB, Dunbar WH, Ewing JW, Johnson CL, Paulos LE: Arthroscopic meniscal repair evaluated with repeat arthroscopy. Arthroscopy 2(1):14–20, 1986.
20. Scapinelli R: Studies on the vasculature of the human knee joint. Acta Anat 70:305, 1968.
21. Scott GA, Jolly BL, Henning CE: Combined posterior incision and arthroscopic intra-articular repair of the meniscus. J Bone Joint Surg 68-A:847–861, 1986.
22. Shrive N: The weight-bearing role of the menisci of the knee. J Bone Joint Surg 56-B(2):381, 1974.
23. Stone RG, Miller G: Discoid lateral meniscus: Diagnosis and treatment (abstr). Arthroscopy 2(2):113, 1986.
24. Sutton JB: Ligaments: Their Nature and Morphology. 2nd ed. London, MK Lewis, 1897.
25. Walker PS, Erkman MJ: The role of the menisci in force transmission across the knee. Clin Orthop 109:184–192, 1975.
26. Wirth CR: Meniscus repair. Clin Orthop 157:153–160, 1981.

7

George Pianka
Joseph Combs

Arthroscopic Diagnosis and Treatment of Symptomatic Plicae

The development of synovial membranes in the knee is a complex process of compartmentalization, fusion, and absorption that results in one synovial cavity.[8] In a 6-week embryo, joint structures begin to develop with very rapid changes taking place. Blastemal tissue between the femoral and tibial cartilages is thinned, forming the intermediate zone. Embryonic mesenchyme becomes intra-articular and gives rise to menisci and cruciate ligaments at approximately 8 weeks, while the capsule does not form until 10 to 12 weeks of gestation. The embryonic synovial mesenchyme is solid, as cavities are not developed until the 9th week. Three primitive compartments form in the 9th week, lined by septa of embryonic synovium. The superior femoropatellar compartment and two inferior femorotibial compartments enlarge by proliferation of the synovial mesenchyme. At the end of the 9th week the cavities are lined with synovium and irregular. The process of involution and absorption of the lining tissue eventually leads to a single cavity at 12 weeks of gestation. The persistence of the synovial partitions constitutes the synovial plicae.

The incidence of synovial plicae reported in the literature has ranged from 20 to 60 per cent (Table 7–1). Much of the earlier work is in the Japanese literature where this entity is described and characterized in detail.[1,12,14–16] Mayeda investigated synovial cords in 1918, finding a 21 percent incidence in adult cadaver knees and a 35 percent incidence in

Table 7–1
History/Incidence of Synovial Plicae

1918, Mayeda	Investigated synovial cords
	Examined 100 knees of 55 cadavers—21%,
	63 knees of 37 fetus cadavers—35%
1939, Iino	67 cadaver knees—50%
1948, Mizumachi et al	39 knees—25.6%
1965, Aoki	120 knees—21.6%
1973, Hughston et al	Suprapatellar plica, abstract
1976, Sakakibara	100 knees—45%
	Classified medial plica—A, B, C, D
1978, Patel	72/371 patients—18.9%
	SP—2; MP—38; both—32
1979, Broukhim et al	423 patients, 145 plicae—33%
1981, Munzinger et al	136 knees—45%
1982, Jackson et al	Combined Canadian/Japanese Study
	345 knees, 206 plicae—60%;
	36 "pathologic"—17% (10% of total)

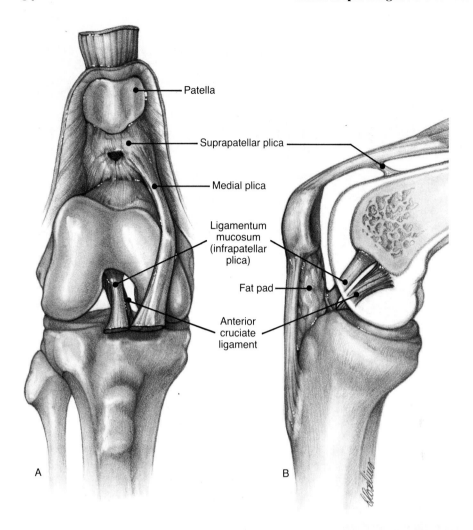

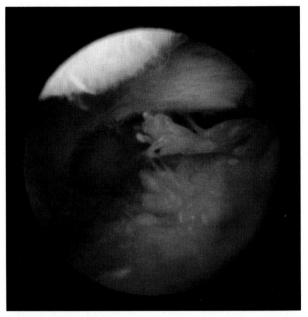

Figure 7–1
Most common sites of plicae.

fetal cadavers.[15] Iino was the first to study these structures systematically, finding them in over 50 percent of the knee joints he studied arthroscopically followed by arthrotomy.[12]

CLASSIFICATION

The three most commonly described synovial plicae are classified according to the site of the membrane from which they arise. The infrapatellar plica is the most common of the three, followed by the suprapatellar and then the mediopatellar plica.[9] These membranes vary in shape, size, and configuration and may coexist in various combinations (Fig. 7–1).

The suprapatellar plica, also known as plica synovialis suprapatellaris, runs transversely and divides the medial and lateral joint compartments from the suprapatellar pouch (Figs. 7–2 and 7–3). Occasionally, there is a communication between the suprapatellar pouch and the remainder of the knee joint through a variably sized, centrally placed diaphragm known as the "porta."[9,11,26] Usually only a remnant of this transverse septum is present as a medial or lat-

Figure 7–2
A crescent-shaped medial suprapatellar fold inserting on the medial wall is the most common appearance of the suprapatellar plica.

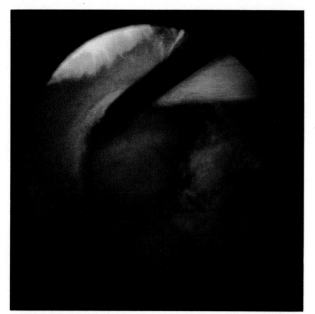

Figure 7–3
A suprapatellar plica probed with a veres needle appears thickened and fibrotic.

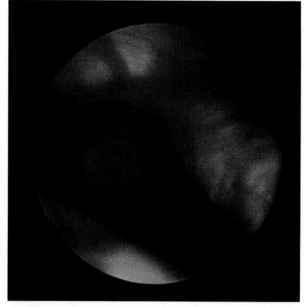

Figure 7–4
A mediopatellar plica coursing above the medial femoral condyle.

eral synovial fold. Most common is the medial suprapatellar fold, which is crescent shaped, originating under the quadriceps and inserting on the medial wall of the joint above the patella. The suprapatellar plica has variable shape, size, and thickness, with its edge being smooth, sharp, or irregular. During flexion of the knee, the plica lies parallel to the femur, whereas in extension it lies transverse to the femur.[10] The suprapatellar plica is thought to be much less clinically significant, unless it is thickened, large, and contiguous with the mediopatellar plica.[19-21] Anatomic dissections have failed to show the suprapatellar plica coming into contact with the medial femoral condyle and rarely with the patella even when symptoms were present.[9,13,26]

The mediopatellar plica, also known as plica synovialis patellaris, medial intra-articular band, Iino's band, plica alaris elongata, synovial shelf, and medial shelf, is a synovial fold that runs along the medial wall of the joint, beginning at or near the suprapatellar plica and coursing obliquely downward, inserting on the synovium covering the infrapatellar fat pad (Figs. 7–4, 7–5, and 7–6). Its many names reflect the variations in configuration of the same structure. The mediopatellar plica may be large, and during knee flexion its free edge tends to impinge on the superior anteromedial portion of the medial femoral condyle, causing articular changes such as erosions and chondromalacia (Figs. 7–7 through 7–15). With greater flexion it may also cause impingement on the medial facet of the patella[9,19,22] (Figs. 7–16 and 7–17). Sakakibara described four types of mediopatellar plica: Type A is a cordlike elevation in

the synovial wall; Type B is a shelflike structure that does not cover the anterior surface of the medial femoral condyle; Type C is a large, shelflike structure that covers the anterior surface of the medial femoral condyle; Type D is similar to Type C, except that there is a split in the insertion into the medial wall[24] (Figs.

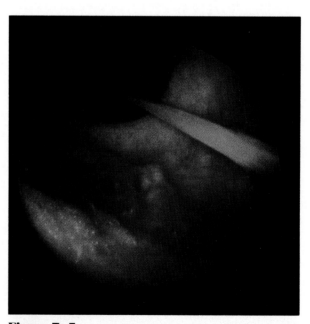

Figure 7–5
Three types of medial plicae are demonstrated: a thickened, fibrotic medial shelf, a crescent synovial fold, and a thin fibrous band.

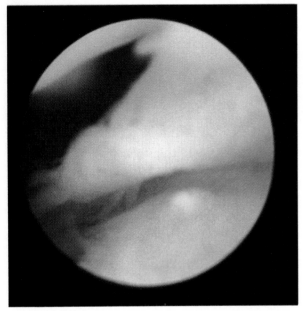

Figure 7–6
A thickened medial plica from chronic repetitive trauma.

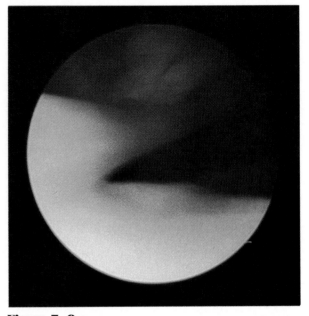

Figure 7–8
In full extension, the plica is seen to lie freely between the patella and medial femoral condyle.

7–18 through 7–20). The mediopatellar plica's bow-string effect on the medial femoral condyle accounts for the great majority of internal derangements of the knee caused by a synovial fold.

The infrapatellar plica, also called plica synovialis infrapatellaris and ligamentum mucosum, is the most common of the synovial folds. It originates from the intercondylar notch of the femur, runs parallel to the anterior cruciate ligament, widening distally, and inserts on the infrapatellar fat pad. It may be in continuity with the anterior cruciate ligament, may be completely separate from it, or may persist as a fenestrated septum. The infrapatellar plica does not cause clinical symptoms but can be of clinical importance during aspiration, arthroscopy, or removal of loose bodies.[9,11]

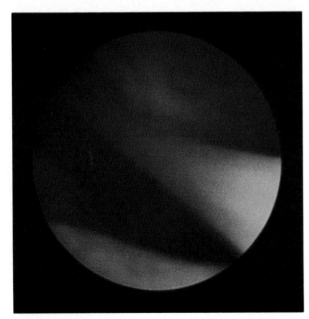

Figure 7–7
Typical appearance of a medial patellar plica.

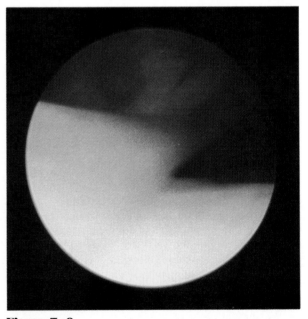

Figure 7–9
In 15 degrees of flexion, the free edge begins to impinge on the medial femoral condyle.

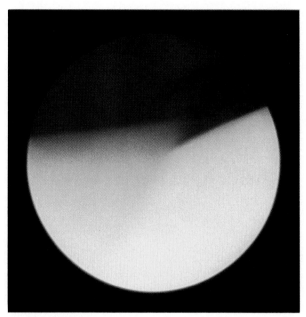

Figure 7–10
In 60 degrees of flexion, there is impingement and friction between the plica and the medial femoral condyle.

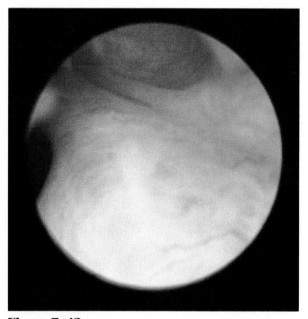

Figure 7–12
A double medial patellar plica consists of a thickened, fibrotic flap and a smaller, thickened synovial fold.

ABNORMAL PLICAE

The majority of synovial folds in the knee joint are asymptomatic. Consisting largely of elastic and areolar tissue, they are constantly changing shape and length during knee flexion and extension.

Initially, there may be inflammation, edema, and thickening of the plica, causing it to become less flexible. This may alter the smooth gliding of the plica along the femoral condyles. An inflammatory synovitis may ensue, causing further thickening and eventual replacement of the elastic tissue with fibrous tissue.[24] Rarely, the plica may become hyalinized and calcified. This sequence of histologic change results in a thickened, white and fibrotic pathologic plica

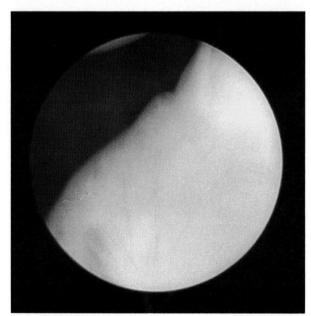

Figure 7–11
Flexion to 90 degrees reveals changes on the anteromedial portion of the medial femoral condyle.

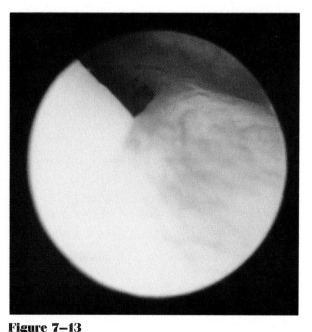

Figure 7–13
At 30 degrees of flexion, the plica impinges on the medial femoral condyle.

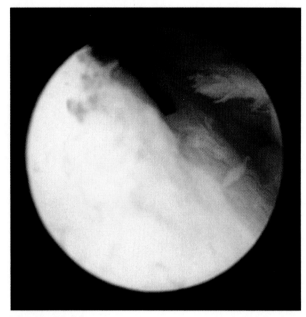

Figure 7–14
At 90 degrees of flexion, erosions and chondromalacia are evident.

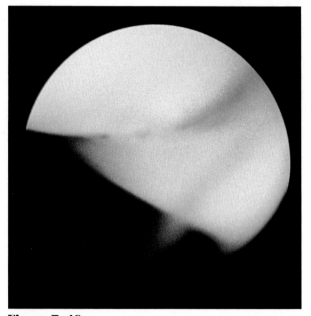

Figure 7–16
A medial plica with patella contact, causing chondromalacia of the patella and lateral displacement.

from a thin, pink, pliable membrane (Figs. 7–21 and 7–22).

Various etiologic factors have been found to lead to this change. Direct or indirect blunt trauma is the most common attributing factor. Strenuous exercise, osteochondritis dissecans, injuries of the meniscus,

and intra-articular osteocartilaginous bodies are other derangements leading to the plica syndrome.[1–3,21] The unpliable plica may snap over the medial femoral condyle, causing pain. The plica may provoke a secondary mechanical synovitis around the margins of the condyles. Repeated irritation and

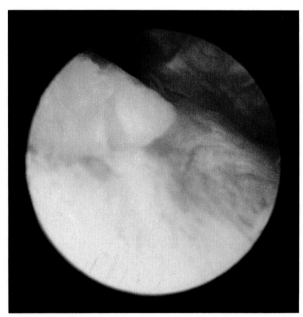

Figure 7–15
Further flexion reveals spur formation and a groove in the anterior portion of the medial femoral condyle.

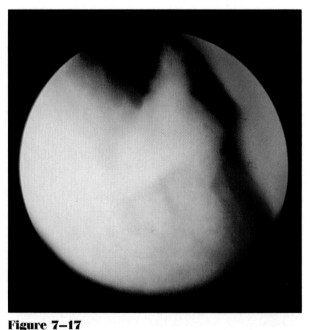

Figure 7–17
The same medial plica as in Figure 7–16, causing chondromalacia at the contact point with the medial femoral condyle.

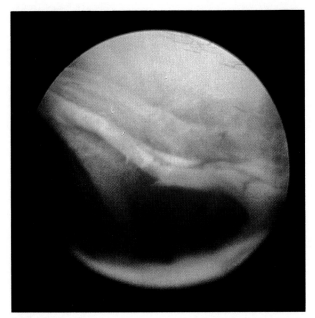

Figure 7–18
A Type A mediopatellar plica, with cordlike elevation in the synovial wall.

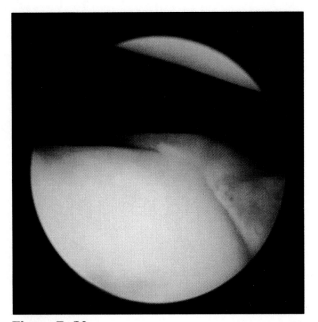

Figure 7–20
A Type C mediopatellar plica covers the anterior surface of the medial femoral condyle.

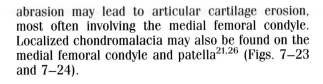

abrasion may lead to articular cartilage erosion, most often involving the medial femoral condyle. Localized chondromalacia may also be found on the medial femoral condyle and patella[21,26] (Figs. 7–23 and 7–24).

SYMPTOMATOLOGY

In a report by Patel, the associated incidence of a mediopatellar plica and chondromalacia of the medial femoral condyle was 40 percent, and chondro-

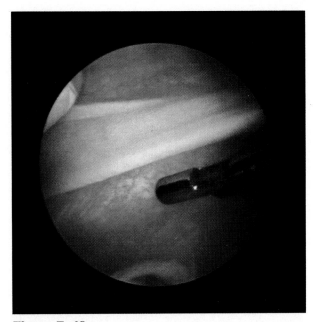

Figure 7–19
A Type B mediopatellar plica, demonstrated by a shelf-like structure that does not impinge on the medial femoral condyle.

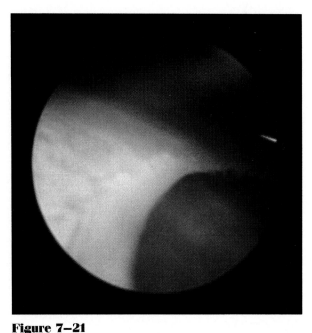

Figure 7–21
The thin, pink, pliable membrane has undergone fibrosis and thickening from inflammation.

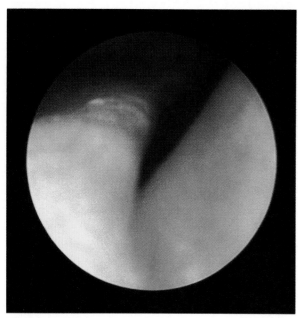

Figure 7–22
The degree of thickening of the membrane can be mild to large.

malacia of the medial facet of the patella was 60 percent.[20] Plica syndrome is the combination of historical and physical findings associated with a pathologic plica. A repetitive process causing synovial inflammation, edema, and fibrosis leads to an inflexible synovial fold that causes a constellation of symptoms and findings. The patient is often a young athlete, male or female, who relates an episode of

blunt or twisting trauma to the knee, followed by pain and sometimes an effusion. A high incidence of mediopatellar plica is found in girls under 20 years of age who have been diagnosed as having chondromalacia or patellofemoral dysplasia.[20] A recent episode of strenuous exercise or a change in footwear or running surface may be present in the history. The symptoms that are exhibited are also found in other internal derangements of the knee, including pain, swelling, clicking, snapping, locking, and giving way (Table 7–2). Athletic activities commonly involved are basketball, bicycling, jogging, and tennis.

The pain is usually intermittent, dull, and aching. Most often, the pain is about the superior aspect of the knee over the femoral condyle. Pain is more severe if localized articular cartilage damage is present secondary to direct repetitive frictional wear.

Activity usually exacerbates the symptoms. Knee flexion, as with stair climbing, causes pain as the knee flexes from 45 to 90 degrees. The pain is often worse after prolonged sitting as the plica is stretched across the femoral condyle. The swelling is often chronic and intermittent, depending on the level of activity. Clicking, snapping, or locking sensations are brought on by activity that causes the plica to bowstring across the femoral condyle during flexion and extension.[17] Locking may be present owing to a thickened, inelastic suprapatellar plica that can alter the patella's course in the intercondylar groove, also causing patellar malalignment and subsequent chondromalacia.[9] Jackson and associates proposed that pannus formation on the medial femoral condyle, caused by the plica, may contact the anterior horn of the medial meniscus with the knee in extension, or

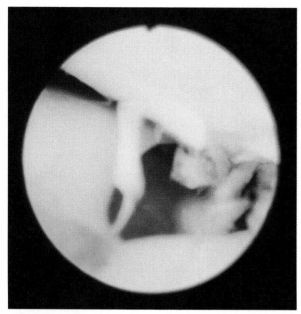

Figure 7–23
Grade III articular changes due to a mediopatellar plica impinging on the medial facet of the patella.

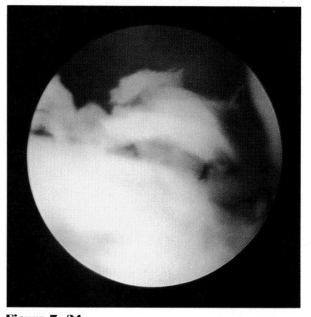

Figure 7–24
Chondromalacia with Grade III changes on the medial femoral condyle.

Table 7–2
Clinical Parameters of Medial Plicae

	BROUKHIM ET AL[5]	HARDAKER ET AL[9]	MUSE ET AL[18]
	25 Patients	69 Patients (73 knees)	42 Patients (51 knees)
Pain, medial femoral condyle	100%	94% (65)	59% (38)
chief complaint	100%	100%	92% (47)
Swelling	12% (3)	59% (41)	67% (34)
or			
effusion	—	11% (9)	20% (10)
Snapping	100%	67% (46) subj.	78% (40) subj.
		57% (39) exam	
Pseudolocking	N/R		35% (18)
Palpable	N/R	16% (11)	67% (34)
band			
Atrophy	N/R	64% (44)	N/R
Instability	0	7% (5)	N/R
Trauma, specific		48% (33)	41% (21)
nonspecific	100%	38% (26)	59% (31)
Response	0	17% (12)	0
to treatment			

N/R, not reported.

the plica may impinge on the edge of the meniscus in varying degrees of flexion and result in medial joint line pain.[14]

Examination of the knee may or may not reveal an effusion. A relatively constant finding is localized tenderness on the medial femoral condyle or a tender, bandlike structure palpable under the medial retinaculum. A mediopatellar plica can be palpated along the medial femoral condyle paralleling the medial border of the patella. A palpable or audible snap may be elicited during brisk flexion and extension of the knee, which may be confused with a positive McMurray's sign, making it difficult to differentiate from a meniscal lesion if there is also joint line tenderness.[19,21] The most common incorrect diagnoses made in people with a pathologic plica are chondromalacia patella and meniscus tears. Other diagnoses include ligament strain, bursitis, contusion, and osteochondritis dissecans.[9]

Imaging studies have thus far played a limited role in the diagnosis. Plain roentgenograms may be helpful only if they show osteocartilaginous bodies or osteochondritis dissecans. Arthrography has been shown to be of value in delineating plicae using cross-table anteroposterior and tangential views.[2] Ultrasound may also be of value as a noninvasive method of identifying a plica, achieving a 92 percent sensitivity.[6] Synovial folds have been demonstrated by computed tomography combined with double-contrast arthrography.[4]

TREATMENT

Treatment of asymptomatic plicae can be either nonoperative or operative. Conservative treatment has met with partial success. Rest, anti-inflammatory agents, local heat, hamstring stretching, and pro-

gressive resistive exercises were more successful in a population with an average age of 21.5 years and symptoms for less than 3 months. Repetitive trauma was the usual cause for development of the plica syndrome. On the other hand, a group of patients with blunt or twisting trauma, an average age of 28.5 years, and symptoms for 6 months did not respond to conservative therapy.[9] After 12 weeks of failed conservative therapy, a patient may become a candidate for arthroscopic evaluation.

Arthroscopy has introduced a means of not only verifying the clinical diagnosis but also initiating surgical treatment with a minimum of morbidity. Other causes for internal derangement can be realized and treated simultaneously. Treatment results with arthrotomy and arthroscopy with section and excision of the plica have been very successful, ranging from 70 to 92 percent[5,9,17–19] (Table 7–3). Hardaker and associates showed excellent results in 53 patients after arthrotomy and excision of the synovial plica while three of eight patients who had arthroscopically released plicae underwent arthrotomy owing to persistent symptoms.[9] Jackson and colleagues reported a 70 percent significant improvement or complete relief in 69 patients treated with arthroscopic section.[7] Muse and coworkers showed a 92 percent complete relief or only mild pain in 51 arthroscopically treated knees; they recommend complete resection to decrease the incidence of recurrent pain.[18] This recommendation is given by many workers who have had similar findings.[7,13,17,19]

TECHNIQUES

In gaining access to the various plicae arthroscopically, certain maneuvers are helpful. In the suprapatellar plica, a standard inferolateral portal into a fully

Table 7–3
Treatment Results

Broukhim et al[5]	25 patients (6–10 months)
	    sectioned—16—complete
	              5—marked improvement (84%)
	              4—no improvement

Hardaker et al[9]	73 knees (69 patients) mean 19 months (3–68 months)
	    conservative—12—improved
	              8—5/8 improved
	           53—good to excellent

Munzinger et al[17]	15 knees (15 patients) average of 19 months (12–36 months)
	    section/excision—12—good
	              3—fair
	              0—poor

Jackson et al[14]	69 patients (1–6 years) section/excision—70% significantly improved, complete relief

Muse et al[18]	51 knees (42 patients) average of 26 months
	    resection—66% unrestricted activity
	           26% strenuous activity with mild pain
	           6% strenuous activity limited by pain
	           2% no strenuous activity

extended knee may produce resistance upon introduction of the blunt trocar. Gentle pressure may produce a "pop" indicating penetration of the membrane with advancement of the obturator into the suprapatellar pouch.[25] A basket forceps or scissors is used to resect the septum through a superolateral portal. Resection is performed from the medial and lateral synovial walls and completed using a high-speed synovial resector. On the medial patellar plica the inferolateral portal is initially used to identify the pathology, and a superolateral portal is used to resect the plica in a similar fashion to the suprapatellar plica. The arthroscope is then replaced in the superolateral portal, which usually shows a large portion of the plica inserting on the infrapatellar fat pad that needs to be resected. Occasionally the medial plica can be visualized only from the superior portal. The infrapatellar plica is not pathologic in itself but may have to be resected to improve visualization or gain access to loose bodies. An inferomedially placed basket forceps, scissors, or motorized shaver can be used to resect the plica, also known as the ligamentum mucosum. Emphasis is made on not resecting normal synovial membranes whose presence does not correlate with the clinical signs and symptoms.[25] Multiple plicae variants require adequate arthroscopic skills for visualization and resection (Figs. 7–25 through 7–30).

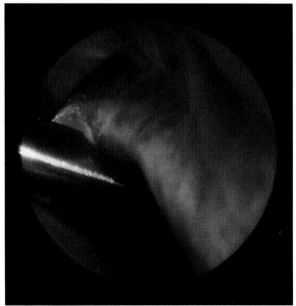

A   B

Figure 7–25
A and *B*, A fibrous shelf in the suprapatellar pouch may be resected using manual instruments.

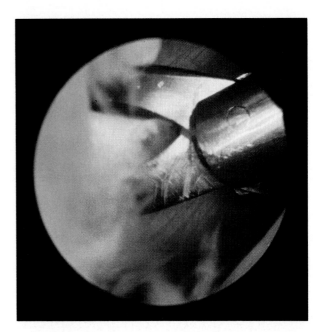

Figure 7–26
Cutting a medial plica through a superolateral portal.

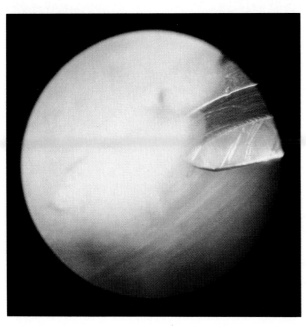

Figure 7–27
A full-thickness cut through a medial plica using scissors.

Figure 7–28
A fibrous band in the patellofemoral joint.

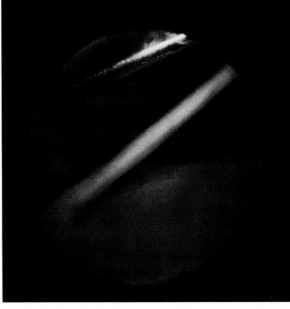

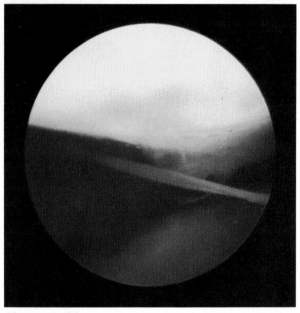

Figure 7–29
A transverse fibrous band across the patellofemoral joint.

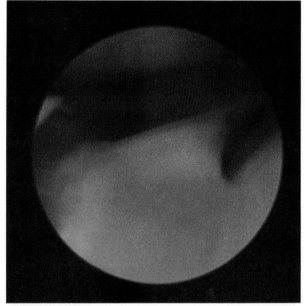

Figure 7–30
Extrusion of a medial meniscus that resembles a plica.

References

1. Aoki T: A case of internal derangement of the knee due to so-called shelf. J Jap Orthop Assoc 39:933, 1965.
2. Aprin M, Shapiro J, Gershwind M: Arthrography (plica views). Clin Orthop 183:90, 1984.
3. Bick EM: Surgical pathology of synovial tissue. J Bone Joint Surg 12:33–44, 1930.
4. Boven F, DeBoeck M, Portliege R: Synovial plicae of the knee on computed tomography. Radiology 147(3):805, 1983.
5. Broukhim B, Fox JM, Blazina ME, Del Pizzo W, Hirsh L: The synovial shelf syndrome. Clin Orthop 142:135–138, 1979.
6. Derks WMJ, De Mooge P, Van Linge B: Ultrasonographic detection of the patellar plica in the knee. J Clin Ultrasound 14:355–360, 1986.
7. Gillquist J: A new modification of the technic of arthroscopy of the knee joint. Acta Chir Scand 142:123, 1976.
8. Gray DJ, Gardner E: Prenatal development of the human knee and superior tibiofibular joints. Am J Anat 86:235, 1950.
9. Hardaker WT, Whipple TL, Bassett FM: Diagnosis and treatment of the plica syndrome of the knee. J Bone Joint Surg 62A:221, 1980.
10. Harty M, Joyce JJ III; Synovial folds in the knee joint. Orthop Rev 7:91–92, 1977.
11. Hughston JC, Stone M, Andrews JR: The suprapatellar plica: Its role in internal derangement of the knee. J Bone Joint Surg 55A: 1318, 1973.
12. Iino S: Normal arthroscopic findings of the knee joint in adult cadavers. J Jap Orthop Assoc 14:467–523, 1939.
13. Jackson RW: The impact of arthroscopy on the management of disorders of the knee. J Bone Joint Surg 57A:1116, 1975.
14. Jackson RW, Marshall DJ, Fujisawa Y: The pathologic medial shelf. Orthop Clin North Am 13:307, 1982.
15. Mayeda T: Ueber das Strangartige Gebilde in der Kniegelenkohle (chorda cavi articularis genu). Mitteil Med 21:507–553, 1918.
16. Mizumachi S, Kawashima W, Okamura T: So-called synovial shelf in the knee joint. J Jap Orthop Assoc 22:1, 1948.
17. Munzinger M, Ruckstuhl J, Scherrer M, Gschwend N: Internal derangement of the knee joint due to pathologic synovial folds: The mediopatellar plica syndrome. Clin Orthop 155:59, 1981.
18. Muse GL, Grana WA, Mollingsworth S: Arthroscopic treatment of medial shelf syndrome: Arthroscopy. J Arth Rel Surg 102:67, 1983.
19. Patel D: Arthroscopy of the plicae—Synovial folds and their significance. Am J Sports Med 6:217, 1978.

20. Patel D: Plica as a cause of anterior knee pain. Orthop Clin North Am 17(2):273, 1986.
21. Pipkin G: Lesions of the suprapatellar plica. J Bone Joint Surg 32A:363, 1950.
22. Pipkin G: Knee injuries: The role of the suprapatellar plica and suprapatellar bursa in simulating internal derangement. Clin Orthop 74:161, 1971.
23. Reid GD, Glasgow M, Gordon DA, Wright TA: Pathological plica of the knee mistaken for arthritis. J Rheumatol 7:573, 1980.
24. Sakakibara J: Arthroscopic study on Iino's band. J Jap Orthop Assoc 50:513, 1976.
25. Schonholtz GJ, Magee CM: The synovial plica of the knee joint. Contemp Orthop 12(2):31, 1986.
26. Tasker, T, Waugh W: Articular changes associated with internal derangement of the knee. J Bone Joint Surg 64B: 486, 1982.

8

Vincent J. Vigorita
Synovial Disorders

NORMAL SYNOVIUM: MICROANATOMY AND FUNCTION

The synovium forms when a primitive mesenchyme cavitates, forming a recognizable joint space at about 8 weeks of embryonic life (Fig. 8–1).

At maturation, the synovium appears pale pink in color and architecturally covers all surfaces of the joint space, excluding the articular cartilage and fibrocartilage of the meniscus. However, the synovium does cover peripheral aspects of the meniscus, and synovial intima-type cells do coat parts of the cruciate ligamentous insertions. Only in abnormal conditions does the synovium encroach upon the surface of articular cartilage, a change classically seen in the reddish "pannus" or inflammatory synovial invasion of the articular cartilage in rheumatoid arthritis.

The villous appearance of synovium is not necessarily abnormal but rather nonspecific and may be seen in a broad range of conditions. In general, traumatic synovitis and degenerative joint disease (osteoarthritis) are attended by edematous change and mild villous hypertrophy. Inflammatory arthritis (classically rheumatoid arthritis) shows a dramatically reddish hyperplastic synovium with fibrinous exudation characterized by abundant tan fibrinous loose bodies called rice bodies.

Normally, the synovium appears smooth and transparent but turns thick, dull, and opaque with pathologic change. With hemorrhage, it becomes obviously bloody but in chronic hemarthrosis turns a reddish brown, owing to hemosiderin deposition and the release of iron from red blood cells, or even, in severe cases, a dark purple. The appearance of reddish purple synovium indicates bleeding and may be seen in trauma, bleeding disorders such as hemophilia, and pigmented villonodular synovitis. Whereas in ochronosis (alkaptonuria) the synovium may appear a dull gray, fibrocartilage and articular cartilage will be discolored black. Darkening or blackening may also be seen when there is extensive release of metallic debris. White foci in the synovium usually indicate gout (urate deposition), pseudogout (calcium pyrophosphate crystal deposition), or soft tissue calcifications (deposits due to trauma or calcinosis syndromes). Cement debris may also lead to pallor.

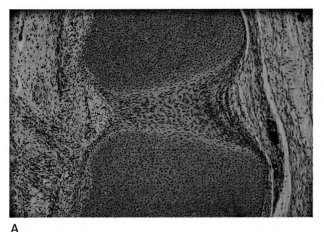

A

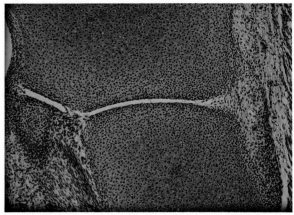

B

Figure 8–1

Embryonic joint showing evolution of primitive mesenchyme (*A*) into a joint space (*B*) at about 8 weeks of intrauterine life.

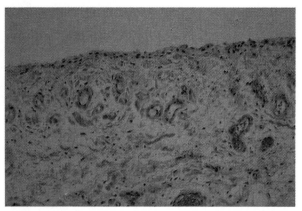

Figure 8–2

Normal synovium. The most superficial zone (or intima) is a 1- to 2-cell layer of synoviocytes below which is a fibrovascular zone (subintima) containing fibroblasts, histiocytes, and mast cells.

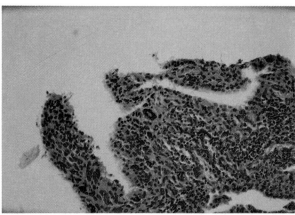

Figure 8–4

Hypertrophy of synovial cells may lead to multinucleated giant cells as in this example of a Grimley-Sokoloff giant cell associated with rheumatoid arthritis. The similarity to the unrelated tuberculous Langhans giant cell is striking.

Microanatomic Structure

The synovium consists of a thin layer of synovial cells or synoviocytes, the intimal layer, above a richly fibrovascular zone, the subintimal layer, that contains arterioles, fat, and other connective tissue cells such as fibroblasts, histiocytes, and occasionally mast cells (Fig. 8–2). This loose connective tissue zone layer becomes gradually more fibrous at capsular insertions. The intimal zone consists of an admixture of cell types broadly classified as those demonstrating macrophage function (synovial A cells) and those more synthesizing in function (synovial B cells). Ultrastructural studies demonstrate abundant mitochondria, Golgi apparatus, vacuoles, lysosomes, phagosomes, vesicles, and surface undulations—characteristics suited to macrophage activity in type A cells; and rough endoplasmic reticulum, free ribosomes, and smoother profiles—characteristics suited to synthetic activity in type B. As might be expected, synoviocytes may be "intermediate" in nature, featuring organelle functions of both type A and type B. Recently, some evidence supports the existence of other cells, such as antigen-type cells (HLA-DR, Ia-like). Although the synovial cells lack desmosomes or tight junctions, characteristic of epithelial tissue, the complexity of this cell structure is evident in the changes seen in various pathologic states. Hyperplasia may be limited to a mild increase in intimal cell number (Fig. 8–3) or there may be dramatic change, including large, bizarre cells such as the Grimley-Sokoloff giant cells (Fig. 8–4) or even striking mucin-producing cells (Fig. 8–5). In this latter condition (mucinous hypertrophy of the synovium), the copious amount of material secreted testifies to the potential capacity of this membrane.

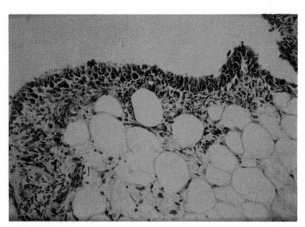

Figure 8–3

Hyperplastic synovium. The synoviocyte layer (intima) shows increased size and numbers of cells.

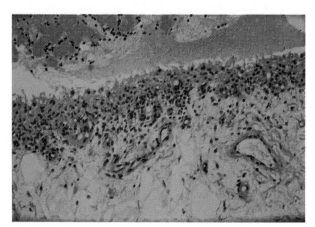

Figure 8–5

Synovial hyperplasia with mucinous appearance, illustrating the synthetic potential of synovial cells.

The fibrovascular subintimal layer is the zone containing the ubiquitous fibrohistiocytic cells and the zone infiltrated by lymphocytes and plasma cells in rheumatoid arthritis. The various components of the synovial subintima explain the source of tumors reported in the knee, such as:

Hemangiomas (arterioles)

Hemangiopericytomas (the pericyte of the arteriole)

Fibromas (fibroblast)

Leiomyomas (smooth muscle of arteriole wall)

Lipomas, Hoffa's disease (fat)

Pigmented villonodular synovitis (PVNS) (fibrohistiocyte)

The etiology of the rare malignant tumors arising near joints, called synovial sarcoma and epithelioid sarcoma, is less well known. These latter tumors are highly malignant and are characterized by aggressive and destructive local growth and metastatic potential.

Functions of the Synovium

The functions of the synovium are best appreciated by understanding the characteristics of its cellular components and microarchitectural structure. For example, the synovial A cells are suited to phagocytic (or macrophage) activity and ingest native or foreign material, such as hemosiderin in chronic bleeding conditions (hemophilia) or iatrogenically introduced substances (gold in the treatment of rheumatoid arthritis). The phagocytic potential of the synovium is probably best illustrated by the marked foreign body giant cell and histiocytic reaction in some cases of loosened prostheses (Fig. 8–6) or in the resorption of bone and cartilage debris in rapidly destructive joint disease or neuropathic joints (Fig. 8–7). On the other hand, the synovial B cell is suited to synthetic function and most characteristically secretes the hyaluronate-protein of synovial fluid. However, more than likely, both type A and type B cells appear to have secretory and phagocytic potential. Other functions in conjunction with the vascular and lymphatic systems of the synovium include the regulation of movement of physiologically important proteins and electrolytes.

IRON SYNOVITIS: HEMARTHROSIS AND HEMOPHILIA

Considering the rich vascularity of the subintimal layer of the synovium, microscopic bleeds from normal daily use of the joint may be expected. In fact, a few red blood cells are considered normal in joint fluid analysis. Trauma to the knee, however, is often accompanied by significant hemarthrosis, an important association since bleeding—or perhaps more specifically the release of iron from ruptured red blood cells—stimulates clinically significant synovial change, i.e., a synovitis characterized by pain and swelling.

In chronic hemarthrosis, iron will accumulate in the synovium. Histopathologic localization includes both the synovial intimal cells (Fig. 8–8) and histiocytic cells of the subintimal zone (Fig. 8–9). Experimental evidence suggests that iron adversely affects synovial function. Chronic hemarthrosis, for example, actually may increase the synthetic function of the otherwise macrophagic synovial type A cell. Hemophilia represents this situation in a clinical extreme.

Classically, hemophilia A is characterized by inadequacy of factor VIII. It primarily affects males, with

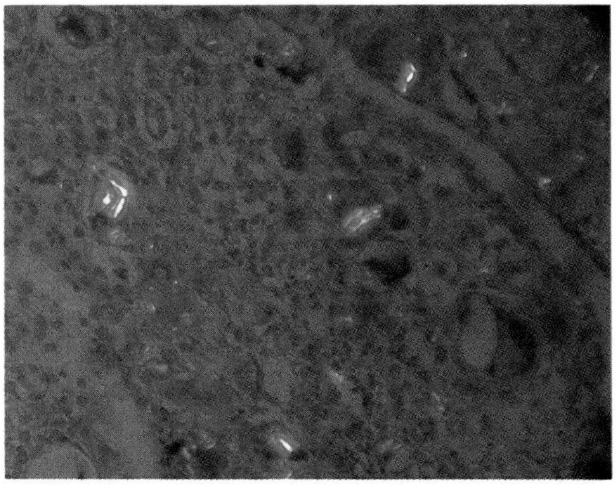

Figure 8–6
Intracytoplasmic refractile particles engulfed by synovial phagocytes illustrate the macrophagic potential of the synovium. (Polarized light microscopy.)

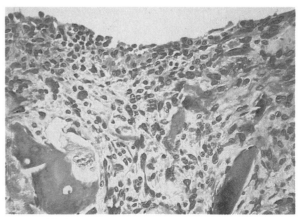

Figure 8–7
Phagocytic synovial function is also evident in bone and cartilage debris resorbed in cases of rapidly destructive joint disease.

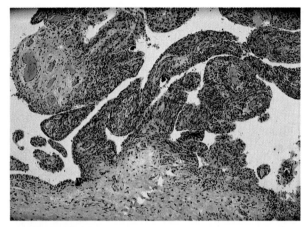

Figure 8–8

The bleeding-induced iron accumulation in the synovium is often localized to the superficial intimal layer of synoviocytes.

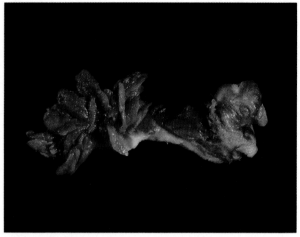

Figure 8–10

Hemarthrosis induces a brownish pigmentation of the synovium with an often villous hyperplasia (left).

substantial intra-articular bleeds into the joints, especially the knees. Grossly, the joint becomes brown (Fig. 8–10). Synovial hyperplasia is significant, iron accumulation in the joint profound, and secondary destruction of the articular surface and bone dramatic. The use of factor VIII concentrates as therapy has slowed considerably the progression of arthropathy but, unfortunately, created one of the significant early-risk groups for the acquired immune deficiency syndrome (AIDS). Large tumor-like masses of blood-coagulum sealed off by fibrous tissue may ensue, termed pseudotumor of hemophilia, and should be removed surgically if possible. Although in its clinical extreme hemophilia represents an inexorable vicious cycle, the hemarthrosis associated with trauma is obviously less significant. However, chronic bleeding of whatever etiology will lead to iron-associated synovial change (iron synovitis). At what point this becomes clinically significant is unclear. It is of interest that experimental models of hemarthrosis pathologically mimic hemophilia more than pigmented villonodular synovitis, which, as will be discussed later, is associated with iron secondarily.

ARTHRITIS

Degenerative Joint Disease (DJD) Versus Rheumatoid Arthritis (RA)

Although a broad range of disorders may give rise to arthritis, de novo arthritis may be readily classified into two groups: degenerative joint disease (osteoarthritis) and rheumatoid arthritis. They are distinct etiologically, clinically, roentgenographically, and pathologically (macroscopically and microscopically).

Whereas both degenerative joint disease (osteoarthritis) and rheumatoid arthritis commonly involve the knee, there are significant differences in the primary component of the joint involved. Notwithstanding recent experimental interest in synovial tissue modulation of cartilage destruction by substances such as catabolin (interleukin-1), the synovium in degenerative joint disease appears, at least initially, an innocent bystander—with the brunt of damage initially involving the articular cartilage (fibrillation and eventual denudement) and secondly the bone (subchondral cyst formation and sclerosis with marginal new bone formation or osteophytosis). Although the synovium may show hyperplasia, this is usually minimal and nonspecific (Fig. 8–11). Rarely

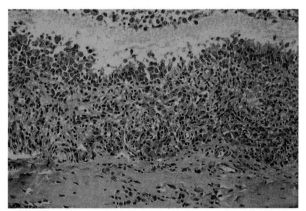

Figure 8–9

Iron may also localize in the fibrocytic zone. Here the intracellular accumulation of hemosiderin is markedly distinct from the synovial lining cells.

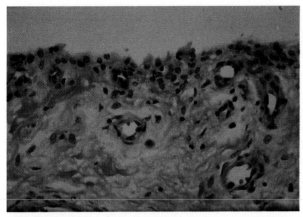

Figure 8–11
Synovial hyperplasia of the synovium in degenerative joint disease is moderate, noninflammatory, and nonspecific.

does inflammation reach the extent seen in rheumatoid arthritis. In acute RA the synovium shows the most significant pathology. Infiltrated by lymphocytes and plasma cells, the synoviocytes become hyperplastic and the surface exudes a fibrinous exudate. Changes in the articular cartilage are truly secondary as the pannus, or inflammatory synovium, invades the surface of the joint, causing chondrolysis, eventual cartilage denudement, and, in chronic cases, the appearance of a secondary degenerative phenomenon. However, both chondrolysis and osteoporosis characterize rheumatoid arthritis, thus distinguishing it clearly from degenerative joint disease.

This distinction is evident in laboratory diagnosis and monitoring. The inflammatory changes in rheumatoid arthritis are discernible in elevated sedimentation rates and positive rheumatoid factors (an elevated immunoglobulin protein, usually IgM, circulating in the serum). There is no equivalent useful laboratory monitor for degenerative joint disease.

DEGENERATIVE JOINT DISEASE (OSTEOARTHRITIS, DJD)

DJD is classically a painful joint condition initially associated with relief at joint rest and later with pain throughout activity, usually increasing with age and commonly involving the knees, especially in obese individuals or those with significant previous traumatic damage.

There is no specific laboratory abnormality in DJD. Radiographic changes in the knees initially show joint space narrowing and subchondral sclerosis. Eventually new bone forms at the margins of articular cartilage (osteophytosis), which may give rise to villous synovial hypertrophy and metaplasia leading to chondro-osseous loose bodies.

Variants of DJD include an inflammatory type,

characterized by more lymphocytic infiltration and hyperplasia of the synovium, and a rapidly destructive joint process that shows accelerated clinical and roentgenographic joint damage correlated pathologically by extensive cartilage and bone debris throughout the joint.

RHEUMATOID ARTHRITIS

Rheumatoid arthritis is classically a chronic, symmetric, persistent arthritis that often affects the knees and may be associated with systemic symptoms and rheumatoid nodules (classically subcutaneous). Its etiology remains obscure, but laboratory studies and familial history suggest both immunologic and genetic factors in its expression. Most patients with rheumatoid arthritis have a circulating protein in their blood, usually IgM, which is the basis for the "rheumatoid factor test," a nonspecific but often useful serologic test in corroborating the clinicopathologic diagnosis. Atypical infections may trigger an as yet undetermined genetic predisposition. The presence of rheumatoid factor and elevated sedimentation rates correlate well with the characteristic synovial changes of a hyperemic synovial tissue (Fig. 8–12) infiltrated by a pronounced lymphocyte and plasma cell infiltration (Fig. 8–13), often producing a fibrinous exudate (Fig. 8–14). The latter proteinaceous exudation may override the articular bone surfaces of the joint, often creating tan friable bodies (rice bodies) (Fig. 8–15).

Treatment

Treatment of rheumatoid arthritis is initially directed at inducing remission of the characteristic lymphoplasmacytic inflammatory response and maintaining joint function. Salicylates, other nonsteroidal anti-inflammatory agents, gold, antimalarial drugs, penicillamine, corticosteroids, and cytotoxic drugs have all been used prior to surgical synovectomy, which may provide temporary articular cartilage salvage, and/or joint replacement. Chondrolysis and osteoporosis are two significant changes associated with rheumatoid arthritis.

Variants

Other disorders have been associated with rheumatoid-like inflammatory joint disease, but these "rheumatoid variants," such as psoriatic arthritis, Reiter's syndrome, and the arthritides associated with colitis, show less inflammatory synovial changes, vary in clinical progression of disease, and usually are not associated with a positive rheumatoid factor.

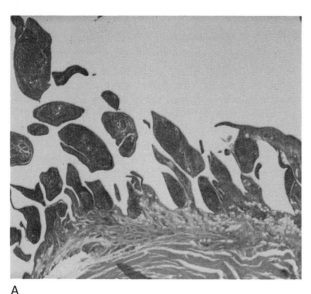

A

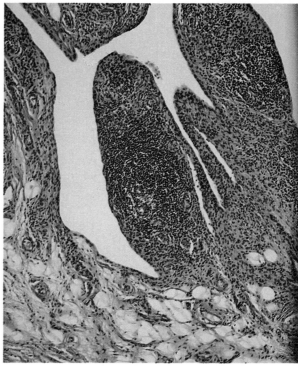

B

Figure 8–12

A and *B*, In rheumatoid arthritis, the synovium becomes hyperplastic and swollen by a lymphocyte and plasma cell infiltration mimicking lymphoid proliferation in other immune conditions.

CRYSTAL-INDUCED SYNOVITIS

There are essentially two synoviotropic crystal deposition disorders of the knee: gout and CPDD (calcium pyrophosphate deposition disease, chondrocalcinosis, or pseudogout). Although the two are often considered together, they are quite distinct etiologically, clinically, and pathologically (Table 8–1).

Gout

Classically this is a severe and painful monarthritis of the first metatarsophalangeal joint, but virtually any joint or part of the body may be affected. The knee is not an uncommon site. In general, gout should be suspected in painful episodes of arthritis in one or more joints of the lower extremity with the

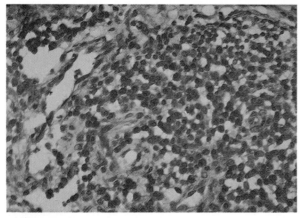

Figure 8–13

At higher magnifications, the lymphoid follicles in the thickened villi are usually peripherally associated with plasma cells—the IgM-producing cells of the rheumatoid factor or "latex fixation" laboratory test.

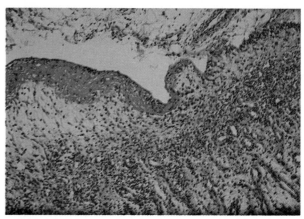

Figure 8–14

A fibrinous exudate is produced that coats the synovial surface.

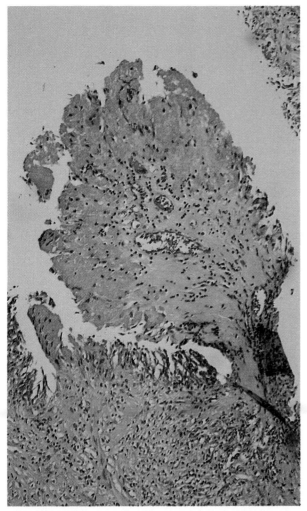

Figure 8–15

Initially produced by synovial cells, this fibrinous material may fall off into the joint, as demonstrated in this photomicrograph. The resultant synovium fills with soft, tannish "rice bodies."

patient showing significant if not complete improvement between episodes. Although the diagnosis should be suspected with elevated serum uric acid (roughly >8.0 mg/dl in men and >6.5 mg/dl in women), normouricemic episodes of gout are well documented.

It is characterized by attacks of severe pain lasting up to several days. The joint may appear erythematous and the patient ill with chills and fever. Initially, radiographs are unremarkable with only soft tissue swelling. With progressive attacks and more urate crystal deposition, tophi, which are granulomatous aggregates of crystals, accumulate in the joint tissue, causing discrete radiolucent marginal erosions of the articular bone (Fig. 8–16). Despite significant bone destruction, joint preservation may be well maintained until late in the disease.

Gout is most often a primary disorder of purine metabolism or an abnormality in the excretion of uric acid. In only rare cases is an underlying enzyme defect uncovered. About 10 per cent of cases are secondary, resulting from overproduction or impaired excretion of uric acid. Obesity, alcoholism, diuretic therapy, and cancer chemotherapy (especially of lymphoproliferative disorders) are frequently observed clinical correlates. Indomethacin, other nonsteroidal anti-inflammatory drugs, colchicine, and allopurinol or probenecid have all been used.

The intraoperative appearance of gout is dramatic: on cut section, tophi show chalk-white aggregates of a soft texture (Fig. 8–17). Microscopically, in tissue the crystal aggregates are surrounded by a marked mononuclear and giant cell inflammatory reaction (Fig. 8–18). Surgical removal of large tophi may improve joint function. Confirmation requires demonstration of the crystals, which can be done utilizing compensated polarized light microscopy. This technique requires a light microscope, polarizing lenses, and a red compensator filter. Fluid aspirated from the joint is submitted to the laboratory in a test tube;

Table 8–1
Synoviotropic Crystal-Associated Disorders

	GOUT	*PSEUDOGOUT*
Crystal	Sodium urate	Calcium pyrophosphates
Radiograph	*Early:* Soft tissue swelling *Later:* Radiolucent erosions around the edges of articular cartilage	Fine, radiopaque, linear deposits in the meniscus and articular cartilage
Frequency of occurrence in knee	Common	Very common; increases with age in DJD
Laboratory studies	Elevated serum uric acid	None
Crystal character with polarized light	Needle-shaped	Rhomboid
Crystal character with compensated polarized light	Parallel yellow; perpendicular blue	Parallel blue; perpendicular yellow
Birefringence	Negative	Positive

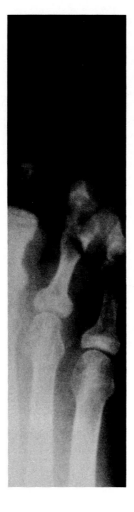
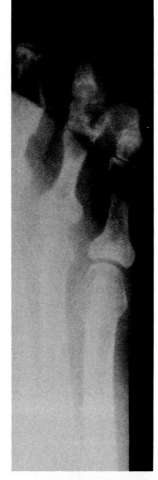

Figure 8–16
  Radiographs in chronic to-phaceous gout show marked bone erosions at the rim of articular bone. This is a classic foot radiograph.

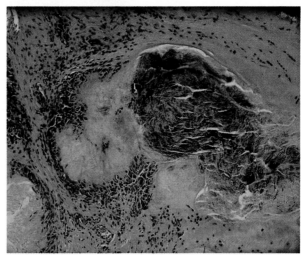

Figure 8–18
  Microscopically, the tophus is a large deposit of crystals surrounded by a marked mononuclear and giant cell reaction. In routine tissue fixation, the urate crystals will dissolve in the aqueous formalin solution. Here crystals are shown undissolved (brown, right). In the usual processing the pathologist relies on the inflammatory reaction around vague pinkish-white zones (left) to diagnose the condition. (Hematoxylin & eosin stain.)

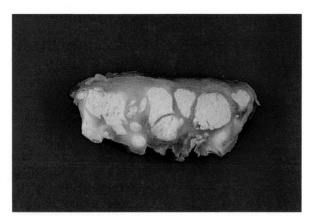

Figure 8–17
  Gouty tophi appear grossly as chalk-white, circumscribed deposits similar to rare calcinosis deposits. In gout, the deposits have a pastelike consistency.

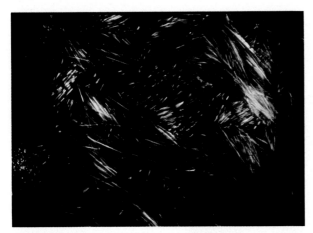

Figure 8–19
With polarized light, gout crystals are seen to be fine, slender, needle-like, and brilliantly refractile.

Figure 8–20
With the use of polarized light and a first order red compensator filter, crystals appear yellowish-pink or blue. The red compensator has an orientation marker. Sodium urate crystals appear yellow (or pink) when oriented parallel to the marker and blue when oriented perpendicular to the marker. By convention this is considered negatively birefringent.

the fluid is centrifuged and the sediment spread onto a glass slide for microscopic examination (Figs. 8–19 and 8–20.)

Calcium Pyrophosphate Deposition Disease
(CPDD, Pseudogout, Chondrocalcinosis)*

CPDD is a polyarticular deposition of calcium pyrophosphate crystals in fibrocartilage, articular cartilage, and synovial tissue in the knee, hip, symphysis pubis, wrist, and intervertebral disc. Anatomic studies have demonstrated a predilection for the fibrocartilage of the meniscus and the synovium and less so for the superficial zones of the articular cartilage.

Although CPDD may be seen microscopically in at least 15 per cent of osteoarthritic knees examined at joint replacements, the characteristic white, flecklike deposits observed intraoperatively are seen less frequently.

The prevalence of CPDD in degenerative joint disease is consistent with the accumulation of pyrophosphates by release from articular cartilage. Since chondroid metaplasia has been observed with deposits of calcium pyrophosphate, local activation of certain enzymes, such as alkaline phosphatase or inorganic pyrophosphatases, leading to inactivation of

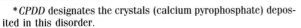

*CPDD designates the crystals (calcium pyrophosphate) deposited in this disorder.

Pseudogout refers to the occasional painful occurrence of CPDD-induced arthritis mimicking gout.

Chondrocalcinosis refers to the fine linear radiopaque densities seen in the joint spaces of involved cases.

calcification inhibitors, may be important. It is significant that symptomatic arthritis due specifically to CPDD is unusual and much less common than gout. CPDD is usually less painful than gout but shares similarities of exacerbation during surgery, and relief between episodes. Joints, especially the knees, are bilaterally and symmetrically involved. Radiographs show fine, radiopaque linear densities appearing along the joint space (Fig. 8–21). This has been shown to be in the meniscus, articular and synovial tissue, and superficial articular cartilage. However, unlike the case in gout, the clinically apparent disease does not necessarily correlate with the extent of roentgenographically detectable disease. Microscopically the crystals are rhomboidal, less birefringent, and less inflammatory than in gout (Figs. 8–22 through 8–25). Treatment is directed at relief during painful attacks and includes salicylates, indomethacin, and other nonsteroidal anti-inflammatory agents.

SYNOVIAL CHONDROMATOSIS
(Synovial Osteochondromatosis)

The synovium, capable of undergoing metaplasia to cartilage in a broad range of conditions including trauma and degenerative joint disease, may produce multiple cartilaginous and chondro-osseous loose

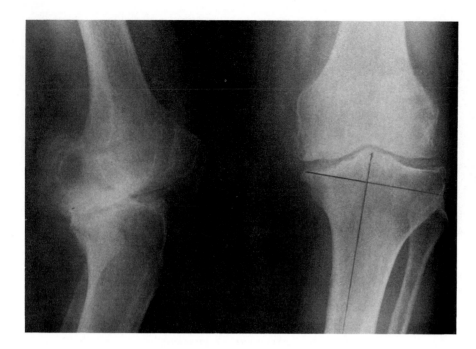

Figure 8–21
Radiograph of this osteoarthritic knee displays the granular radiopaque densities of calcium pyrophosphate.

bodies throughout the joint. This latter condition, synovial chondromatosis (synovial osteochondromatosis), is best characterized as a benign tumorous proliferation. Initially embedded in the synovium, the nodules may dislodge from the synovium and become free loose bodies ranging in number from a few to hundreds.

Synovial chondromatosis is a monoarticular condition of the third, fourth, and fifth decades of life with predilection for the knee. It is usually associated with swelling and may be associated with pain, limitation of motion, and occasionally clicking or locking. Radiographically, the condition is easily recognized if the cartilaginous bodies have undergone calcification or ossification, which they often do (Fig. 8–26). The numerous radiopaque densities range in size from a millimeter to centimeters, varying considerably in

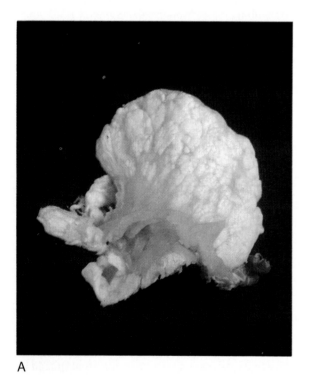

A

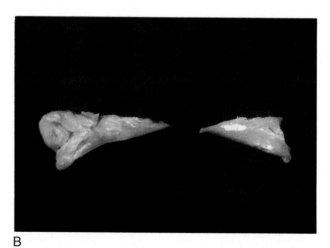

B

Figure 8–22
CPDD (pseudogout) crystals appear white and often as fine, flakelike deposits. *A*, The synovium is thoroughly coated. *B*, Affected menisci show linear white streaks as in this one removed at knee replacement for osteoarthritis.

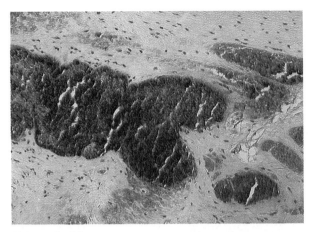

Figure 8–23

Unlike sodium urate crystals, calcium pyrophosphate crystals appear as purple depositions on routine tissue processing. The lack of an inflammatory response is in contrast to that of gout. (Hematoxylin & eosin stain.)

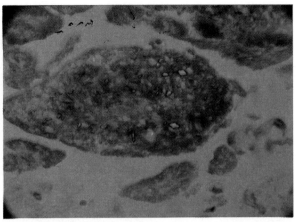

Figure 8–25

With the red compensator filter, CPDD crystals are classically blue when parallel to the red filter orientation and yellow or pink when perpendicular—an observation frequently cited but less often actually observed. By convention, this is considered positively birefringent.

the extent of calcification. Arthrography is useful in diagnosing the noncalcified bodies. Grossly the synovium shows flakelike bodies, or it may possess an irregular nodular contour. Whitish or translucent bluish-gray nodules, ranging greatly in size and shape, may be more obviously attached on the membrane or floating in the joint space (Fig. 8–27).

Histopathologic differences of these bodies have supported a distinction between a secondary synovial chondromatosis associated with degenerative joint disease and a primary synovial chondromatosis not associated with any underlying disorder (Figs. 8–28 through 8–31). The loose bodies in the secondary condition classically may show more organized cellular growth such as layers of calcification. However,

in primary synovial chondromatosis a more disorganized growth of cartilage cells is often apparent.

Surgical removal of all the nodules is important in preventing recurrence.

If the chondro-osseous bodies are entirely free loose bodies within the joint, a thorough cleaning of the joint may suffice. However, the disorder may involve chondro-osseous change within the synovial subintimal connective tissue, a fact that may require total synovectomy to prevent recurrence.

In very rare instances, chondrosarcomas may arise in the setting of synovial chondromatosis. They are characterized by extracapsular involvement and should be distinguished from a de novo primary synovial chondrosarcoma of the joint.

PIGMENTED VILLONODULAR SYNOVITIS (PVNS)

Although sometimes considered an inflammatory reaction, PVNS is a tumorous proliferation of stromal mononuclear and multinucleated giant cells of fibrohistiocytic origin. The nodular growth pattern, the occasionally observed mitotic activity of the stroma, the relative lack of inflammatory cells, and the ability to erode local tissue support the classification of PVNS as a tumor. The name is fitting for only some of the lesions. PVNS may show little pigmentation, is often a solitary nodular growth with little villous hyperplasia, and, as mentioned, shows little inflammatory activity.

The joint fluid color is variable, ranging from normal to brownish-red. The synovium may appear diffusely pigmented or, more commonly, focally so. The

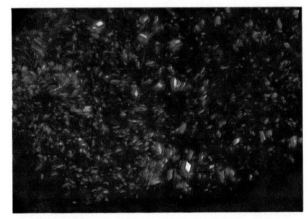

Figure 8–24

Calcium pyrophosphate crystals are less refractile on polarized light and have a rectangular or rhomboid shape.

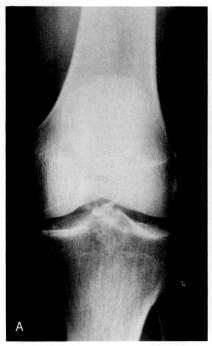
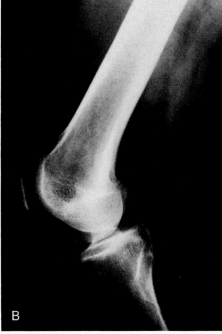

Figure 8–26
A and *B*, The presence of multiple loose bodies typical of primary synovial chondromatosis is obvious if the lesions are calcified or ossified, as shown in a case involving the knee. Noncalcified chondroid bodies may require arthrography for preoperative detection.

pigment is due to both hemosiderin accumulation from microscopic synovial hemorrhage (brown) and aggregations of lipid-laden macrophages (yellow) in the periphery of expanding nodules. Hyperplastic and pigmented changes mimicking those of chronic hemarthrosis in the adjacent synovium are secondary in nature and do not represent the lesion proper.

At least five clinical types of PVNS are identified in the knee (Figs. 8–32 through 8–36):
   (1) loose body,

   (2) a localized nodule (pedunculated or embedded in the synovium),
   (3) aggregates of nodules confined to one compartment,
   (4) a truly diffuse involvement of the synovium, and
   (5) synovial PVNS extending into bursa.
   Localized nodular and nodular aggregate types are the most common types of PVNS.
   Typically, PVNS is a monoarticular arthritis usually

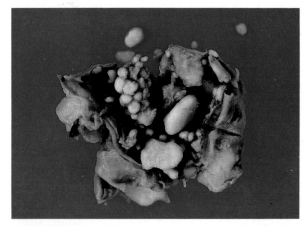

Figure 8–27
Primary synovial chondromatosis appears intraoperatively as whitish bodies, attached or freely floating, varying widely in size and shape.

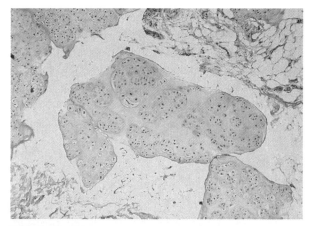

Figure 8–28
The classic microscopic appearance is that of proliferating chondrocytes; the macroscopic nodules are mimicked by the microscopic chondrocytic aggregation.

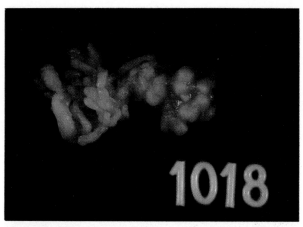

Figure 8—29

In traumatic knees or degenerative joint disease, the synovium may undergo chondroid or chondro-osseous metaplasia, as seen in this nodular growth (right).

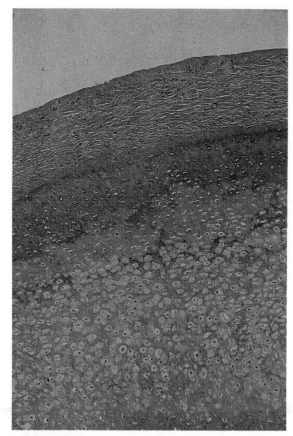

Figure 8—31

In chondromatosis associated secondarily with joint disease, the layers of calcification may appear quite distinct, as seen in this microscopic transection of a radiopaque loose body.

observed in the early and middle adult period, rarely at the extreme ends of life. Symptoms may be gradual in onset. Clinically, patients may present with discomfort or pain. Swelling, stiffness, locking, or even instability of the knee may occur. Torsion of a pedunculated nodular form of PVNS has been associated with the unusual clinical presentation of acute pain.

The most common x-ray findings in the knee are soft tissue swelling (Figs. 8—37 and 8—38). Arthrograms may best demonstrate the nodules as discrete pitting defects. Bone changes are less frequent but may include erosions and degenerative changes.

The treatment of PVNS is surgical. If an isolated

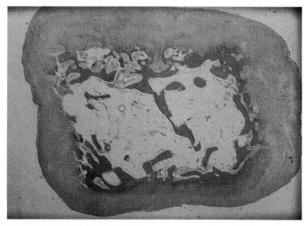

Figure 8—30

These transformations may be purely cartilaginous or mixtures of cartilage and bone. An osseous fibrocartilaginous loose body is shown.

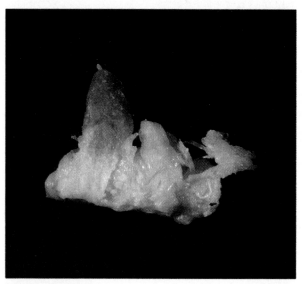

Figure 8—32

The fact that pigmented villonodular synovitis (PVNS) is usually a focal intra-articular growth is supported by this tan villous nodule of PVNS, an incidental finding in a knee joint replacement.

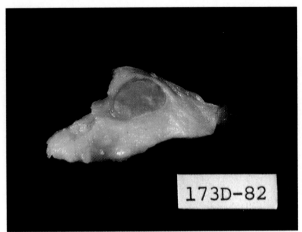

Figure 8–33
Another example of a small, solitary nodule of PVNS. The localization below the glistening translucent synovium gives credence to the origin of PVNS in the fibrohistiocytic cell population of the subintimal zone.

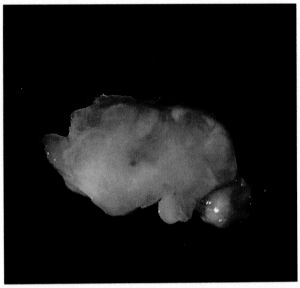

Figure 8–35
On cross-section, the nodules of PVNS usually show that the pigment is peripheral. Here the central silk-colored region of collagenous stroma is surrounded by a rim of yellow (lipid-laden macrophages or xanthoma cells) and brown (hemosiderin) pigment.

loose body or nodule is confirmed, arthroscopic surgical excision may be attempted. However, the propensity of the lesions to recur (in up to one third of cases) requires careful examination of the remainder of the joint to exclude multiple foci. Smaller nodules may be missed, embedded as they are in the subintimal synovial layers.

The diffuse form of PVNS is more problematic and requires total synovectomy (Figs. 8–39 through 8–41). If not removed, PVNS will continue to grow and erode into the articular bone. Bursal PVNS also requires adequate surgical excision and may extend deeply into surrounding soft tissue.

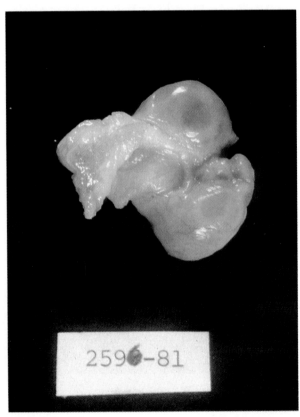

Figure 8–34
PVNS may be seen as an intra-articular loose body. The pale tan (chicken liver) color is characteristic.

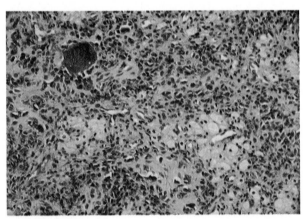

Figure 8–36
Microscopically, the collagenous stroma is awash in mesenchymal mononuclear and giant cells. Inflammation is sparse. Xanthomatous cells are usually focal in distribution (bottom).

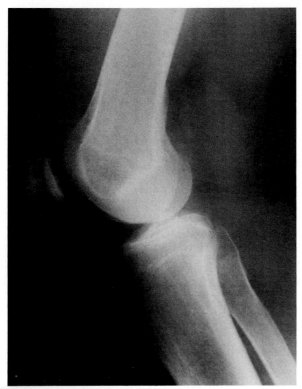

Figure 8–37
PVNS in the knee may show only soft tissue swelling and less commonly bone erosion or degenerative changes.

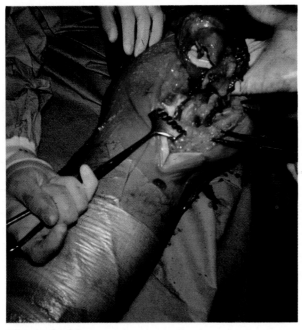

Figure 8–38
PVNS may involve the joint extensively, as seen in this truly villonodular proliferation. Recurrences are seen in at least a third of diffuse cases. (Courtesy of Dr. Barry Walsh.)

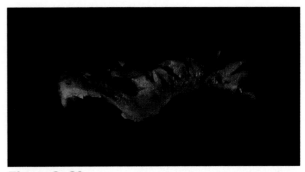

Figure 8–39
The diffuse type of PVNS is characterized grossly by tan or brown pigmentation. Here the synovial villi are thickened and the synovial intima is lifted off its fibrous floor as the lesion proliferates laterally and upward.

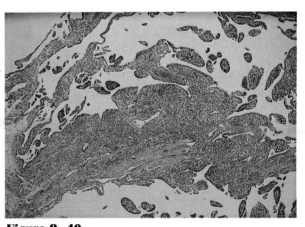

Figure 8–40
The villous hypertrophy of the synovium is evident as the mesenchymal proliferation engorges the synovium.

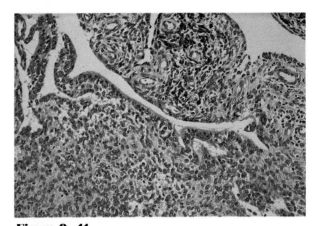

Figure 8–41
A higher microscopic view of PVNS synovium shows hemosiderin accumulation around capillaries (upper right) in contrast to the hyperplastic synoviocytes (center) and proliferating cellular lesion (below, left).

ACKNOWLEDGMENT

The assistance of Claudette Hickey in manuscript preparation is gratefully acknowledged.

Specific References

1. Cooper NS, Soren A, McEwen C, Rosenberger JL: Diagnostic specificity of synovial lesions. Hum Pathol 12:314–328, 1981.
2. Felson DT, Anderson JJ, Naimark A, Walker AM, Meenan RF: Obesity and knee osteoarthritis. Ann Intern Med 109:18–24, 1988.
3. Flandry F, Hughston JC: Current Concepts Review: Pigmented villonodular synovitis. J Bone Joint Surg 69:942–949, 1987.
4. Gardner DL: Structure and function of connective tissue and joints. In Scott JT (ed): Copeman's Textbook of Rheumatic Diseases. 6th ed. Edinburgh, Churchill-Livingstone, 1986, pp 207–209, 229–241.
5. Hamilton A, Davis RI, Nixon JR: Synovial chondrosarcoma complicating synovial chondromatosis. J Bone Joint Surg 69A:1084–1088, 1987.
6. Hasselbacher P: Structure of the synovial membrane. Clin Rheum Dis 7(1):57–69, 1981.
7. Howie CR, Smith GD, Christie J, Gregg PJ: Torsion of localized pigmented villonodular synovitis of the knee. J Bone Joint Surg 67B:564–566, 1985.
8. Markel SF, Hart WR: Arthropathy in calcium pyrophosphate dihydrate crystal deposition disease. Arch Pathol Lab Med 106:529, 1982.
9. Milgram JW: Synovial osteochondromatosis: A histopathologic study of thirty cases. J Bone Joint Surg 59:792–801, 1977.
10. O'Rahilly R, Gardner E: The embryology of movable joints. In Sokoloff L (ed): The Joints and Synovial Fluid. Vol I. New York, Academic Press, 1978, pp 49–103.
11. Rao AS, Vigorita VJ: Pigmented villonodular synovitis (giant cell tumor of the tendon sheath and synovial membrane). J Bone Joint Surg 66A:76–94, 1984.
12. Sledge CB: Developmental anatomy of joints. In Resnick D, Niwayama G (eds): Diagnosis of Bone and Joint Disorders. Vol 1. Philadelphia, WB Saunders, 1981, pp 2–18.
13. Vernon-Roberts B: Structure and function of joints. In Currey HLF (ed): Mason and Currey's Clinical Rheumatology. 4th ed. Edinburgh, Churchill-Livingstone, 1986, pp 1–15.
14. Villacin AB, Brigham LN, Bullough PG: Primary and secondary synovial chondrometaplasia. Hum Pathol 10:439, 1979.

General References

1. Beary JF, Christian CL, Sculco TP (eds): Manual of Rheumatology and Outpatient Orthopedic Disorders: Diagnosis and Treatment. Boston, Little, Brown, 1981.
2. Hirohata K, Morimoto K, Kimura H: Ultrastructure of Bone and Joint Diseases. 2nd ed. Tokyo, Igaku-Shoin, 1981.
3. Rodman GP, Schumacher HR, Zvaifler NJ (eds): Primer on the Rheumatic Diseases. 8th ed. Atlanta, Arthritis Foundation, 1983.
4. Sokoloff L (ed): The Joints and Synovial Fluid. Vol 1. New York, Academic Press, 1978.

9

James A. Rand

Arthroscopic Diagnosis and Management of Articular Cartilage Pathology

The orthopedist must frequently deal with joint injuries and arthrosis. Management of this pathology requires a knowledge not only of the surgical options available but also the normal physiology and response to injury of the periarticular soft tissues, bone, and articular cartilage. The limited capacity for repair of mature articular cartilage must be considered in formulating a treatment plan. Iatrogenic injury to articular cartilage must be avoided.

NORMAL CARTILAGE

The gross morphologic appearance of articular cartilage suggests a homogeneous simple structure that provides a surface for joint motion. However, articular cartilage is a highly complex, specialized structure that performs several important functions. Articular cartilage may be considered as composed of two basic components: cells (chondrocytes) and extracellular matrix. The cell volume of mature articular cartilage is less than that of other tissues, accounting for 5 per cent or less of the tissue volume.[6,54] The cells of articular cartilage are not in direct contact with each other.[6] Articular cartilage is devoid of nerves, blood vessels, and lymphatics.[4] The avascular nature of articular cartilage means that the chondrocytes must rely upon diffusion of nutrients for their maintenance.[54,56,103] Anaerobic metabolic pathways are well developed in the chondrocytes to allow their metabolic activity for synthesis of the matrix components.[54] Nutrition may account for the inverse relationship between cartilage thickness and cell density in mammalian tissues.[102]

The matrix components of articular cartilage give cartilage its mechanical properties. The cartilage matrix is composed of two component groups: tissue fluid and structural macromolecules.[6] The fluid component of the matrix constitutes 70 per cent of its volume,[54] primarily water with small proteins and metabolites.[6] The high water content is essential for the special mechanical characteristics of cartilage. The fluid component of cartilage is not contained by a membrane.[6] The volume of water and its behavior are determined by interaction with the complex macromolecules of the matrix.[6] The high water content and the complex interaction of water with the macromolecules provide a resiliency to the matrix allowing it to resist compression, restore shape after deformation, and contribute to joint lubrication.[6,102]

The structural macromolecules of articular cartilage consist of fibrillar and nonfibrillar components.[6] The fibrillar portion consists of collagen. Collagen constitutes 50 per cent of the tissue dry weight.[6] The collagen is Type II and is unique to hyaline cartilage, nucleus pulposus, and vitreous body.[6,54] Collagen provides tensile strength and form for the tissue. Proteoglycans make up the other major part of the ground substance. Other noncollagenous components are proteins and glycoproteins. Proteoglycans constitute 40 per cent of the dry weight of the cartilage and form the major macromolecules of the ground substance.[6,54] Proteoglycans consist of 95 per cent polysaccharides and 5 per cent proteins.[6] The predominant types of polysaccharides are chondroitin sulfate, keratin sulfate, and hyaluronic acid.[6,54] Proteoglycans consist of either monomers or aggregates.[6]

The proteoglycan subunit or monomer consists of a central protein core to which are attached the polysaccharides (Fig. 9–1).[6] Aggregates consist of a hyaluronic acid filament to which multiple monomeric

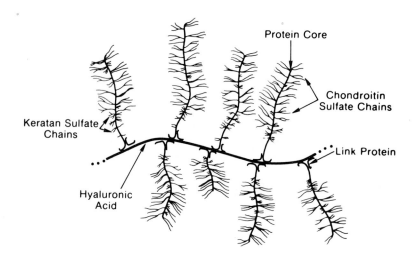

Figure 9–1

Proteoglycan structure. (Reproduced with permission from Buckwalter JA: The fine structure of human intervertebral disc. *In* American Academy of Orthopaedic Surgeons: Symposium on Idiopathic Low Back Pain. St. Louis, CV Mosby, 1982.)

subunits are attached. Aggregates form from the extracellular noncovalent association of the molecules. Link proteins stabilize the association between monomers and hyaluronic acid. The high content of anionically charged groups in the polysaccharides contributes to the unique properties of bonding water and the tendency of adjacent proteoglycan chains to repel each other. Proteoglycans fill a large volume, giving cartilage its resiliency and stiffness to compression. The collagen component of cartilage gives cartilage its tensile stiffness. As load is applied to articular cartilage, water is forced from the loaded area. As the proteoglycans are forced together, the cartilage becomes stiffer and more resistant to compression. Once the load is removed, water is returned to the cartilage and the preloaded state is resumed. This mechanism helps distribute loads, reduce stresses, and provide resiliency and stiffness to the cartilage.[6] Articular cartilage serves as an important load-absorbing layer in the knee subjected to impact loading.[37]

Articular cartilage thickness in the human knee averages 3.7 ± 0.8 millimeters on the lateral and 4.0 ± 0.8 millimeters on the medial femoral condyle. The thickness of articular cartilage gradually diminishes toward the peripheral portion of the joint surface. An increase in thickness of articular cartilage is seen in patients who have an increased body weight.[34]

Articular cartilage has four layers or zones proceeding from the surface to the subchondral bone. The layers are (1) superficial or tangential, (2) transitional, (3) deep or radial, and (4) calcified cartilage (Fig. 9–2).[6,14,54,107] The superficial zone is the thinnest zone and has a high collagen content.[107] A thin layer devoid of cells lies adjacent to the joint.[6] The superficial zone acts as a tension-resisting layer and helps maintain the integrity of the articular cartilage.[107] The transitional zone has a much larger volume than the superficial zone. Proteoglycans are less strongly bound in the transitional than in the superficial zone.[6] The deep or radial zone forms the largest part of articular cartilage. The zone of calcified cartilage separates the hyaline cartilage from the subchondral bone. Collagen fibers from the radial zone penetrate into the calcified cartilage. The various zones have differing functions.[6] The superficial zone primarily resists shear. The transitional zone provides a medium for stress distribution from one of shear at the surface to compression deeper in the tissue.[6,72] The radial zone helps distribute loads and resist compression. The calcified cartilage anchors the articular cartilage to the subchondral bone.

Lubrication of the articular surface may occur by glycoproteins and water between the surfaces providing boundary or "weeping" lubrication.[60,82] Hyaluronic acid in synovial fluid appears to be important in the lubrication of periarticular soft tissues.[80,82]

RESPONSE TO INJURY

Injuries to articular cartilage may be separated into those that act primarily on the matrix and those that produce mechanical disruption.[6] Of course, secondary mechanical damage may follow matrix injury, and matrix digestion from proteolytic enzymes may follow mechanical injury. The extent of articular cartilage damage will depend upon the nature of the injuring force and the ability of the cartilage to resist or respond to the injury. In most tissues, injury causes tissue necrosis followed by a vascular-mediated inflammatory response and finally repair. The avascularity of articular cartilage prevents a vascular response to injury unless the subchondral bone is penetrated. Adult cartilage is able to respond to injury. Chondrocytes are capable of cell division and DNA synthesis.[57] Articular chondrocytes are capable of altering the rate of proteoglycan synthesis in response to a variety of physical and pathologic states.[57] Therefore, the potential for chondrocyte participation in the repair process exists.

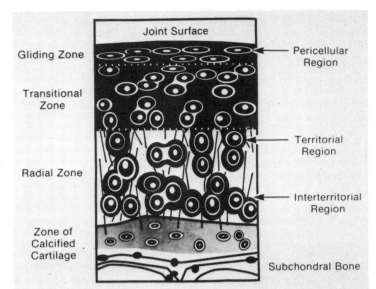

Figure 9–2
Four zones of articular cartilage. (Reproduced with permission from Buckwalter JA: Articular cartilage. *In* AAOS Instructional Course Lectures. St. Louis, CV Mosby, 1983, pp 349–370.)

Matrix degradation of articular cartilage occurs from the release of proteolytic enzymes that attack proteoglycans. Human leukocytes possess enzymes that can penetrate articular cartilage and degrade matrix proteoglycans.[6] In septic arthritis, proteolytic enzymes can degrade the ground substance (Fig. 9–3).[17] Once the collagen fibrils are exposed, mechanical damage to the joint surface may occur.[17] If the damage to the proteoglycans is arrested early, restoration of the lost proteoglycans is possible.[6] Once advanced destruction has occurred, repair is no longer possible.

Mechanical injury may be a single event or repetitive. Blunt trauma or penetrating injuries may occur. The response of the articular cartilage to mechanical injury will depend upon the type, extent, location, and duration of application of the injuring force. An osteochondral fracture would be an acute single injury whereas joint overload from malalignment would result in repetitive injury (Fig. 9–4). Differing responses may be expected depending upon the type of injury. The maturity of the patient, the depth of injury, the duration of injury, and treatment provided will affect the healing response. Two potential mechanisms of repair exist, depending upon the depth of injury: (1) extrinsic repair, and (2) intrinsic repair.[103]

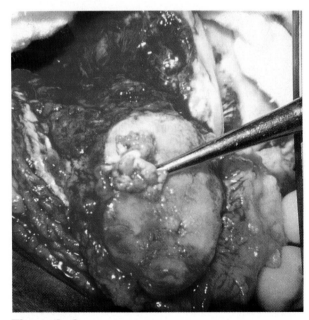

Figure 9–3
Granulation tissue invading a patellar articular surface that has a chronic (1 month) septic arthritis.

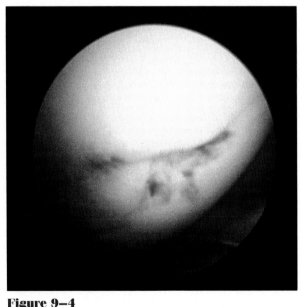

Figure 9–4
An acute chondral fracture to subchondral bone of the medial femoral condyle.

Intrinsic repair depends upon synthesis of matrix by surviving chondrocytes adjacent to the injury site to fill the defect.[103] In humans, superficial defects in articular cartilage are not ordinarily repaired.[14,79] However, Redfern's canine studies suggest that wounds in articular cartilage are capable of healing by intrinsic repair from the cut surfaces.[85] Lacerations of hyaline cartilage, either perpendicular or tangential to the surface, follow a similar course.[6] Lacerations disrupt the collagen fibril network and kill a few chondrocytes. Cells adjacent to the injury site divide and synthesize new matrix. The avascular environment limits nutrients to the chondrocytes. Since there is no inflammatory response, the repair process is short lived.[6]

Intrinsic repair of superficial lacerations of articular cartilage has been supported by observations of cartilage flow into the defect as well as matrix production by the cartilage cells.[62] In an immature canine model, superficial defects in the femoral condyle filled with cartilage and were covered by a superficial cell layer. In three of ten cases in which the lesion was peripherally located and had a vertical wall, complete repair of the defect was observed. Hyaline cartilage was found in these defects.[7] In an adult rabbit patellar model following superficial laceration, there were loss of matrix, superficial fibrillation, increased proteoglycan synthesis, and cell clusters.[62] Similar findings are observed in osteoarthritis. The superficial lacerations remained localized to the traumatized area of the articular cartilage through the 34-week study period.[62] No repair of superficial lacerations was observed in either immature or mature dogs up to 66 weeks following injury.[20] In immature rabbits, there was increased metabolic activity of the chondrocytes adjacent to the defect with matrix production, but the defect was not filled by the repair reaction.[28] The new matrix that was formed was absent by 2 years, probably related to abrasion by joint movement.[30] Over the two years of the study, there was no progression to diffuse osteoarthritis.[30] In summary, superficial articular cartilage lacerations will not significantly heal, but progression to diffuse osteoarthritis appears unlikely. Prevention of iatrogenic articular cartilage injury during arthroscopic surgery is essential, as repair of the superficial scuffing is unlikely to occur.

Extrinsic repair depends upon new connective tissue gaining access to the surface of the articular cartilage. New connective tissue may arise from synovium or from exposure of subchondral bone by full-thickness injuries.[103] Following full-thickness lacerations to bone, a fibrin clot fills the defect. The fibrin clot is replaced by granulation tissue and subsequently by fibrous tissue.[20,55,56] The fibrous tissue gradually undergoes metaplasia into fibrocartilaginous tissue (Fig. 9–5).[20,55,56] In adult rabbits, the ability for repair of a full-thickness defect is variable, ranging from none to complete healing.[49] The ability

to heal the defect appears to be unique to the individual animal, with both knees within an individual displaying a similar response.[49] In immature dogs, 27 of 30 full-thickness defects were repaired with fibrocartilaginous tissue, with only three having complete repair with hyaline cartilage.[7] In mature or immature dogs, full-thickness defects of the femoral condyles displayed complete healing by 16 weeks, with formation of a new subchondral bone plate by 66 weeks.[20] Subchondral bone violation and functional stress were felt to be important in the repair process.[20] In mature and immature rats, the process of repair appears similar with fibrocartilaginous healing of the full-thickness defect.[47] In rabbits, fibrocartilaginous repair tissue has filled drill holes through exposed subchondral bone and fused with the surrounding rim of articular cartilage.[63] The reparative cartilage was most frequently focal rather than a continuous sheet (Fig. 9–6).[63]

The durability of the repair tissue induced by extrinsic repair has been an area of concern. In the rabbit, the cartilaginous material that is present at 2 to 4 months is gradually replaced by fibrous tissue by 12 months.[69] Fibrocartilage is not as durable as hyaline cartilage and, with time, undergoes fibrillation. The increasingly fibrous texture of the repair tissue probably results from a loss of proteoglycan rather than a change in collagen type.[29] The size of the full-thickness defect is important. Healing of a 3-millimeter but not a 9-millimeter defect occurred in an equine model.[15] In the rabbit, the repair tissue is primarily hyaline cartilage, Type II collagen, but there is

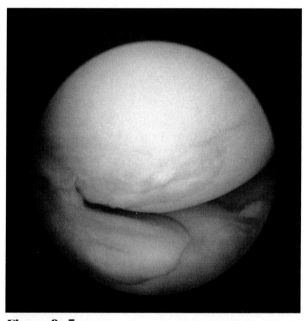

Figure 9–5
Fibrocartilaginous repair of a full-thickness defect of the medial femoral condyle 1 year after injury.

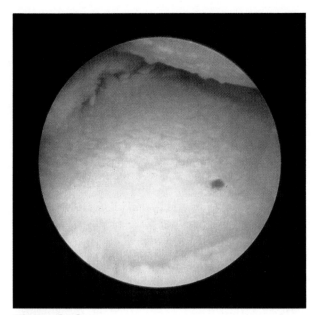

Figure 9–6
Fibrocartilaginous resurfacing of the medial tibial condyle as focal plaques.

some Type I collagen characteristic of fibrocartilage.[29] However, other investigators have found only Type II collagen typical of articular cartilage.[11]

Full-thickness loss of cartilage over an extensive area of bone is a severe problem. If multiple drill holes are made into the subchondral bone of rabbit models, repair tissue growing in from the holes must grow across the exposed bone surface.[69] Although the tissue is initially hyaline in appearance, it becomes fibrous with time and undergoes fibrillation.[69] A pathologic review of 32 intra-articular fractures revealed the repair tissue arising from the subchondral bone with only fibrous tissue bridging the clefts in the articular cartilage.[66] The articular chondrocytes did not significantly contribute to the repair response.[66]

Blunt trauma to the knee occurs frequently. The knee hitting the dashboard of an automobile receives high-energy injury to the articular cartilage. Using a drop tower device on human articular cartilage, the critical limit for maintenance of structural integrity of the articular cartilage was found to be a stress of 25 newtons per square millimeter.[87] Donahue subjected a canine patellar model to blunt trauma. He noted changes similar to osteoarthritis in the zone of calcified cartilage, consisting of cellular clones, vascular invasion, and a decrease in proteoglycans.[21] What is the mechanism linking blunt mechanical injury to the articular cartilage with biochemical changes? A four-fold increase in arachidonic acid, which is a precursor in prostaglandin synthesis, was observed in articular cartilage following blunt trauma. Mechanical trauma may damage the cell membrane, releasing arachidonic acid, which is converted to prostaglandin E. The prostaglandins result in the release of proteases that degrade the proteoglycan matrix of the articular cartilage, leading to cartilage destruction.[12]

The effect of repetitive impulse loading upon articular cartilage has been investigated. In a canine model subjected to repetitive blunt trauma, there was necrosis of the cartilage and underlying bone, which gradually separated from the remainder of the condyle.[86] Radin and associates found that repetitive impulse loading for 40 minutes per day for only 1 week in the rabbit resulted in a 20 per cent increase in subchondral bone stiffness and a 17 per cent decrease in proteoglycans.[81] These results were interpreted as a primary bone response from trauma with secondary early metabolic changes in the articular cartilage. Repetitive overuse plus peak overloading in a rabbit model damaged the superficial articular cartilage layer, exposing the underlying matrix with cell cluster formation, fibrillation, and subchondral bone thickening.[19] These results suggest a simultaneous injury to the articular cartilage and bone, possibly leading to late osteoarthritis. An increase in prostaglandin E was found, suggesting a role of prostaglandins in articular cartilage damage.

REHABILITATION

The optimal postoperative rehabilitation for healing of articular cartilage defects must be considered in terms of associated soft tissue and bony injuries. What is the effect of immobilization, motion, or compression applied across the articular surface? Articular cartilage nutrition depends upon diffusion of nutrients from the synovial fluid, and joint motion appears to aid in this process. Nine weeks' immobilization of the rabbit knee resulted in a fixed contracture that required ten times more torque to extend the knee than in controls.[110] Although there is no change in collagen in the periarticular soft tissues, there is loss of water and proteoglycans. Immobilization does not stimulate new collagen synthesis. Motion of the joint inhibits contractures by stimulating proteoglycan synthesis, ordering new collagen fibers, and preventing anomalous cross-linking in the matrix. In the human knee, immobilization results in progressive contractures of the periarticular tissues and intra-articular adhesions.[24] There is degeneration of the articular cartilage in areas of direct articular cartilage contact. Thompson and associates found that compression across an immobilized rabbit knee for 4 weeks resulted in a gradual decrease in articular cartilage thickness, chondrocyte cloning, and changes in collagen architecture.[106] Forced immobilization of a rabbit knee for 6 days or longer resulted in varying necrosis, from a superficial lesion to a full-thickness defect of the articular cartilage of the two opposing joint surfaces.[94] Three days was the shortest period of compression that resulted in a demonstrable articular cartilage lesion. Immobilization interfered with the diffusion of nutrients from the synovial fluid into the articular cartilage.

Therefore, postoperative rehabilitation is important for optimal healing of cartilage lesions. A full-thickness articular cartilage defect in the rat will resurface with fibrocartilage in the presence of active joint function but fill only with fibrous tissue if immobilized.[47,48] Full-thickness articular cartilage defects subjected to little shearing stress displayed greater healing than those subjected to high stresses.[100] However, in a canine model, no difference in healing was observed of a full-thickness articular cartilage defect between normally utilized, exercised, or immobilized joints.[27] Continuous passive motion in the immature or adult rabbit resulted in the formation of hyaline cartilage in 52 per cent of the full-thickness defects, compared with 9 per cent of those with active use or 8 per cent of immobilized knees at 3 weeks.[96,97] Healing of the defects was observed in 44 per cent of the continuous passive motion group compared with 5 per cent of those with active motion or 3 per cent in the immobilized group.[97] At 1 year, the superiority of the repair tissue in the continuous passive motion group was maintained.[95] Therefore, postoperative immobilization should be avoided whenever feasible in clinical management.

Perichondrial grafts have been studied as a technique to improve resurfacing of articular defects.[23,74,76] Engkvist and associates placed perichondrial grafts into the glenoid cavity of rabbits that were denuded of articular cartilage.[23] Newly formed articular cartilage was found on the bone up to 8 weeks after grafting. Perichondrial grafting to the metacarpophalangeal joint of a human patient was successful in forming cartilage at 4-month follow-up.[23] In a canine model, rib perichondrial grafts were capable of resurfacing the patella with cartilage, but by 1 year the cartilage demonstrated degenerative changes.[22] Rib perichondrial resurfacing of a rabbit patella resulted in satisfactory repair in 50 per cent of the animals at 6 to 12 weeks.[2] A mixture of Type I and Type II collagen was found in the regenerated cartilage. In a rabbit, tibial periosteal grafts transplanted to the femoral condyle resulted in regeneration of hyaline-like cartilage originating from the periosteal graft.[91–93] Immobilization of the joint was found to inhibit chondrogenesis.[92] Continuous passive motion has been demonstrated to aid chondrogenesis. Free intra-articular periosteal grafts in a rabbit model formed cartilage in 8 per cent of the immobilized group, compared with 56 per cent in the continuous passive motion group.[75]

In an adolescent rabbit model, tibial perichondrial grafting to a 3.5-millimeter osteochondral defect in the femoral condyle was studied.[76] At 5 weeks, hyaline cartilage was the predominant tissue in 10 per cent of the defects treated by immobilization, inter-

mittent active motion, or controls, compared with 70 per cent of the knees treated by continuous passive motion. Bonding of the new cartilage to the surrounding tissues was better in the continuous passive motion group. A 1-year follow-up of perichondrial grafting to full-thickness defects in the patellar groove of adolescent rabbits revealed degenerative changes in 57 per cent of the group that was immobilized, 73 per cent of those with active intermittent motion, and 22 per cent in the group with continuous passive motion.[74] The percentage of hyaline cartilage in the three groups was not significantly different.

DIAGNOSIS OF ARTICULAR CARTILAGE INJURY

Diagnosis of articular cartilage injury requires a high index of suspicion by the attending physician. In purely cartilaginous injuries, the radiographs may be normal. Arthroscopy is an excellent but invasive technique for evaluation of the articular surface of many joints. Interpretation of the arthroscopic findings can be difficult. Lesions ranging from softening of the articular surface to full-thickness defects may be present, but determination of the time of occurrence of the injury and of the ultimate prognosis is difficult. Double-contrast arthrography can be used to evaluate large defects but is inadequate for definition of small defects. Magnetic resonance imaging (MRI) of articular cartilage is a noninvasive technique that may be helpful in some cases. Using a 0.35 tesla coil, 18 of 22 known hyaline cartilage defects were identified in cadaver knees.[109] Seven of nine 1-millimeter-deep lesions were identified, compared with 15 of 16 3-millimeter lesions. MRI was insensitive for the detection of surface and texture changes without loss of cartilage substance, compared with arthroscopy. Using a 1.5 tesla coil and T2-weighted images, only defects of 3 millimeters or larger could be consistently identified.[33] In both series, an intra-articular effusion or saline improved contrast for detection of cartilage lesions. Therefore, arthroscopy remains the most accurate technique in evaluating articular cartilage pathology.

Clinical Management

Management of articular cartilage injury may be nonoperative or operative. Nonoperative management consists of patient education, physical therapy, and anti-inflammatory medication. Education to avoid repetitive impact loading and overstress of the damaged joint is essential. Muscle rehabilitation will provide dynamic stabilizers to assist in control of joint instability. Reduction of body weight will decrease the forces acting across weight-bearing joints. Nonsteroidal anti-inflammatory agents will aid in the relief of symptoms. These agents, such as salicylates, may inhibit degradative enzyme release by interfering with prostaglandin release.[12] In a prospective study of recurrent patellar dislocations treated either with or without aspirin, 3 gm/day, 13 of 17 showed no chondromalacia at subsequent surgical exploration.[13] This compares with 2 of 23 controls.

CHONDRAL AND OSTEOCHONDRAL FRACTURES

Traumatic injuries to the joint may result in fractures involving both bone and articular cartilage. Experimental studies of the healing response of chondral injuries have resulted in recommendations concerning management. Trauma to the articular surface may create three stages short of complete fracture: (1) splitting at the tidemark; (2) depression of cartilage into bone; and (3) fissuring of cartilage and bone in a vertical plane.[50] Repair of full-thickness defects occurred by granulation tissue from the subchondral bone with fibrocartilage but not hyaline cartilage formation.[50] In the human, large defects fill with fibrous tissue or fibrocartilage whereas small defects heal with fibrocartilage or hyaline cartilage.[8] The healing of lesions varying from a pure cartilaginous separation to a large osteochondral fracture with differing degrees of detachment was studied in

an immature rabbit model.[104] A partially detached large osteochondral fragment was found eventually to fuse with the condyle. A small osteochondral fragment might fuse with the condyle, remain as a pedunculated fragment, or become a loose body. Complete detachment of a large fragment resulted in a defect in the condyle that healed by hyaline cartilage but with deformity. An intracartilaginous cleavage healed by enchondral ossification.[70] The fixation of osteochondral fractures affects healing.[1] If the fragments were adequately fixed, the fragments united; if the fragments were not rigidly fixed, nonunion occurred with necrosis of the bone but viable cartilage. The quality of reduction of an intra-articular fracture in rabbits affects the results.[70] Inadequate reduction or adequate reduction without compression of a cartilage fracture resulted in healing only by fibrocartilage.[70] Fractures that were reduced and fixed with compression healed by hyaline cartilage.

Chondral and osteochondral fractures are easily confused with other injuries such as meniscal tears. The diagnosis of an articular cartilage fracture is often missed; in one report, an incorrect diagnosis was made in 27 of 34 patients.[35,71] Osteochondral fractures are most frequently a disorder of adolescence whereas partial-thickness chondral injuries occur most commonly in the fourth decade (Fig. 9–7).[44] Full-thickness chondral separations into or to subchondral bone have vertical margins, whereas

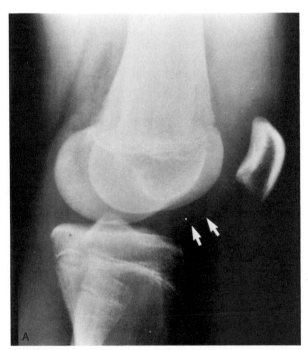
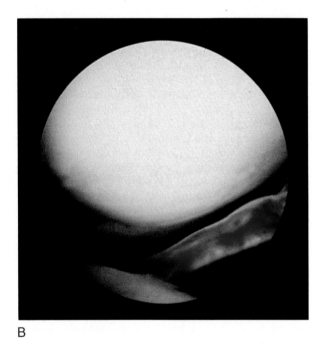

A   B

Figure 9–7

A, Lateral radiograph and B, arthroscopic appearance of lateral femoral condyle of an acute osteochondral fracture. The fracture fragment lies in the lower right position of the photograph. (Reproduced with permission from Rand JA: Arthroscopy and articular cartilage defects. In Whipple TL [ed]: Arthroscopic Surgery Desk Reference. Redondo Beach, CA, Bobit Publishing Company, 1986, pp 129–144.)

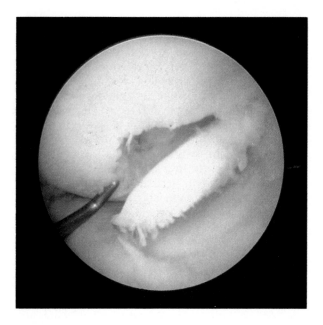
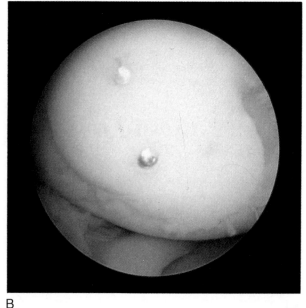

B

Figure 9–8

  A, Arthroscopic appearance of osteochondritis dissecans on the weight-bearing surface of the medial femoral condyle. *B*, After reduction and fixation with Kirschner wires.

partial-thickness chondral injuries have oblique margins.[44] Chondral injuries are most frequently located on the medial femoral condyle.[31,36,44] Removal of the chondral fragment is the recommended management, but recovery is often prolonged.[36] Patients with chondral fractures usually have normal radiographs, no effusion, and are skeletally mature. In contrast, patients with osteochondral fractures have a calcified fragment, a defect on radiographs, and hemarthrosis and are adolescents.

  Osteochondral fractures involving the weight-bearing surface of the joint may result from direct injury or by indirect means by combined rotatory and compression forces.[46,67] A vertically applied force results in compaction; a tangentially applied force results in shear; and traction by a ligament results in avulsion.[73] Exogenous shearing forces create peripheral chondral fractures whereas endogenous forces result in centrally located lesions.[46] A rotatory stress in an adolescent followed by a snap and an acute hemarthrosis often indicates an osteochondral fracture.[46,59,73] Radiographically, the displaced fragment appears as a thin calcified fragment or may not be visible (Fig. 9–7).[59,73] A frequent location of the fracture is the weight-bearing surface of the lateral femoral condyle.[59] Separation of the fracture in the adult is between the calcified and uncalcified cartilage, leaving the osteochondral junction undisturbed, whereas in the adolescent the fracture occurs through the subchondral bone because of little calcified cartilage.[46] Early treatment of osteochondral fractures, especially if they involve the weight-bearing surface, should be by replacement of large frag-

ments.[46,59,73] Fixation may be by pins (Fig. 9–8), Smillie nails, bone pegs (Fig. 9–9), or screws (Fig. 9–10), but the internal fixation device must not protrude into the joint where it may impinge on the opposing joint surface.[41,46,73] Small or comminuted fragments may be excised and the bed trephined.[73] If the diagnosis is delayed, the fragments undergo resorptive changes, proliferation of new cartilage, and degenerative cartilage calcification. Therefore, fragments diagnosed after a prolonged time from injury are not suitable for replacement and will need to be excised.[67]

  Another etiology of osteochondral fractures is related to patellar dislocations (Fig. 9–11).[25,64,71,90,105] The mechanism of injury is impingement of the medial patellar facet against the lateral femoral condyle upon reduction of the dislocation, leading to an osteochondral fracture of either the patella or femur.[64] Another rare mechanism of injury is a direct blow to the dislocated patella, striking the lateral femoral condyle.[25] Osteochondral fractures complicate 5 per cent of all acute dislocations of the patella.[90] Treatment of the fractures is similar to other osteochondral fractures, combined with treatment of the patellar dislocation.[90,105]

ARTICULAR CARTILAGE LESIONS

  Localized lesions of articular cartilage damage are frequently encountered during arthroscopy. The etiology of these lesions and their management remain

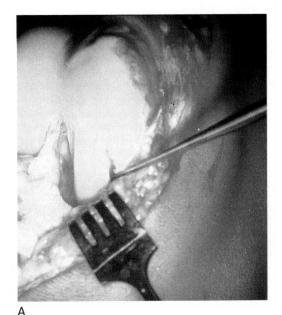

A

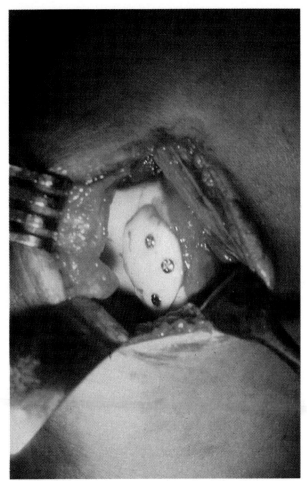

Figure 9–10
Osteochondral fracture of the lateral femoral condyle
fixed with screws. The screws *must* be removed prior to
beginning motion to prevent damage to the opposing tibial
articular cartilage.

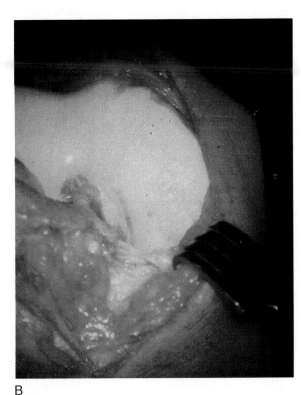

B

Figure 9–9
A, Acute osteochondral fracture of the medial
femoral condyle. *B,* After reduction and fixation
with bone pegs.

controversial. Outerbridge classified changes in the
articular cartilage into four grades: (1) softening and
swelling of articular cartilage (Figs. 9–12 and 9–13);
(2) fragmentation and fissuring in an area 0.5 inch or

less (Fig. 9–14); (3) fragmentation and fissuring in
an area greater than 0.5 inch in diameter; and (4)
erosion of cartilage exposing bone (Fig. 9–15).[78]

The etiology of articular cartilage damage can be
trauma, nutritional, or errors of metabolism.[99] Sud-
den direct or indirect trauma is the etiology of osteochondral fractures. The role of repetitive minor
trauma is controversial. Certainly malalignment with
chronic repetitive overload will lead to articular cartilage degeneration. However, the exact role of repetitive heavy use of the joint is unclear. In a study of
coxarthrosis, the incidence (3 per cent) was the
same in laborers or white collar workers.[51] The importance of joint motion for articular cartilage nutrition has been emphasized. Immobilization will lead
to articular cartilage degeneration. Disorders that
lead to deposition of abnormal substances in the articular cartilage, such as ochronosis or pseudogout,

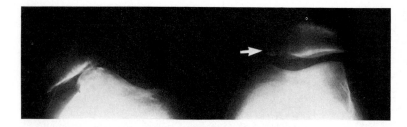

Figure 9–11

Merchant radiograph of a dislocated right patella and an old dislocation of the left patella with an old osteochondral fracture (arrow). (Reproduced with permission from Rand JA: Arthroscopy and articular cartilage defects. *In* Whipple TL [ed]: Arthroscopic Surgery Desk Reference. Redondo Beach, CA, Bobit Publishing Company, 1986, pp 129–144.)

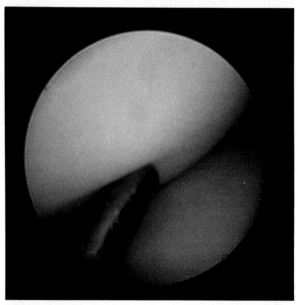

Figure 9–12

Softening articular cartilage of the medial femoral condyle, with the intact surface demonstrated by a blunt probe.

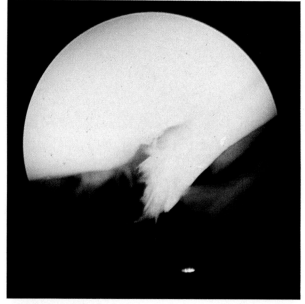

Figure 9–14

A localized area of cartilage fragmentation on the medial facet of the patella.

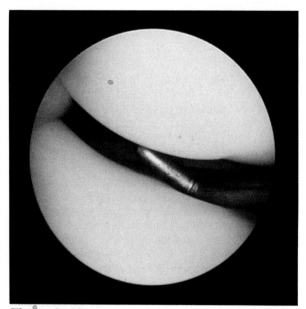

Figure 9–13

Blister formation on a medial femoral condyle, with intact articular cartilage.

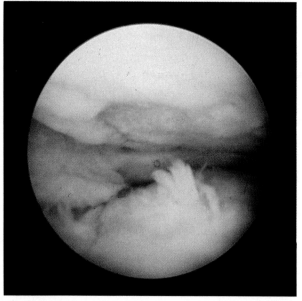

Figure 9–15

Extensive erosion with exposure of bone on the medial femoral and tibial condyle 10 years after medial meniscectomy.

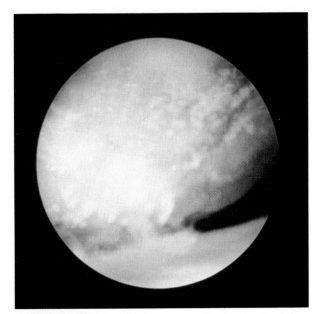

Figure 9–16
Calcium pyrophosphate deposition and secondary osteo-arthritis of the medial femoral condyle.

will lead to articular cartilage degeneration (Fig. 9–16). Synovial disorders, such as rheumatoid arthritis, may directly attack and destroy articular cartilage (Fig. 9–17). Recurrent hemorrhage into the joint may result in articular cartilage injury (Fig. 9–18). The relationship between meniscal tears and articular cartilage lesions has been controversial. In a review of 350 knees, no relationship was identified between articular cartilage lesions and either meniscal or anterior cruciate tears.[9]

Arthroscopic evaluation of articular cartilage should begin with a complete examination of the joint to look for associated lesions, such as meniscal or ligament tears. Utilization of a blunt probe will allow palpation of areas of articular cartilage softening before a defect in the articular surface exists (Fig. 9–19). Palpation of areas of fibrillation will allow definition of the depth of injury and its extent. The use of carbon dioxide as a medium for arthroscopy may help define areas of early articular cartilage damage (Fig. 9–20).

Treatment of localized articular cartilage lesions should be conservative. Trimming of articular cartilage flaps that were loose and unstable was beneficial in 40 of 50 knees followed from 18 to 36 months.[38] Of 275 knees treated by debridement of a variety of articular cartilage lesions, 76 per cent had satisfactory results at 26 months' follow-up.[99] However, the more advanced the articular cartilage lesion, the less likely is the patient to benefit from the procedure. Gentle debridement with basket forceps and a side-cutting low-speed shaver is the best technique. Some of the beneficial effects of debridement may well result from the lavage of the knee during the arthroscopic procedure with elimination of loose fragments of articular cartilage, resulting in a decrease in synovitis.[77] In patellar lesions, the results of localized shaving and debridement diminish with the extent of pathology and duration of follow-up.[77] It is undesirable to be so aggressive in debridement of a partial-thickness lesion that a full-thickness defect is created. A pathologic review of patellas treated by open debridement to bone found no significant repair arising from articular chondrocytes and only fibrous pannus from the subchondral bone.[65]

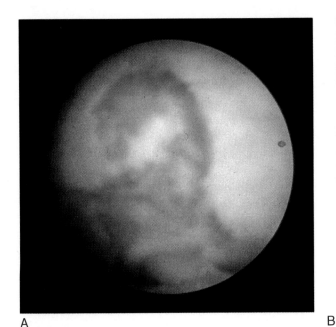

A

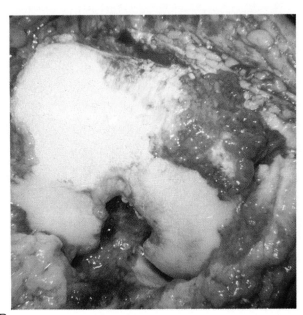

B

Figure 9–17
A synovial pannus from rheumatoid arthritis on the medial femoral condyle. *A*, Arthroscopic appearance. *B*, At arthrotomy.

IATROGENIC CARTILAGE INJURY

Although arthroscopy has allowed improved diagnosis and management of many intra-articular problems, its widespread usage has led to articular cartilage injury in some patients. The arthroscopist must always remain aware of the relationship between surgical instruments and the articular cartilage to prevent iatrogenic injury (Fig. 9–21).

The physiologic effects of the irrigation medium upon articular cartilage during arthroscopy may be important, especially in prolonged operative procedures. An in vitro comparison of saline, Ringer's lactate, and Ham F12 solution was performed. Incorporation of $^{35}SO_4$ as an indicator of proteoglycan synthesis was greater in those specimens exposed to Ringer's lactate compared with saline.[84] Since saline is highly electrically conductive, water as an irrigating medium has been recommended for electrosurgery during arthroscopy. In the rabbit, irrigation with water resulted in damage to the superficial zone of articular cartilage.[58] The control knees irrigated with saline showed some increase in cellular fragility, but no overt damage. Therefore, an isotonic solution that is physiologic, such as Ringer's lactate, appears to have fewer detrimental effects on articular cartilage than do nonisotonic solutions.

High-energy devices are being utilized in arthroscopic surgery. Both electrosurgery and lasers have been designed for arthroscopic use. Electrosurgery was initially devised for lateral retinacular release but is now being utilized for meniscal resection.[68] Inadvertent contact between the cutting electrode and articular cartilage will result in necrosis, the extent of which depends upon the power utilized (Fig. 9–22).[83] The lowest possible power setting should be selected. The application of a laser to meniscal tissue results in a limited depth of meniscal injury.[108] However, accurate aiming of the laser beam to avoid injury to the articular surface can be difficult.

DEBRIDEMENT

Debridement procedures may be accomplished by open or arthroscopic means. Loose bodies may be removed, degenerative menisci excised, fibrillated articular cartilage shaved, osteophytes removed, and exposed bone drilled or abraded.

Open debridement operations were popularized by Pridie and Magnuson.[39,40,53] Magnuson reported that fibrocartilage would resurface areas of bone that were debrided.[53] A series of 62 knees followed for a mean of 6.5 years following Pridie's debridement operation with drilling of exposed bone revealed objectively satisfactory results in 64 per cent.[39] Fibrocartilage was documented at the site of drilling of eburnated bone. Contraindications to this procedure were angular deformity and instability.[40] Indications for debridement included patellofemoral arthritis, nonrheumatoid panarthritis, and focal osteoarthritis. Arthroscopic techniques of debridement (abrasion arthroplasty) of exposed bone have demonstrated resurfacing of the bone by fibrocartilage (Fig. 9–23).[42,43] Seventy-four of ninety-five patients noted

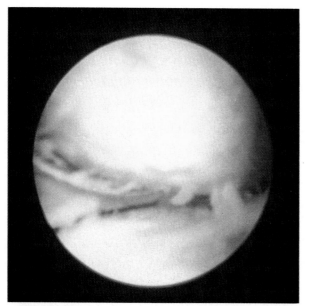

Figure 9–18
Degeneration of the articular cartilage of the medial compartment of the knee in a 9 year old boy with hemophilia.

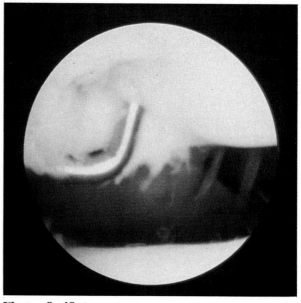

Figure 9–19
Use of the probe to evaluate the extent of cartilage damage of an osteochondral fracture of the patella.

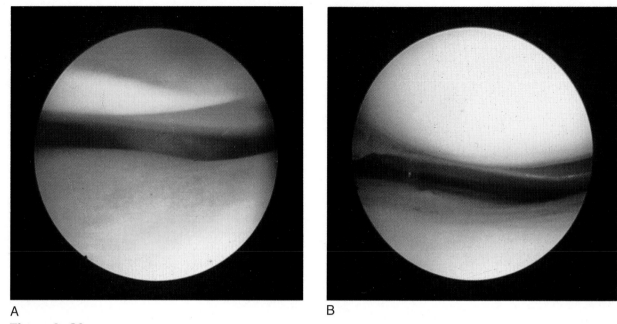

A   B

Figure 9–20
Arthroscopic appearance of a normal medial compartment of a knee in *A*, saline and *B*, carbon dioxide.

symptomatic improvement 2 years after abrasion, and 50 per cent had an increase in the joint space.[43] Integrity of the fibrocartilage has been found for up to 6 years. Eighty per cent of 55 knees followed for an average of 22 months showed symptomatic improvement following abrasion arthroplasty.[10] Friedman and associates reported 110 patients treated by arthroscopic debridement for degenerative joint dis-

ease; 73 had abrasion of exposed bone. They found improvement in 60 per cent; 34 per cent were unchanged; and 6 per cent were worse.[26] Arthroscopic debridement of meniscal tears and osteophytes in 69 knees followed for 1 year revealed satisfactory results in 84 per cent.[101]

Whether or not arthroscopic debridement will provide satisfactory long-term results will require fur-

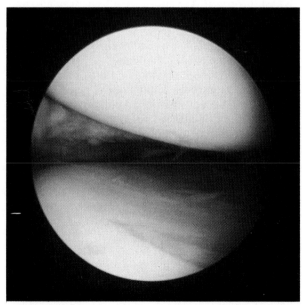

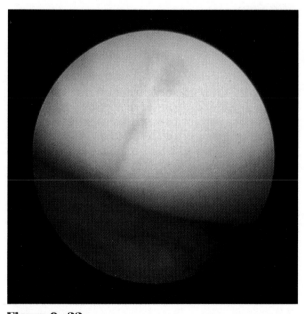

Figure 9–21
Superficial cartilage lacerations of the medial tibial condyle following arthroscopic medial meniscectomy.

Figure 9–22
Lacerated articular cartilage of the medial tibial condyle from an electrocautery used for arthroscopic meniscectomy.

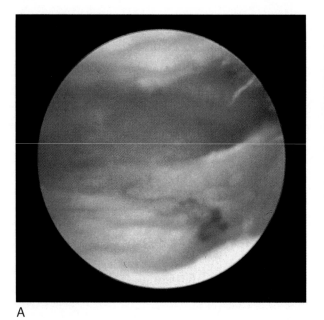

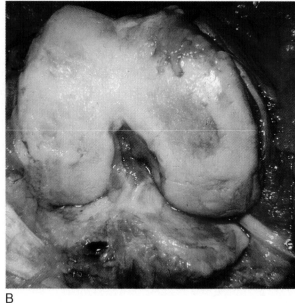

A   B

Figure 9–23

A, Abrasion of the medial tibial condyle to expose a vascular supply. *B*, Regenerative fibrocartilage of the lateral femoral condyle 1 year after abrasion arthroplasty.

ther investigation. Simple shaving of fibrillated articular cartilage cannot be expected to induce a healing response in the cartilage and should be limited to areas with unstable articular cartilage. Since the majority of individuals with symptomatic osteoarthritis of the knee have angular deformities and many have secondary instability, selection of patients for debridement procedures must be carefully performed.

CARTILAGE TRANSPLANTATION

Cartilage transplantation with autografts or allografts to localized defects has provided variable results. The problems associated with cartilage grafting include a suitable donor, attachment of the graft to the recipient site, graft incongruity, prolonged nonweight bearing, and fixation of the graft that will allow early knee motion to provide nutrition to the graft and prevent articular cartilage degeneration.

Clinical studies of autografts using the patella or nonweight-bearing portion of the femoral condyles have revealed short-term satisfactory results (Fig. 9–24).[16,88] In an immature rabbit model, thin allografts were resorbed, medium-thickness grafts were preserved, and thick cartilage grafts with bone underwent necrosis.[98] In a canine model, a comparison of allografts and autografts revealed slight degeneration but preservation of viable articular cartilage in both groups. There was more synovitis and a low-

grade inflammatory response in the allograft group.[89] In immature rabbits, allografts of intact cartilage and intact growth plate grafts produce better results than in ungrafted defects or in arthritic joints.[3] Cultured chondrocytes were able to provide some repair of defects in arthritic knees.[3] Small-segment allografts have been unpredictable. Twenty-six of 78 small-fragment grafts have required further surgery and 17 of 37 bipolar grafts for unicompartmental osteoarthritis have required revision surgery.[32] The best results achieved were 75 per cent satisfactory at 3.8 years in patients with a traumatic injury.[61] Subsequent revascularization has been felt to be the major cause of failure.

Four of twelve allografts for tibial plateau fractures failed at 2 years.[52] Survival of articular cartilage following allograft transplantation appears to be limited, with fibrocartilage replacing most of the hyaline cartilage.[5,32] A pathologic study of 42 failed allografts revealed fragmented donor cartilage with degenerative changes but some areas of viable cartilage.[45] Fibrous pannus was found to be growing over and resorbing articular cartilage in 17 of the 44 specimens.[45] Numerous microfractures in the cancellous bone portion of the graft were identified, with replacement of donor by host bone.[45] Czitrom and associates concluded that allografts (1) are best for traumatic injuries; (2) are poorly suited for primary osteoarthritis, osteonecrosis, osteochondritis dissecans, or patients taking steroids; (3) are best performed on a single side of the joint; and (4) must have malalignment corrected prior to allograft transplantation.[18]

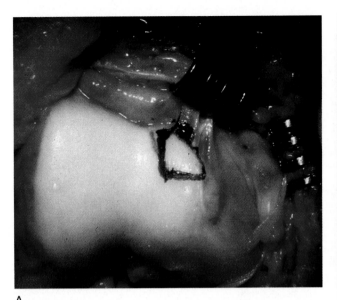

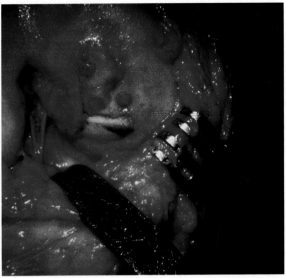

A   B

Figure 9–24

A, Donor site of articular cartilage from the medial trochlea of the femur. *B,* Recipient site on the medial femoral condyle. The adjacent area of osteochondritis dissecans has been fixed with bone pegs. (Reproduced with permission from Rand JA: Arthroscopy and articular cartilage defects. *In* Whipple TL [ed]: Arthroscopic Surgery Desk Reference. Redondo Beach, CA, Bobit Publishing Company, 1986, pp 129–144.)

Summary

In summary, articular cartilage injuries are frequent but difficult problems to manage. Arthroscopy has improved the diagnosis of articular cartilage lesions at early stages in the disease process. The ability to diagnose articular cartilage lesions and to remove articular cartilage mechanically should not induce the surgeon to perform excessively aggressive treatment. The limited repair capabilities of articular cartilage must be considered and iatrogenic damage must be avoided.

References

1. Aichroth P: Osteochondral fractures and their relationship to osteochondritis dissecans of the knee. J Bone Joint Surg 53B:448–454, 1971.
2. Amiel D, Coutts RD, Abel M, Stewart W, Harwood F, Akeson WH: Rib perichondral grafts for the repair of full-thickness articular cartilage defects. J Bone Joint Surg 67A:911–920, 1985.
3. Aston JE, Bentley G: Repair of articular surfaces by allografts of articular and growth plate cartilage. J Bone Joint Surg 68B:29–34, 1986.
4. Bollet AJ, Nance JL: Biochemical findings in normal and osteoarthritic articular cartilage. II. Chondroitin sulfate concentration and chain length, water and ash content. J Clin Invest 45(7):1170–1177, 1966.
5. Brown KLB, Cruess RL: Bone and cartilage transplantation in orthopaedic surgery. J Bone Joint Surg 64A:270–277, 1982.
6. Buckwalter JA: Articular cartilage. AAOS Instructional Course Lectures, 32:349–370, 1983.
7. Calandruccio RA, Gilmer WS: Proliferation, regeneration, and repair of articular cartilage of immature animals. J Bone Joint Surg 44A(3):431–455, 1962.
8. Campbell CJ: The healing of cartilage defects. Clin Orthop 64:45–63, 1969.
9. Casscells S: The torn meniscus, the torn anterior cruciate ligament, and their relationship to degenerative joint disease. Arthroscopy 1:28–32, 1985.
10. Chandler EJ: Abrasion arthroplasty of the knee. *In* Whipple TL (ed): Arthroscopic Surgery Desk Reference. Redondo Beach, CA, Bobit Publishing Company, 1986, pp 145–153.
11. Cheung MS, Cottrell WH, Stephenson K, Nimni ME: In vitro collagen biosynthesis in healing and normal rabbit articular cartilage. J Bone Joint Surg 60A:1076–1081, 1978.

12. Chrisman OD, Ladenbauer-Bellis IM, Panjabi M, Goeltz S: The relationship of mechanical trauma and the early biochemical reactions of osteoarthritic cartilage. Clin Orthop 161:275–284, 1981.

13. Chrisman OD, Snook GA, Wilson TC: The protective effect of aspirin against degeneration of human articular cartilage. Clin Orthop 84:193–196, 1972.

14. Collins DH: The Pathology of Articular and Spinal Diseases. London, Edward Arnold and Company, 1949.

15. Convery FR, Akeson WH, Keowin GH: The repair of large osteochondral defects. Clin Orthop 82:253–262, 1972.

16. Crova M, Gallinaro P, Lorenzi GL: Osteochondral transplant in the surgical treatment of osteochondrosis of the knee. Ital J Orthop Traumatol 3:273–281, 1977.

17. Curtiss PM: Cartilage damage in septic arthritis. Clin Orthop 64:87–90, 1969.

18. Czitrom AA, Langer F, McKee N, Gross AE: Bone and cartilage allotransplantation. Clin Orthop 208:141–145, 1986.

19. Dekel S, Weissman SL: Joint changes after overuse and peak loading of rabbit knees. *In vivo.* Acta Orthop Scand 49:519–528, 1978.

20. DePalma AF, McKeever CD, Subin DK: Process of repair of articular cartilage demonstrated by histology and autoradiography with tritiated thymidine. Clin Orthop 48:229–242, 1966.

21. Donohue JM, Buss D, Oegema TR, Thompson RC: The effects of indirect blunt trauma on adult canine articular cartilage. J Bone Joint Surg 65A(7):948–957, 1983.

22. Engkvist O: Reconstruction of patellar articular cartilage with free autologous perichondrial grafts. Scand J Plast Reconstr Surg 13:361–369, 1979.

23. Engkvist O, Johansson SH, Ohlsen L, Skoog J: Reconstruction of articular cartilage using autologous perichondrial grafts. Scand J Plast Reconstr Surg 9:203–206, 1975.

24. Enneking WF, Horowitz M: The intra-articular effects of immobilization on the human knee. J Bone Joint Surg 54A(5):973–985, 1972.

25. Frandsen PA, Kristenson H: Osteochondral fracture associated with dislocation of the patella: Another mechanism of injury. J Trauma 19:195–197, 1979.

26. Friedman MJ, Berasi CC, Fox JM, DelPizzo W, Snyder SJ, Ferkel RD: Preliminary results with abrasion arthroplasty in the osteoarthritic knee. Clin Orthop 182:200–205, 1984.

27. Frost GE: Cartilage healing and regeneration. J South Afr Vet Assoc 50:181–187, 1979.

28. Fuller JA, Ghadially FN: Ultrastructural observations on surgically produced partial thickness defects in articular cartilage. Clin Orthop 86:193–205, 1972.

29. Furukawa T, Eyre DR, Koide S, Glimcher MJ: Biochemical studies on repair of cartilage resurfacing in experimental defects in the rabbit knee. J Bone Joint Surg 62A:79–89, 1980.

30. Ghadially FN, Thomas I, Oryschak AF, Lalonde JM: Long-term results of superficial defects in articular cartilage: A scanning electron-microscopic study. J Pathol 121:213–217, 1977.

31. Gilley JS, Gelman MI, Edson DM, Metcalf RW: Chondral fractures of the knee. Radiology, 138:51–54, 1981.

32. Gross AE, McKee NH, Prutzker KPH, Langer F: Reconstruction of skeletal deficits at the knee. Clin Orthop 174:96–106, 1983.

33. Gylys-Morin VM, Hajek PC, Sartoris DJ, Resnick D: Articular cartilage defects: Detectability in cadaver knees with MRI. Am J Roentgenol 148:1153–1157, 1987.

34. Hall FM, Wyshak G: Thickness of articular cartilage in the normal knee. J Bone Joint Surg 62A:408–413, 1980.

35. Hermans GPN: Endogenous osteochondral fractures in the knee joint. Acta Orthop Belg 48:495–503, 1982.

36. Hopkinson WJ, Mitchell WA, Curl WW: Chondral fractures of the knee. Am J Sports Med 13:309–312, 1985.

37. Hoshino A, Wallace WA: Impact-absorbing properties of the human knee. J Bone Joint Surg 69B:807–811, 1987.

38. Hubbard MJS: Arthroscopic surgery for chondral flaps in the knee. J Bone Joint Surg 69B:794–796, 1987.

39. Insall JN: Intra-articular surgery for degenerative arthritis of the knee. J Bone Joint Surg 49(2):211–228, 1967.

40. Insall J: The Pridie debridement operation for osteoarthritis of the knee. Clin Orthop 101:61–67, 1974.

41. Johnson EW, McLeod TL: Osteochondral fragments of the distal end of the femur fixed with bone pegs. J Bone Joint Surg 59A:677–679, 1977.

42. Johnson LL: Healing of human articular cartilage: An arthroscopic view. Orthop Trans 5:400, 1981.

43. Johnson LL: Arthroscopic abrasion arthroplasty. Historical and pathologic perspectives: Present status. Arthroscopy 2:54–69, 1986.

44. Johnson-Nurse C, Dandy DJ: Fracture-separation of articular cartilage in the adult knee. J Bone Joint Surg 67B:42–43, 1985.

45. Kandel RA, Gross AE, Gand A, McDermott AGP, Langer F, Pritzker KPH: Histopathology of failed osteochondral shell allografts. Clin Orthop 197:103–110, 1985.

46. Kennedy JC, Grainger RW, McGraw RW: Osteochondral fractures of the femoral condyle. J Bone Joint Surg 48B:436–440, 1966.

47. Kettunen K: Effect of articular function on the repair of a full thickness defect of the joint cartilage. Ann Chir Gynecol Fenn 52(4):627–642, 1963.

48. Kettunen K, Rokkanen P: The repair of a full thickness articular defect. Ann Chir Gynecol Fenn 62:166–168, 1963.

49. Key JA: Experimental arthritis: The changes in joints produced by creating defects in the articular cartilage. J Bone Joint Surg 13:725–739, 1931.

50. Landells JW: The reactions of injured human articular cartilage. J Bone Joint Surg 39B(3):548–562, 1957.

51. Lindburg H, Danielson LG: The relation between labor and coxarthrosis. Clin Orthop 191:159–161, 1984.

52. Locht RC, Gross AE, Langer F: Late osteochondral allograft resurfacing for tibial plateau fractures. J Bone Joint Surg 66:328–335, 1984.

53. Magnuson PB: Technique of debridement of the knee joint for arthritis. Surg Clin North Am 24:249–266, 1946.

54. Mankin HJ: The articular cartilages: A review. AAOS Instructional Course Lectures 19:204–224, 1970.

55. Mankin HJ: The reaction of articular cartilgae to injury and osteoarthritis. (First of two parts.) N Engl J Med 291:1285–1291, 1974.

56. Mankin HJ: The reaction of articular cartilage to injury and osteoarthritis. (Second of two parts.) N Engl J Med 291:1335–1340, 1974.

57. Mankin HJ: Current concepts review. The response of articular cartilage to mechanical injury. J Bone Joint Surg 64A:460–465. 1982.

58. Marshall GJ, Snyder SJ, Kirchen ME, Sweeney JR: The effect of water, surgical saline, and buffered saline on synovial and articular cartilage of rabbit knees. Presented at 31st Annual Meeting, Orthopaedic Research Society, 1985, p 295.

59. Matthewson MM, Dandy DJ: Osteochondral fractures of the lateral femoral condyle. J Bone Joint Surg 60B:199–202, 1978.

60. McCutchen GW: Boundary lubrication by synovial fluid: Demonstration and possible osmotic explanation. Fed Proc 25:1061–1068, 1966.

61. McDermott ACP, Langer F, Pritzker KPH, Gross AE: Fresh small fragment osteochondral allografts. Clin Orthop 197:96–102, 1985.

62. Meachim G: The effect of scarification on articular cartilage in the rabbit. J Bone Joint Surg 45B:150–161, 1963.

63. Meachim G, Roberts C: Repair of the joint surface from subarticular tissue in the rabbit knee. J Anat 109:317–327, 1971.

64. Milgram JW: Tangential osteochondral fracture of the patella. J Bone Joint Surg 25:271–280, 1943.

65. Milgram JW: Injury to articular cartilage joint surfaces. Chondral injury produced by patellar shaving. Clin Orthop 192:168–173, 1985.

66. Milgram JW: Injury to articular cartilage joint surfaces: II. Displaced fractures of underlying bone. Clin Orthop 206:236–247, 1986.

67. Milgram JW, Rogers LF, Miller JW: Osteochondral fractures: Mechanisms of injury and fate of fragments. Am J Roentgenol 130:651–658, 1978.

68. Miller GK, Dickason JM, Fox JM, Blazina ME, Del Pizzo W, Friedman MJ, Snyder SJ: The use of electrocautery for arthroscopic subcutaneous lateral release. Orthopedics 5:309–314, 1982.

69. Mitchell N, Shepard N: The resurfacing of adult rabbit articular cartilage by multiple perforations through the subchondral bone. J Bone Joint Surg 58A(2):230–233, 1976.

70. Mitchell N, Shepard N: Healing of articular cartilage in intra-articular fractures in rabbits. J Bone Joint Surg 62A(4):628–634, 1980.

71. Morscher E: Cartilage-bone lesions of the knee joint following injury. Reconstr Surg Traumat 12:2–26, 1971.

72. Mow VC, Lai WM: Some surface characteristics of articular cartilage—I. A scanning electron microscopy study and a theoretical model for the dynamic interaction of synovial fluid and articular cartilage. J Biomech 7:449–456, 1974.

73. O'Donoghue DM: Chondral and osteochondral factures. J Trauma 6:469–481, 1966.

74. O'Driscoll SW, Keeley FW, Salter RB: Durability of regenerated articular cartilage produced by free autogenous periosteal grafts in major full thickness defects in joint surfaces under the influence of continuous passive motion. J Bone Joint Surg 70A:595–606, 1988.

75. O'Driscoll SW, Salter RB: The induction of neochondrogenesis in free intra-articular periosteal autografts under the influence of continuous passive motion. J Bone Joint Surg 66A:1248–1257, 1984.

76. O'Driscoll SW, Salter RB: The repair of major osteochondral defects in joint surfaces by neochondrogenesis with autogenous osteoperiosteal grafts stimulated by continuous passive motion. Clin Orthop 208:131–140, 1986.

77. Ogilvie-Harris DJ, Jackson RW: The arthroscopic treatment of chondromalacia patellae. J Bone Joint Surg 66B:660–665, 1984.

78. Outerbridge RE: The etiology of chondromalacia patellae. J Bone Joint Surg 43B:752–757, 1961.

79. Paget J: Healing of cartilage. Clin Orthop 64:7–8, 1969.

80. Radin EL: The physiology and degeneration of joints. Sem Arthritis Rheum 2(3):245–257, 1972–1973.

81. Radin EL, Ehrlich MG, Chernack R, Abernathy P, Paul IL, Rose RM: Effect of repetitive impulse loading on the knee joint of rabbits. Clin Orthop 131:288–293, 1978.

82. Radin EL, Paul IL: A consolidated concept of joint lubrication. J Bone Joint Surg 54A:607–616, 1972.

83. Rand JA, Gaffey TA: Effect of electrocautery on fresh human articular cartilage. Arthroscopy 1:242–246, 1985.
84. Reagan BF, McInerny VK, Treadwell BV, Zarins B, Mankin HJ: Irrigating solutions for arthroscopy. J Bone Joint Surg 65A:629–631, 1983.
85. Redfern P: On the healing of wounds in articular cartilage. Clin Orthop 64:4–6, 1969.
86. Rehbein F: Die Entschung der Osteochondritis dissecans. Arch Dtsch Chir 265:69–114, 1950.
87. Repo RV, Finlay JB: Survival of articular cartilage after controlled impact. J Bone Joint Surg 59A(8):1068–1076, 1977.
88. Rinaldi E: Treatment of osteochondritis dissecans and cartilaginous fractures of the knee by osteo-cartilaginous autografts. Ital J Orthop Traumatol 8:17–21, 1982.
89. Rodrigo JJ, Sakovich L, Travis C, Smith G: Osteocartilaginous allografts as compared with autografts in the treatment of knee joint osteocartilaginous defects in dogs. Clin Orthop 134:342–349, 1978.
90. Rorabeck CM, Bobechko WP: Acute dislocation of the patella with osteochondral fracture. J Bone Joint Surg 58B:237–240, 1976.
91. Rubak JM: Reconstruction of articular cartilage defects with free periosteal grafts: An experimental study. Acta Orthop Scand 53:175–180, 1982.
92. Rubak JM, Poussa M, Ritsilä V: Chondrogenesis in repair of articular cartilage defects by free periosteal grafts in rabbits. Acta Orthop Scand 53:181–186, 1982.
93. Rubak JM, Poussa M, Ritsilä V: Effects of joint motion on the repair of articular cartilage with free periosteal grafts. Acta Orthop Scand 53:187–191, 1982.
94. Salter RB: The effects of continuous compression on living articular cartilage. J Bone Joint Surg 42A(1):31–49, 1960.
95. Salter RB, Minster RR, Clemonds N, Bogach E, Bell RS: Continuous passive motion and the repair of full thickness articular cartilage defects—A one year follow-up. Orthop Trans 6:266–267, 1982.
96. Salter RB, Simmonds DF, Malcolm BW, Rumble EJ, MacMichael D: The effects of continuous passive motion on the healing of articular cartilage defects—An experimental investigation in rabbits (abstr). J Bone Joint Surg 57A(4):570–571, 1975.
97. Salter RB, Simmonds DF, Malcolm BW, Rumble EJ, MacMichael D, Clements ND: The biological effect of continuous passive motion on the healing of full thickness defects in articular cartilage. J Bone Joint Surg 62A:1232–1251, 1980.
98. Sengupta S, Lumpur K: The fate of transplants of articular cartilage in the rabbit. J Bone Joint Surg 56B(1):167–177, 1974.
99. Shahriaree H: Chondromalacia. In Whipple TL (ed): Arthroscopic Surgery Desk Reference. Redondo Beach, CA, Bobit Publishing Company, 1986, pp 115–127.
100. Sokoloff L: Repair of Articular Cartilage in the Biology of Degenerative Joint Disease. Chicago, University of Chicago Press, 1969, pp 61–69.
101. Sprague NF: Arthroscopic debridement for degenerative knee joint disease. Clin Orthop 160:118–123, 1981.
102. Stockwell RA: Cell density, cell size, and cartilage thickness in adult mammalian articular cartilage. J Anat 108:584–585, 1971.
103. Stockwell RA, Meachim G: The chondrocytes. In Freeman MAR (ed): Adult Articular Cartilage. New York, Grune and Stratton, 1973.
104. Tallqvist G: The reaction to mechanical trauma in growing articular cartilage. Acta Orthop Scand (Suppl) 53:1–112, 1962.
105. Thije JHT, Firma AJ: Patellar dislocation and osteochondral fractures. Netherl J Surg 38:150–154, 1986.
106. Thompson RC, Bassett CA: Histological observations on experimentally induced degeneration of articular cartilage. J Bone Joint Surg 52A:435–443, 1970.
107. Weiss C, Rosenberg L, Helfet AJ: An ultrastructural study of normal young adult human articular cartilage. J Bone Joint Surg 50A:663–671, 1968.
108. Whipple TL, Caspari RB, Meyers JF: Laser energy in arthroscopic meniscectomy. Orthopedics 6:1165–1169, 1983.
109. Wojtys E, Wilson M, Buckwalter K, Braunstein E, Martel W: Magnetic resonance imaging of knee hyaline cartilage and intra-articular pathology. Am J Sports Med 15:455–463, 1987.
110. Woo SL-Y, Matthews JV, Akeson WH, Amiel D, Covery FR: Connective tissue response to immobility. Arthritis Rheum 18(3):257–264, 1975.

10

Ronald P. Karzel, Jr.
Marc J. Friedman

Arthroscopic Diagnosis and Treatment of Cruciate and Collateral Ligament Injuries

As both skill in arthroscopy and interest in reconstruction of the cruciate ligaments have increased, arthroscopic reconstruction of the cruciate ligaments has become increasingly common. In this chapter, we discuss potential advantages of arthroscopic reconstruction, principles of arthroscopic repair and reconstruction of the anterior cruciate ligament and posterior cruciate ligament, with emphasis on the technical factors leading to a good result. Finally, we briefly review literature results regarding such reconstructions and point to possible future developments.

ADVANTAGES OF ARTHROSCOPIC RECONSTRUCTION

The most obvious advantage of arthroscopic cruciate repair is the avoidance of an arthrotomy. This results in smaller incisions and improved cosmesis. More important, the avoidance of a large parapatellar incision probably reduces the risk of patellofemoral tracking abnormalities, reduces the chance of injury to the infrapatellar branches of the saphenous nerve, minimizes articular cartilage desiccation, allows earlier range of motion, and may diminish the loss of proprioceptive feedback that has been noted after arthrotomy.[11] Arthroscopy allows excellent visualization for diagnosis and treatment of associated intra-articular pathology, such as meniscal tears. The intercondylar attachment site on the femur can be better visualized by arthroscopy than by arthrot-

omy. Finally, the graft can be directly visualized arthroscopically as the knee is moved through a range of motion to check for impingement of the graft on the anterior femur.

No published studies have directly compared complications and results of ligament reconstructions performed arthroscopically versus those performed by arthrotomy. Gillquist and Odensten studied arthroscopic reconstruction versus "mini-arthrotomy" and concluded that arthroscopic reconstruction was less desirable.[20] They found no difference in rehabilitation time or postoperative quadriceps strength between the groups. The arthroscopically treated group had an average operation time 30 minutes longer than the mini-arthrotomy group. In addition, these investigators felt that notchplasty could not be performed as reliably through the arthroscope. They concluded that the mini-arthrotomy technique was preferable. However, the mini-arthrotomy they performed was only 4 cm long and did not involve dislocation of the patella. The mini-arthrotomy technique allowed an open notchplasty but still relied extensively on arthroscopic technique for graft placement. Also, the drawbacks of longer operative time and incomplete notchplasty would be expected to improve with experience. Their study, therefore, should not be viewed as indicating that a more traditional arthrotomy technique is preferable to arthroscopic technique. Their study does re-emphasize, however, the importance of careful, thorough notchplasty, whether performed open or arthroscopically.

DECISION MAKING IN LIGAMENT RECONSTRUCTION

An 18 year old high school football player comes to the sports clinic with a history of a knee injury 48 hours previously. He sustained a noncontact rotary stress to the knee when cutting on a pass play. He felt a pop at the time of injury, followed by knee pain and immediate swelling. Examination discloses a large effusion, 2+ Lachman and anterior drawer examinations with a soft end point, and medial joint line tenderness; a pivot shift cannot be elicited because of pain. The parents and athlete state the patient has received several scholarship offers to play football, and want to give him "a normal knee again." At this point, the physician faces several important decisions regarding further patient management.

Studies have pointed out the high likelihood of a complete anterior cruciate ligament (ACL) tear with this injury, as well as associated meniscal injury.[8,10,19,25,29] Therefore, some clinicians advocate examination under anesthesia and arthroscopy in the acute situation for "high-risk" patients.[9] This approach makes the most sense if one believes that acutely repairing an ACL will be a viable procedure, negating the possibility of future reconstruction. Unfortunately, clinical and biomechanical studies generally have shown that a repaired ACL without augmentation does not have significantly improved function over those not repaired, and that the results deteriorate over time.[12,14,33] We believe that acute repair is a useful procedure only when the ligament avulses bone from the attachment site. This is a rare injury and can often be seen on radiography. Thus, acute arthroscopy cannot be justified solely on the basis of the possibility of acute repair.

Likewise, some recommend arthroscopy in the acute situation to rule out associated pathology, especially to the menisci. With the increasing accuracy of the magnetic resonance imaging (MRI) scan in diagnosing meniscal injuries, especially the more common medial ones, there may be less justification for this approach.

Our current procedure is to perform an examination under anesthesia and arthroscopy during the acute situation for only those patients who are candidates for ACL reconstruction. This decision must be individualized for each patient after complete discussion with the patient about the potential risks and benefits of the operation, as well as the extensive rehabilitation that will be required. Factors to consider include age, degree of initial instability, athletic ability, willingness to alter lifestyle, motivation to undergo rehabilitation, and social circumstances such as ability to remain out of work during rehabilitation. The presence of severe laxity with loss of secondary restraints (Grade 3 or 4 instability) likely will lead to functional instability in the future and favors immediate ACL reconstruction to prevent further injury to the knee.[35] Likewise, an associated collateral ligament injury, a peripheral meniscal tear that may be repaired, or coexisting patellofemoral instability may be indications for ACL reconstruction. In an athletic young patient such as the one presented here, the decision will probably be made to reconstruct the ACL. In this case, we then would proceed to examination under anesthesia and arthroscopy without any further diagnostic testing. At that time, meniscal pathology can be identified and repaired or resected. Following the correction of associated knee pathology, the ACL is primarily reconstructed.

In older, less active patients with less instability, a decision may be reached that the knee should not be primarily reconstructed. In these cases, we do not advocate immediate arthroscopy. Rather, the knee is aspirated to remove the hemarthrosis. This improves patient comfort and allows for a more accurate knee examination. The patient then undergoes an MRI scan to rule out associated pathology. If meniscal pathology is discovered, arthroscopy is performed for correction of the problem. If the tear appears to be peripheral on the MRI scan, further discussion of the possible need for ACL reconstruction may be held again with the patient prior to surgery. If the MRI scan is negative for associated pathology, no arthroscopy of the knee is performed acutely. A rehabilitation program is begun and the patient is followed. Those who continue to have significant disabling instability then may be candidates for delayed ACL reconstruction.

Most of our ACL reconstructions are performed arthroscopically. Contraindications to arthroscopic reconstruction are extensive capsular disruption (evidenced by varus or valgus instability with the knee in full extension) or complete knee dislocation. If the capsular structures are torn, extravasation of irrigation fluid may occur and lead to neurovascular compromise. Also, if ligament damage is extensive, open arthrotomy will be required to repair all the involved structures. If a dislocation has occurred, an arteriogram must be obtained to rule out arterial injury prior to any surgical procedure. Although a concomitant anterior cruciate and medial collateral ligament injury may be an indication for ACL reconstruction, this may still be performed arthroscopically if capsular damage is not extensive. An arthroscopic ACL reconstruction is done and the MCL injury is treated with bracing. Shelbourne has shown that patients treated this way have results better than do those treated by reconstruction of both the ACL and MCL.[40]

A controversial aspect of ACL reconstructions is the choice of graft material to use in reconstruction. Patellar tendon has been shown biomechanically to have the greatest strength. In addition, the bone on either end of the graft allows for rapid and strong incorporation into the bone tunnels.[31] By using screw fixation of the graft, early motion and weight bearing are possible. This graft has become our procedure of choice in the young male athlete, in larger patients, and in situations of chronic instability with loss of secondary restraints. The patellar tendon graft has the disadvantages of requiring a larger scar, the possible complication of patellar tendon rupture, and possibly increasing patellofemoral problems postoperatively. A patellar tendon allograft minimizes these problems but has potential problems of disease transmission and possible immune reaction.

In an attempt to reduce some of these problems, the pes tendons may be used as a graft. The semitendinosus, or semitendinosus and gracilis tendon, is most commonly used. Since the semitendinosus is somewhat variable in size, we prefer to use both tendons. By forming a double loop of both tendons, a graft of substantial size is obtained. This graft may be obtained through a smaller incision than the patellar tendon graft. Studies have shown no loss of knee flexion power after use of this graft,[28] and the knee extensor mechanism is not disturbed. Graft harvesting is quicker, and thus tourniquet time is reduced. We currently use this graft in lighter patients, especially women, in whom cosmesis is important and the functional demands on the knee will be less. This graft is excellent in the acute situation in which secondary restraints are still present. The main disadvantages are the weaker graft strength and less secure fixation of the graft to the bone initially.

Prosthetic ligament replacement is appealing, since most of the disadvantages of the autogenous reconstructions are eliminated. Rehabilitation can be rapid due to the high graft strength. Unfortunately, current prosthetic ligament materials have been disappointing, with a high incidence of breakage and synovitis compared with autogenous grafts.[21] They are presently indicated only in a revision of a previously failed autogenous graft.

Another controversial aspect of ACL reconstruction is the role of extra-articular versus intra-articular stabilization. Studies have shown deterioration in results over time if only extra-articular reconstruction is used.[24] However, some researchers state that extra-articular reconstruction must be performed to "protect" the intra-articular repair during maturation of the graft.[1,4] Others believe that the ACL is the "central pivot" for knee rotation and that intra-articular ACL reconstruction alone is sufficient.[37] We favor the latter approach. In addition to the standard tests for ACL stability, the presence of anterolateral rotatory instability is sought by tests such as the pivot shift. If significant anterolateral rotatory instability is present, this favors primary ACL reconstruction. No initial extra-articular augmentation is needed. By following technical principles such as careful isometric positioning, stresses on the graft are reduced. Extra-articular reconstruction is reserved for those rare cases with significant global instability.

POSTERIOR CRUCIATE LIGAMENT RECONSTRUCTION

In contrast to the situation with the ACL, long-term studies of the effect of surgical reconstruction of the posterior cruciate ligament (PCL) have been inconsistent. Although some studies suggest good results after surgical treatment,[3,6] a large recent study of PCL injuries demonstrated the benefit of conservative therapy alone.[7,34] We presently repair the PCL primarily only in those with bone avulsions (a rare injury), or in those with extensive initial instability, such as associated posterolateral rotatory instability, as evidenced by the reverse pivot shift test. Otherwise, the patient is rehabilitated with an emphasis on quadriceps strengthening. Surgical reconstruction is reserved for those with persistent instability despite rehabilitation.

APPLIED ANATOMY AND TECHNICAL ASPECTS OF ACL RECONSTRUCTION

Basic arthroscopic anatomy is well described in this text in Chapter 5. In this section, we review several important technical aspects of anterior cruciate ligament reconstruction in general and discuss the pertinent anatomy.

Diagnosis and Repair of Associated Pathology

An important first step in ligament reconstruction is examination of the knee under anesthesia. In addition to determining the status of the ACL by the anterior drawer and Lachman and pivot shift tests, the collateral ligaments and secondary restraints should also be evaluated carefully. Comparison should be made between the injured knee and the normal knee. If there is significant gross ligamentous instability and probable rupture of the posterior capsule, as evidenced by opening of the knee joint to varus or valgus stresses in full extension, then arthroscopy may be contraindicated to prevent fluid extravasation into the soft tissues and possible neurovascular compromise. In such a case, arthrotomy will be required for repair of the multiple ligamentous instabilities. Otherwise, the next step is arthroscopic evaluation of the joint.

The arthroscope is inserted through the anterolateral portal and a systematic examination of the knee joint is performed. The cruciate ligaments are evaluated (Fig. 10–1). An anterior cruciate ligament that appears grossly intact should be checked carefully for signs of hemorrhage or laxity to palpation indicative of a partial ACL tear. If a complete tear is noted, the location most commonly will be a midsubstance interstitial tear (Fig. 10–2). Such tears commonly

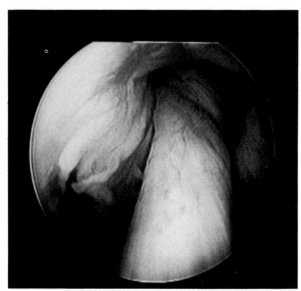

Figure 10–1
Arthroscopic view of normal anterior and posterior cruciate ligaments.

occur after a hyperextension injury, which ruptures the ACL at the apex of the notch. These tears usually are not amenable to repair. In more chronic ACL injury, the proximally ruptured ACL may heal to the posterior cruciate ligament (Fig. 10–3). Since the ACL heals in a nonanatomic position, these patients will have increased laxity to examination, but an end point often will be noted. When making a decision about whether to reconstruct the ACL, these patients should be treated using the same criteria as for those patients with an absent ACL.

Tears of the posterior cruciate ligament also may be evaluated arthroscopically. Visualization of the PCL usually requires passage of the arthroscope through the intercondylar notch with the scope in the anterolateral portal. As the arthroscope is slowly withdrawn out of the notch, the PCL is visualized (Fig. 10–4). A posteromedial portal also may be created to allow better visualization. A recent concept is that injuries of the knee in hyperflexion may lead to interstitial tears of the PCL, which again are not repairable. A less common mechanism of PCL injury is posterior subluxation with direct trauma to the anterior tibia. Patients with this injury may be more likely to sustain a periosteal avulsion of the PCL (Fig. 10–5).[13] Avulsion-type tears have good potential for healing if repaired acutely.

There is a high incidence of associated pathology with anterior cruciate ligament tears.[32] The knee, therefore, should be carefully evaluated, both by inspection and also by using a probe to detect any subtle abnormalities. Particular attention should be directed to the posterior horn of the medial meniscus, which is frequently injured. By passing the arthroscope through the intercondylar notch, the pos-

teromedial corner of the knee, including the posterior horn of the meniscus, and any loose bodies can be visualized. The technique of arthroscopic repair or resection of menisci has been well discussed elsewhere in the text and will not be repeated here. Two technical factors that should be noted are that we prefer to do the initial arthroscopic procedures with the tourniquet deflated. This allows greater working time for later cruciate reconstruction and minimizes the chance of postoperative quadriceps weakness. If a peripherally torn meniscus is noted, sutures should be placed at this time. If the pes tendons will be used for the ACL reconstruction, they should be harvested *before* repairing the medial meniscus. However, these sutures should not be tied until after the anterior cruciate ligament reconstruction is completed.

Notchplasty

An adequate notchplasty is an important part of any ACL reconstruction, whether performed arthroscopically or open. After performance of an adequate notchplasty, the posterior and superior intercondylar aspect of the lateral femoral condyle should be well visualized and inspected with a probe. If adequate visualization is not obtained, it will be impossible to place the graft accurately in an isometric position. Notchplasty also must be adequate to prevent impingement of the graft on the anterolateral aspect of the notch as the knee is extended. Such impingement may prevent loss of full knee extension and may also lead to graft rupture. A narrowed intercondylar notch is especially common in patients with chronic ACL

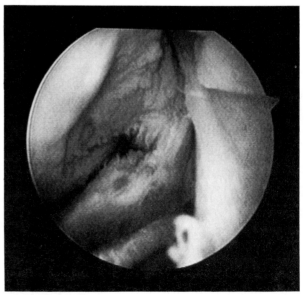

Figure 10–2
Intersubstance tear of anterior cruciate ligament (ACL).

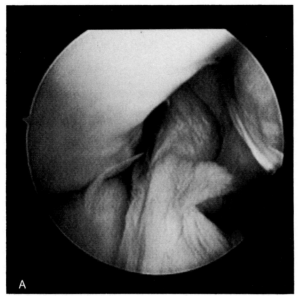

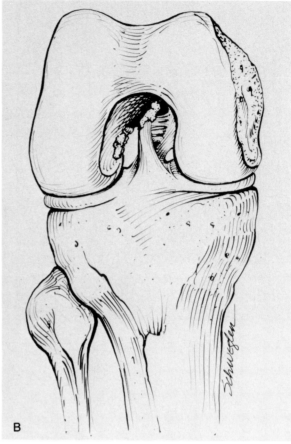

Figure 10-3

  A, An ACL that had previously been torn from the femoral origin and has now reattached itself to the posterior cruciate ligament (PCL) (shown schematically in *B*).

deficiency who have developed osteophytes in the notch.

Notchplasty is performed through the anteromedial portal with the arthroscope positioned in the anterolateral portal. A quarter-inch curved osteotome is inserted first to remove the major portion of the osteophytes from the anterior and superior aspects of the notch. Further bone is removed with an abrasion chondroplasty burr and curettes. Although the anterior aspect of the notch usually can be adequately widened with the knee in approximately 40° of flexion, flexion of the knee to 90° will allow decompression of the posterior and inferior aspects of the notch if necessary. Removal of hypertrophied synovial tissue from the notch also may be necessary to allow complete visualization. However, an attempt is made to leave as much vascularized tissue as possible to allow for possible vascularization of the graft tissue. After notchplasty and debridement have been performed, it should be possible to palpate the posterior aspect of the condyle with a nerve hook. Sometimes a shelf of bone within the notch may falsely mimic the posterior aspect of the notch; palpation

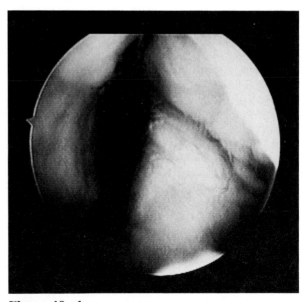

Figure 10-4

  The PCL as visualized with the arthroscope inserted into the notch.

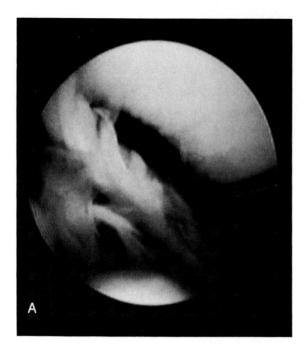

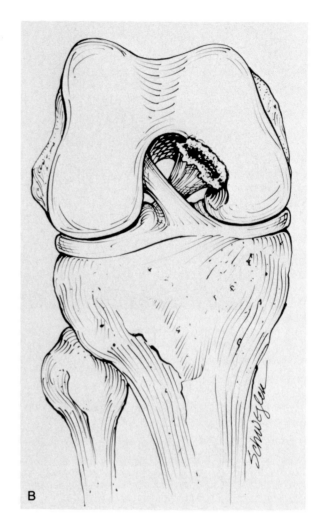

Figure 10–5
Avulsion of the PCL from the femoral origin.

within the notch will reveal bone posterior to this shelf, and further notchplasty may then be performed.

Although Odensten and Gillquist state that a 21-mm notchplasty should be performed in all patients,[32] probably no single notch size is optimal. Rather, sufficient bone should be removed to allow visualization of the posterior aspect of the condyle. After the graft has been placed within the knee, but prior to fixing it in place, the knee should be moved through a full range of flexion and extension while checking for impingement of the graft arthroscopically. Further bone can then be removed as needed to allow graft clearance.

Isometry

Anatomic studies have shown that the normal anterior cruciate ligament fibers form an oval ligament, with different portions of the ligament becoming taut during different degrees of knee flexion and extension. Anatomic studies have described a separate anteromedial bundle that becomes tight as the knee is flexed, and a posterolateral bundle that becomes tight as the knee is extended.[2, 18] In more recent study, investigators were unable to find any separation of the anterior cruciate ligament into discrete bundles.[32] However, the investigators did note that the ligament was twisted through 90° as the knee was flexed from full extension to 90° of flexion, resulting in changes in the lengths and the tensions of different fibers in the ligament as the flexion angle changed. They concluded that there were different functional portions of the anterior cruciate ligament. They found that the most central fibers appeared to have less than 2 mm of excursion through the range of flexion and extension.[32] Unfortunately, present ligament substitutes have fibers that are in a primarily parallel orientation and thus are unable to duplicate the more complex anatomy of the anterior cruciate ligament.[30]

Although the normal mechanics of the ACL, therefore, cannot be duplicated by a graft, reconstruction procedures attempt to place the graft in such a way that changes in the length of the fibers during a range of motion of the knee are minimal. When the ligament graft is placed in such a position, it is considered to be "isometric." The isometricity of the graft substitute is determined by the placement of the drill holes in the femur and tibia. Some investigators recommend locating these isometric points in the direct center of the previous femoral and tibial attachments of the anterior cruciate ligament.[42] Clancy, however, has popularized the concept of eccentric placement of the Kirschner wire guide pins.[31] He recommends placing the tibial guide pin slightly anterior and medial to the tibial insertion of the ACL and the femoral guide pin slightly posterior and superior to the actual origin of the ACL. When the guide pins are then overdrilled using the 10-mm reamer, the margins of the tunnel will coincide with the anatomic center of the ligament. The ACL fibers normally blend slightly with the anterior horn of the lateral meniscus as they insert on the tibia. The anterior horn thus can be used as an anatomic landmark to help find the tibial insertion of the ACL. The femoral origin is located on the lateral wall of the intercondylar notch posteriorly and several millimeters inferior to the superior apex of the notch.

The importance of proper hole placement for achieving isometry in the graft has been emphasized in two recent studies.[32,36] Investigators found that over-the-top placement of the femur was not isometric and produced large changes in graft length and tension as the knee was flexed and extended. The modified over-the-top technique using a femoral bone trough did reproduce normal ACL isometry with minimal graft length and tension changes with knee motion.[36] Anteriorly placed femoral drill holes consistently caused large increases in the length of the graft with knee flexion and a marked loss of tension within the graft as the knee was fully extended. Likewise, when a simulated ACL tear was created and repaired by stapling the proximal end of the ACL stump as far posteriorly as possible, the same loss of tension with extension was noted. Positioning the femoral drill hole posteriorly and superiorly on the lateral femoral condyle allowed for isometric graft placement, but this depended on proper tibial hole position. The best position for the tibial drill hole was found to be anteromedial to the ACL tibial insertion.[36] Too anterior an insertion site on the tibia resulted in lengthening of the graft during knee flexion, whereas too posterior an insertion site resulted in significant shortening of the graft during knee flexion.[32] Placing the tibial hole slightly too far anteriorly was less detrimental than placing the hole posterior to the attachment site.

Clinically, the isometry of the drill holes should be checked prior to insertion of the graft. After guidewires have been passed through the femur and tibia into the desired location intra-articularly, the femoral guide pin is removed. A suture passer is passed from within the joint out through the lateral femoral condyle. A #2 Tevdek suture is placed in the suture passer, which is then pulled back through the femoral condyle intra-articularly. The tibial guide pin is removed, and the suture passer is again passed from external to intra-articular. Using a grasping instrument through the arthroscopic portal, the previously placed intra-articular suture is then passed through the loop in the suture passer, and the passer is pulled out through the tibial tunnel. The femoral end of the suture is clamped and held securely against the lateral edge of the femoral condyle. An isometric testing gauge is passed over the sutures emerging from the tibia and firmly seated in the tibial drill hole (Fig. 10–6). The suture is tightened with the gauge to the desired tension and the spring mechanism is then released. The knee is moved from full extension to 90° of flexion, and the excursion of the suture from the gauge is measured. If isometric placement has been achieved, the excursion should be less than 2 mm and tension should remain constant. If the excursion is more than 2 mm or large changes in tension occur, the placement of the guide pins should be changed and isometry measured again. If the graft is noted to be nonisometric after the larger drill holes have been made, this may be due to the graft being too far anterior on the femur. In this case it is usually necessary to salvage the graft by resorting to an over-the-top position on the femur.

Osseous Tunnel Preparation

After the presumed isometric points have been identified on the tibia and femur, attention must be directed to proper positioning of the tunnels through the bone. Divergence of the femoral and tibial tunnels, in which there is a large angle between the direction of the femoral and tibial tunnels as the knee passes through a range of motion, should be avoided. An acute angle between the graft and the articular surface on the femoral or tibial side is likely to result in wear of the graft as it passes over the sharp bone of the tunnel and may lead to graft failure, especially in prosthetic grafts. The sharpened edges of the tunnel also should be contoured, using either a rasp or abrader to lessen the chance of graft wear. Well-aligned, parallel tunnels will make passage of the graft through the intercondylar notch significantly easier. The size of the tunnel created depends on the graft material used. Generally, the smallest possible tunnel should be used to allow quick healing of the graft to the surrounding bone.[26] The graft can be accurately sized prior to insertion and the appropriate-sized drill holes created.

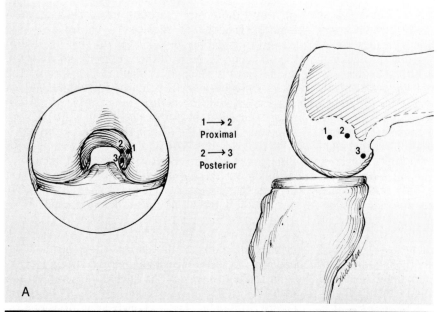

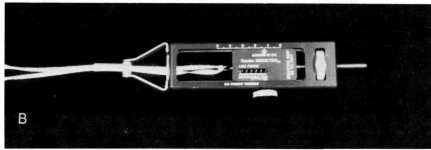

Figure 10–6

A, The attachment site for the ACL on the femur is shown by Point 2 on this diagram. Points 1 and 3 illustrate the effect of moving the holes in a proximal-distal versus an anterior-posterior direction. Point 1 is distal to Point 2; Point 3 is posterior to Point 2. *B,* A commercially available device for determining whether drill holes have been placed isometrically. The tension and excursion of the intra-articular suture can be measured directly.

Tensioning of the Graft

Graft tensioning is an important part of the procedure. If the graft is placed in too great tension, even a small increase in graft length may exceed the yield point of the graft and result in graft failure. In addition, revascularization may be inhibited.[39] On the other hand, if the graft is placed in insufficient tension, there will be a loss of joint stability. The proper amount of tensioning is measured using a commercially available device. Tension is usually adjusted with the knee in a slight amount of flexion. The precise angle for tensioning and the amount of tension applied will vary with the type of substitute used. Work in the cadaver suggests that tensioning approximately 3 to 5 pounds for the patellar tendon, 8 to 10 pounds for the semitendinosus, and 13 to 15 pounds for the iliotibial band gives the best results.[27] Tensioning of prothetic ligaments should be to the manufacturer's specifications. For Gore-Tex, the recommended tension is 20 pounds.

SPECIFIC TECHNIQUES OF ANTERIOR CRUCIATE LIGAMENT RECONSTRUCTION

The previous section discussed general technical aspects common to most types of arthroscopic anterior cruciate ligament reconstruction. In this section, three different techniques of ACL reconstruction are discussed. For each reconstruction, we will emphasize the specific technical aspects that differ from the general technical aspects discussed previously.

Semitendinosus/Gracilis Reconstruction

Standard arthroscopic evaluation, ligamentous examination, and correction of intra-articular pathology are performed arthroscopically as noted above. Likewise, an adequate notchplasty must be done as previously detailed.

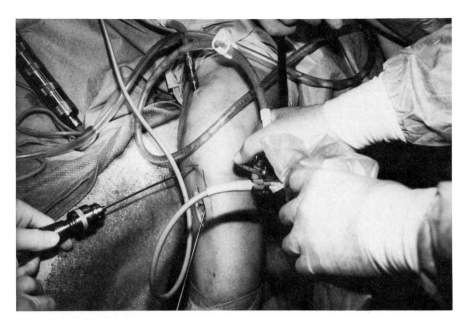

Figure 10–7
A guidewire is placed through an anteromedial puncture and positioned at the appropriate femoral origin site for the ACL reconstruction. (Reprinted from Friedman MJ: Arthroscopic semitendinosus [gracilis] reconstruction for anterior cruciate ligament deficiency. Techniques in Orthopaedics 2(4);74–80 with permission of Aspen Publishers, Inc. © January, 1988.)

A 3- to 5-cm longitudinal incision is made over the lateral femoral epicondylar region, extending proximally from the metaphyseal flair. The iliotibial band is split in line with this incision. The vastus lateralis is identified and retracted superiorly off the bone, using a Taylor retractor. Branches from the superior lateral circumflex vessels are routinely identified in the distal corner of the wound. These are coagulated, and the periosteum overlying the lateral femoral condyle is incised.

With the arthroscope in the anterolateral portal, a nerve hook is passed through the anteromedial portal and used to palpate the posterolateral aspect of the intercondylar notch. As explained previously, a point is chosen just anterior to the posterior femoral cortex at approximately the 11 o'clock position on the right knee or the 1 o'clock position on the left knee. A small defect is created in this area by means of a small curved curette or a small abrader. A smooth guidewire is then passed just above the anteromedial joint line through a small puncture wound separate from the previous arthroscopy portals (Fig. 10–7). A point of insertion is chosen so that the guidewire passes along the medial tibial plateau into the previously determined insertion point on the femur at an appropriate angle. With the guidewire in the hole, the knee is flexed to approximately 120°, and slight varus is applied to the knee (Fig. 10–8). The guidewire is then drilled from inside the knee, aiming for the lateral femoral epicondylar area. This technique allows precise anatomic placement of the drill pin into the femur. Alternatively, one of the commercial femoral drill guides may be used (Fig. 10–9). The drill guide, however, is less accurate on the femoral side. It is usually inserted with the stylus through the anteromedial portal and the arthroscope visualizing through the anterolateral portal.

After careful positioning of the tip of the guide in the appropriate position on the intercondylar notch, the lateral guide sleeve is positioned against the lateral femoral shaft in the region of the metaphyseal flair. The pin is then advanced from outside into the joint. An outrigger attachment with offset holes can be used to change the pin position slightly in an accurate manner (Fig. 10–10). When using the inside-out

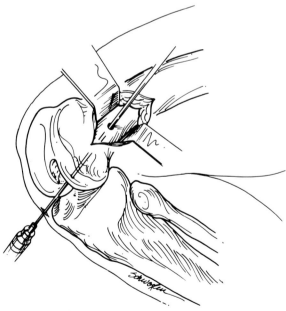

Figure 10–8
The knee is flexed 120°, a varus stress is applied, and the guidewire is drilled out through the lateral femur. (Reprinted from Friedman MJ: Arthroscopic semitendinosus [gracilis] reconstruction for anterior cruciate ligament deficiency. Techniques in Orthopaedics 2(4);74–80 with permission of Aspen Publishers, Inc. © January, 1988.)[15]

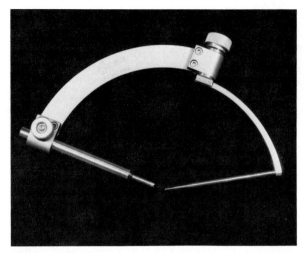

Figure 10-9
One of several commercially available drill guides used to drill the femoral hole from outside in.

technique, the drill is removed after the tip appears on the lateral side of the femur. The guidewire is then pulled back in a retrograde fashion until only the blunt tip of the guidewire is visible in the joint.

A vertical incision is then made 2 cm medial to the tibial tubercle, extending for approximately 7 cm. This incision allows access to the anteromedial sur-

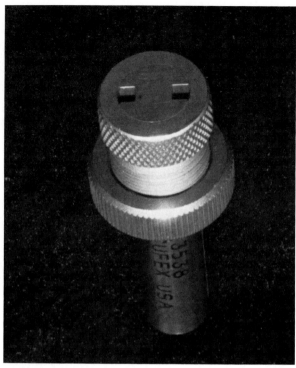

Figure 10-10
A commercially available device that allows for small, reproducible changes in guidewire position.

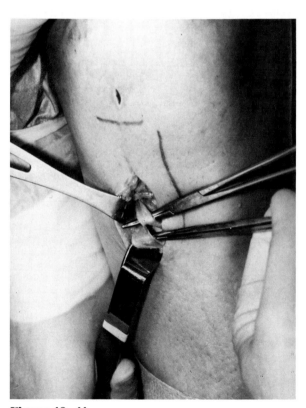

Figure 10-11
The semitendinosus and gracilis tendons are isolated with a right-angle clamp. (Reprinted from Friedman MJ: Arthroscopic semitendinosus [gracilis] reconstruction for anterior cruciate ligament deficiency. Techniques in Orthopaedics 2(4);74–80 with permission of Aspen Publishers, Inc. © January, 1988.)[15]

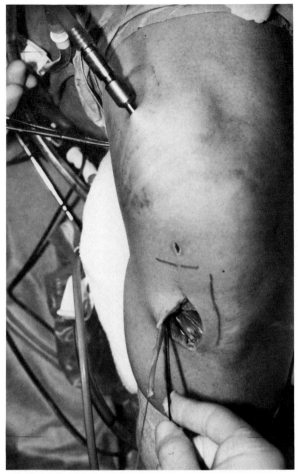

Figure 10–12
The pes tendons are mobilized with the tendon stripper. (Reprinted from Friedman MJ: Arthroscopic semitendinosus [gracilis] reconstruction for anterior cruciate ligament deficiency. Techniques in Orthopaedics 2(4):74–80 with permission of Aspen Publishers, Inc. © January, 1988.)[15]

face of the tibia for placement of the tibial drill hole and harvesting of the pes tendons. The semitendinosus and gracilis tendons are palpated. An incision is made in the deep fascia in a longitudinal direction lateral to the insertion of the tendons. The fascia is retracted and the tendons are localized with a right-angle clamp (Fig. 10–11). Metzenbaum scissors are used to release deep fascial attachments from the tendon in a distal-to-proximal direction. After all the fascial attachments have been released, the tendons are transsected sharply from the tibia. A tendon stripper is placed over the end of the graft, and while tension is maintained on the graft, the tendon stripper is advanced (Fig. 10–12). The thigh is palpated; the tendon stripper should pass up to midthigh level to insure that sufficient graft has been obtained. By gently twisting the tendon stripper at the proper level with graft tension maintained, the graft can be removed easily. Each tendon is harvested sequentially. Generally, a minimum of 30 cm is required to insure

enough length for the double-loop technique. A #1 Tevdek suture is applied in a whipstitch fashion to the ends of the semitendinosus and gracilis grafts. The combined graft is looped and placed in a sizing device to determine the appropriate drill size for the osseous tunnels (Fig. 10–13).

The arthroscope is then reinserted through the anterolateral portal. The tibial drill guide is inserted through the anteromedial portal and positioned anteromedial to the anatomic insertion of the ACL. The external sleeve of the drill guide is placed against the anterior tibial cortex. A guide pin is placed, using the drill guide. The pins are then removed and isometry is checked as noted in the previous section. The tendency is to drill the tibial hole too vertically and thus cause divergence of the femoral and tibial drill holes. A conscious effort should be made to keep the tibial drill hole relatively more horizontal.

After isometry of the drill holes has been checked and found to be appropriate, cannulated drills are drilled from outside in, beginning on the femoral side. Appropriate chamfering of the tunnel edges is performed. The reamers are used in sequential fashion to the size that had been measured directly from the graft. This is done to insure a snug fit in the femoral and tibial tunnels.

A Red Robinson catheter is then passed through the femoral tunnel, grasped with the pituitary inserted through the tibial tunnel, and then pulled out through the tibial tunnel (Fig. 10–14). Dectinel tape is passed through the end of the Red Robinson catheter, which is subsequently pulled back through the tibia and up through the femoral hole. The center of the graft formed by the semitendinosus and gracilis is looped through the loop of Dectinel tape. The tape is pulled back across the joint from the femur to the tibia until the double loops of semitendinosus and gracilis are visible on the tibial side. A 3.2-mm drill is then used to drill a hole slightly distal to the exit tunnel. A 6.5-mm AO cancellous screw with a plastic soft-tissue washer is used to fix the loop of tendon firmly to the tibia (Fig. 10–15). The strongest portion of this graft is toward the previous tendinous tibial end rather than the more proximal muscular end. Since the tibial tunnel is usually somewhat shorter than the femoral tunnel, the loop is placed around the tibial screw, thereby placing the strongest portion of the tendon within the joint. After fixation of the tibia has been accomplished, the knee is moved through a range of motion, under direct arthroscopic visualization, to insure that there is no impingement in the intercondylar notch area. If there is impingement, further notchplasty is performed. If no impingement is seen, the tendon ends protruding from the femoral tunnel are now tensioned. With proper tension applied and the knee held in a 20° posterior Lachman position, double staples are placed in the graft. The iliotibial band is then closed with interrupted Vicryl sutures, and routine skin closure is performed. The patient is placed in a knee brace.

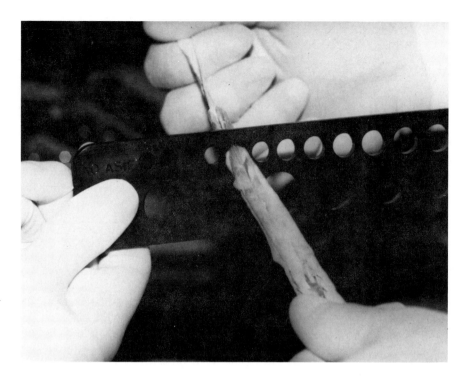

Figure 10–13
The combined pes tendon graft is sized.[15]

Immediately postoperatively, the patient is placed in a brace which allows 30° to 60° of motion for the first week. In the hospital, the patient is in a continuous passive motion machine. The patient returns at 1 week, and the wounds are checked. At that time, the motion is increased in the brace to 20° to 90°. At

4 weeks postoperatively, the patient is allowed to come to full extension passively, using the healthy leg to bring the operated leg into extension. The patient removes the brace and does this two times per day. The patient is also allowed to fully flex the knee passively. At this time, weight bearing is begun. The pa-

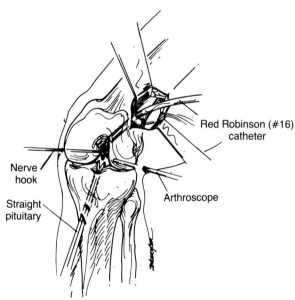

Figure 10–14
A Red Robinson catheter is passed into the femoral tunnel and then pulled out through the tibial tunnel by means of a straight pituitary clamp. (Reprinted from Friedman MJ: Arthroscopic semitendinosus [gracilis] reconstruction for anterior cruciate ligament deficiency. Techniques in Orthopaedics 2(4);74–80 with permission of Aspen Publishers, Inc. © January, 1988.)[15]

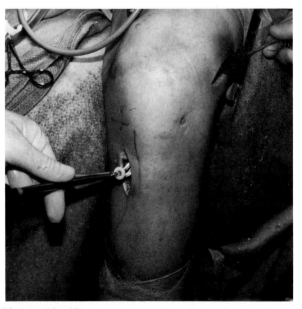

Figure 10–15
The loop of tendon is fixed to the tibia with a 6.5 mm AO cancellous screw and plastic soft tissue washer. (Reprinted from Friedman MJ: Arthroscopic semitendinosus [gracilis] reconstruction for anterior cruciate ligament deficiency. Techniques in Orthopaedics 2(4);74–80 with permission of Aspen Publishers, Inc. © January, 1988.)[15]

tient is allowed to ride a bike and begin quarter squats. No active quad extension of less than 45° is allowed for 3 months. The patient is not allowed to return to competitive athletics until 7 months postoperatively. At that time, the strength of the quadriceps on the operated side, as measured by Cybex testing, should be within 15 per cent of the unoperated quadriceps, and the patient should have a full range of motion. The patient continues to wear a brace for athletic activities.

ACL Reconstruction Using Patellar Tendon

Initial examination of the knee and notchplasty are performed as described previously. The patellar tendon graft is then harvested. To harvest the graft, we use a two-incision technique. A small incision, 2.5 cm in length, is made, extending from the distal pole of the patella proximally. A second incision, 2.5 cm in length, is made 1 cm medial to the tibial tubercle and extended proximally (Fig. 10–16). The skin is undermined in these proximal and distal incisions, and the appropriate-sized bone plug is outlined on the tibial tubercle and on the patella. This corresponds in width to the central one third of the patellar tendon. It is important to make sure that the medial and lateral margins of the patellar tendon are clearly visualized prior to removing the central third of the graft. Approximately 2.5 cm of bone length is used for both the proximal and distal plugs. An oscillating saw is used to remove these bone plugs with the ligament attached. Subcutaneous dissection of the skin bridge between the proximal and distal incision is performed. The tendon is then incised below the skin bridge from distal to proximal, and the patellar bone graft is removed as a single unit (Fig. 10–17, 10–18, and 10–19). Using the two-incision approach results in a smaller scar. Also, the scars are removed from the anterior area of skin directly over the joint line that is subjected to the greatest skin tension with flexion, and this area tends to heal with a less cosmetic scar. After the graft has been harvested, a femoral guide pin is placed into the isometric point on the femur. The stylus of a tibial guide is then placed on the tibial attachment. The same tibial tubercle skin incision is used for placement of the tibial guide outrigger. The drill guide is placed in direct contact with the bone, and the tibial drill hole is made.

Isometric placement is then checked, as noted previously. If placement is satisfactory, the larger cannulated drills are passed sequentially through the tunnel, and chamfering of the tunnel is performed as noted previously. The tunnels are generally overdrilled 1 mm larger than the diameter of the bone plugs that are fashioned on the end of the patellar tendon graft. This allows easier passage of the graft through the drill holes. The bone plugs are carefully

shaped so that they will pass easily through a cannula of the appropriate size. Generally, approximately a 9-mm bone plug is used with a 10-mm hole. Three small drill holes are then made in a longitudinal fashion through the bone plug at each end of the graft. Number 5 Tevdek suture is passed through each hole in a looped fashion. One end of the suture from each loop is marked with a knot.

One of the most difficult technical aspects of ACL reconstruction using patellar tendon graft can be the passage of the graft with its bone plugs through the bony tunnels. As previously mentioned, this passage will be easier if the tunnels have been made relatively parallel and convergent. Passage is also simplified by the use of a plastic sleeve tendon passer (DePuy) (Fig. 10–20). This consists of a loop of tape contained within a closed soft plastic cylinder that comes in a variety of predetermined diameters. The appropriately sized closed end of the tendon passer is passed up through the tibial hole from outside in. The end of the plastic tendon passer is viewed in the joint with the arthroscope in the anterolateral portal. The pituitary forceps is passed through the femoral tunnel from outside to inside. Under arthroscopic visualization the end of the tendon passer is grasped

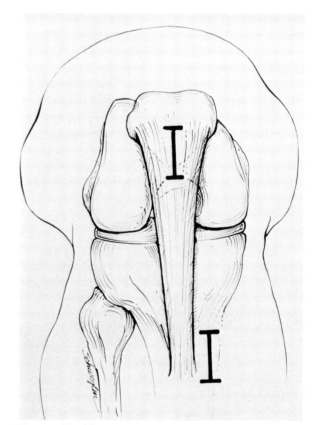

Figure 10–16

To harvest the patellar tendon, a 2.5-cm skin incision is made from the distal pole of the patella extending proximally, and a second incision is made medial to the tibial tubercle.

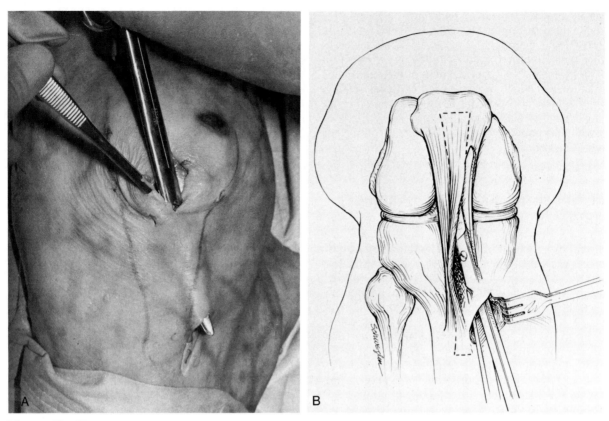

Figure 10–17

A, The skin bridge between the two incision is undermined. *B*, The patellar tendon is then incised at the appropriate width from distal to proximal.

with the pituitary forceps and pulled back through the femoral tunnel until the end is protruding from the femoral cortex. The closed plastic end of the tendon passer is then cut off on the femoral side. The loop of tape is removed. The sutures from the bone plug on one end of the patellar tendon graft are passed through the loop of tape. Tension is applied to the tape by pulling on the free ends that are protruding from the open tibial side of the tendon passer. With gentle tension on the tape protruding through the tibial side, the bony end of the patellar tendon graft is passed into the tendon passer. Since the tendon passer is 1 mm larger in diameter than the graft and since there are no sharp edges on the passer, the graft usually can be smoothly drawn through the plastic tube (Fig. 10–21). The graft is advanced through the joint within the tube until the bony ends of the graft are visible at the outer aspect of the tibial drill hole. With tension maintained on the sutures in the bone plug occupying the femoral tunnel, the plastic sheath of the tendon passer is then slid back distally. After the sheath has been completely removed, the graft is in the proper position within the tunnels. In addition to making passage of the graft through the tunnels easier, the tunnel also helps prevent damage to the intra-articular portion of the graft, which may otherwise occur as the soft tissue is passed over the bony edges of the tunnel.

The femoral end of the graft is then fixed in place within the femoral tunnel using the Kurosaka screw[26] (Fig. 10–22). This is an interference-fit type of fixation. The screw is placed without tapping by introducing it between the wall of the bone plug and the wall of the femoral tunnel. The screw is designed so that the graft remains in the same position while the screw is advanced. The screw should be inserted along the cortical side of the bone plug on the end of the graft. After the screw has been firmly seated, the ends of the sutures from the bony plug are passed through the holes of a plastic button. The ends with the previously placed knot are tied to the ends without the knot over the button as a secondary reinforcement to the fixation. After the firm fixation of the graft in the femoral tunnel has been accomplished, the knee is moved through a range of motion while tension is maintained manually on the tibial side of the graft. If impingement is noted in the region of the notch, further notchplasty is performed at this time. After adequate graft clearance has been obtained, the knee is placed in a 20° posterior Lachman position. The tensioning device is applied to the tibial sutures until the appropriate tension has been ob-

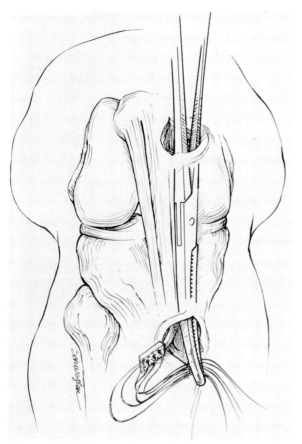

Figure 10–18
After the bone plug has been removed with the attached patellar tendon from the tibial tubercle, sutures are placed through the bone plug and grasped with a curved clamp inserted through the proximal incision.

tained. With the graft held in this position, a second Kurosaka screw is placed to fix the tibial bone plug into the tibial tunnel. The sutures protruding from the tibial tunnel are tied over a plastic button as was done for the femur. The wound is then closed in a similar manner to that described for the pes tendons.

When the Kurosaka screws have been used for fixation of the graft to the bony tunnels, the physical therapy is somewhat more aggressive than that recommended for the semitendinosus graft. The patient is placed initially in a brace allowing 30° to 60° of range of motion. The patient is allowed to remove the brace and passively extend the knee completely out of the brace two times per day. After 1 week, the patient is seen in follow-up, and the brace is increased to 20° to 90° range of motion. Passive extension to 0 degrees extension is continued. At 3 weeks postoperatively, the patient is allowed to begin weight bearing, and full passive motion of the knee is allowed. No competition is allowed for 6 months, again using the criteria outlined in the previous technique.

A common complication after anterior cruciate ligament reconstruction is arthrofibrosis. In our experience, this is more common following patellar tendon graft than with the other graft methods. This may be due to the formation of adhesions between the extensor mechanism and the articular surface, secondary to the dissection of the extensor mechanism. We believe the incidence of this complication can be lessened by isometric placement of the graft and by early motion of the knee. However, when the complication does occur, we believe that early intervention is warranted. If a patient is unable to flex the knee greater

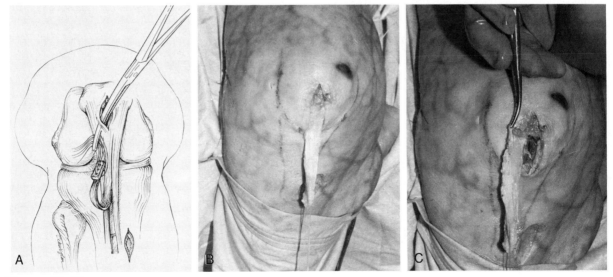

Figure 10–19
A, The graft is pulled proximally beneath the skin bridge out through the proximal incision. *B*, Graft removed from tunnel. The graft remains attached proximally. *C*, The proximal bone plug is then removed to free the graft.

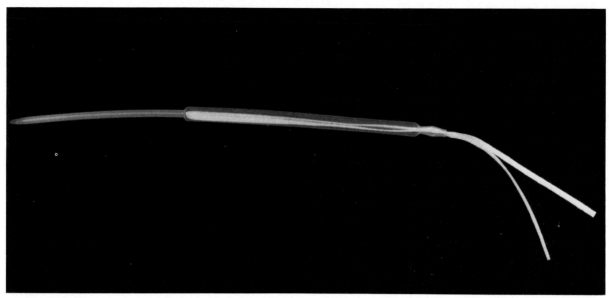

Figure 10–20
A plastic tendon passer (DePuy) that allows easy passage of the graft through the tunnels. The narrow end of the tube is passed through the tibial tunnel and out the femoral tunnel. This end is cut off to expose the tape, which is used to pull the graft back through the plastic sleeve, now located intra-articularly.

than 60° at 2 months after ligament reconstruction, we consider this a sign of arthrofibrosis. We manipulate these patients under anesthesia and usually perform an arthroscopic examination with blunt lysis of the adhesions that are noted. Using this technique, full knee range of motion usually can be obtained perioperatively. The patient is placed in a continuous

passive motion machine overnight and then is discharged with an outpatient CPM machine for the next week. After that, the patient is begun on active range of motion exercises and therapy. We have had good results with this technique, with patients recovering good range of motion with no incidence of rupture of the graft.

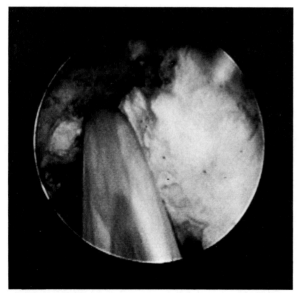

Figure 10–21
The graft is being drawn through the plastic sleeve located within the knee joint. This prevents possible damage to the graft and makes passage through the bony tunnels easier.

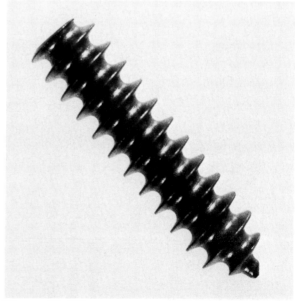

Figure 10–22
The Kurosaka screw gives an interference fit between the bone plug of the graft and the bone tunnel. It is inserted without tapping.

Reconstruction of the ACL Using Gore-Tex

The initial steps in Gore-Tex anterior cruciate ligament reconstruction are those that have already been detailed. Examination of the knee arthroscopically followed by meniscal resection or repair is performed. Adequate notchplasty is performed as detailed previously.

A 5-cm incision is then made 3 cm medial to the insertion of the patellar tendon on the tibial tubercle. The stylus of the tibial drill guide is inserted slightly anterior and medial to the insertion of the anterior cruciate ligament on the tibia. A guidewire is drilled, followed by a 16-mm reamer. The internal and then the external edges of the tunnel are carefully chamfered. An 8-cm incision is made over the lateral femoral epicondylar region extending proximally. The central portion of the iliotibial band is identified and incised longitudinally. The vastus lateralis is retracted superiorly, allowing visualization of the anterolateral surface of the femur. The interval between the iliotibial band superiorly and the biceps femoris is developed by blunt dissection, visualizing the posterolateral capsule and the posterior aspect of the distal femur. A small urologic dilator is then passed from the anteromedial arthroscopic portal into the joint. This is pressed against the posterior capsule and is felt against the palpating finger through the lateral incision. The posterolateral cap-

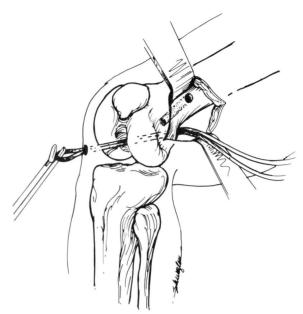

Figure 10—24
Umbilical tape is passed from the posterior side, grasped by a Takahashi clamp inserted through the anteromedial portal, and then pulled out through the portal. The tape is next pulled through the tibial tunnel. (Reprinted from Friedman MJ: Gore-Tex anterior cruciate ligament reconstruction. Techniques in Orthopaedics 2(4):36–43, with permission of Aspen Publishers, Inc. © January, 1988.)[16]

sule is penetrated as high superiorly as possible. The capsular holes are then enlarged progressively with dilators to permit easy passage of the graft.

An AO C clamp is used to drill an oblique tunnel from the superolateral aspect of the femur to the posterolateral surface, with exit of the drill 1 cm medial to the gastrocnemius insertion just above the capsule level (Fig. 10–23). Digital palpation confirms proper positioning of the wire on the posterior femur. A 5/26-inch reamer is then used to overdrill the guidewire. Internal and external chamfering are again performed. An upbiting Takahashi clamp is passed through the anteromedial portal into the knee joint and brought out the posterolateral capsular hole. A leader of umbilical tape is then passed with the pituitary posteriorly until the leader can be grasped by the Takahashi clamp. The clamp holding the tape is then pulled back through the joint and out the anteromedial skin portal (Fig. 10–24). A straight Takahashi clamp is then brought up through the tibial hole into the joint and grasps the leader within the joint. This is pulled back with the clamp out the tibial hole.

A Red Robinson catheter is subsequently passed through the femoral tunnel from the superolateral femur to the posterolateral femur (Fig. 10–25). The leader is inserted into the Red Robinson catheter. A second umbilical tape is then placed as a loop around the end of the umbilical tape secured in the Robinson

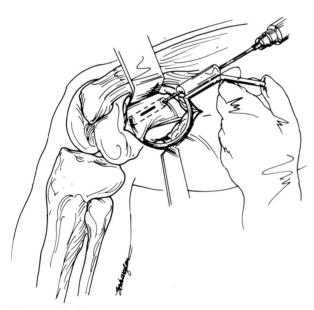

Figure 10—23
A C-clamp is used to drill the tunnel in the distal femur from lateral to posterior. (Reprinted from Friedman MJ: Gore-Tex anterior cruciate ligament reconstruction. Techniques in Orthopaedics 2(4):36–43, with permission of Aspen Publishers, Inc. © January, 1988.)[16]

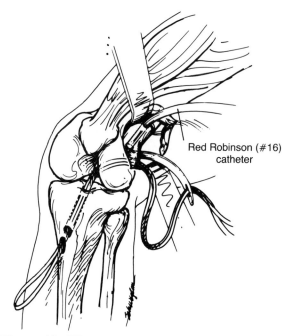

Figure 10–25

A Red Robinson catheter is passed through the extra-articular femoral tunnel, and the ends of the tape are inserted through it. (Reprinted from Friedman MJ: Gore-Tex anterior cruciate ligament reconstruction. Techniques in Orthopaedics 2(4):36–43, with permission of Aspen Publishers, Inc. © January, 1988.)[16]

catheter. The Red Robinson catheter with the two attached tapes is pulled back through the femoral hole. The graft is pulled through the tibia and out the posterolateral capsule, using the second loop of umbilical tape that had been passed. This allows for a more direct pull and affords easier passage through the knee joint than if the loop is used, which passes out the femoral hole. The Gore-Tex is gently sawed back and forth as it is passed through the posterolateral capsule. It is then brought up and out through the lateral femoral condylar tunnel, using the first leader of tape.

A 3.2-mm drill is used to drill a hole for bicortical screw fixation of the loop of Gore-Tex to the lateral femoral surface. The Gore-Tex should deform slightly as the screw is tightened if compression is adequate. The graft is placed under approximately 40 pounds of tension and moved through 20 cycles of flexion and extension. This step ensures that the graft has been snugly positioned within the tibial tunnel and through the exit in the posterolateral capsule.

The knee is now placed in complete extension and the Gore-Tex tensioning device is passed through the hole in the distal end of the graft. Twenty pounds of tension is applied, and a punch is used to make a hole at the appropriate level given by this amount of tension (Fig. 10–26). A 3.2-mm drill and bicortical screw are then used to fix the tibial loop of the Gore-Tex graft. Prior to drilling the 3.2-mm hole, a 1/8-inch

K-wire is used to fix the graft and check the range of motion and stability of the joint. Since this is not an autogenous reconstruction and the permanent prosthesis cannot be expected to stretch out, it is important that full extension to 0° be obtained at this time. If the position is satisfactory, then the tibial loop is fixed with a bicortical screw. The arthroscope is reinserted and extension and flexion carried out to be certain that there is no condylar notch impingement at this time. If there is impingement, further notchplasty is performed until no bony impingement occurs.

Rehabilitation is rapid after a Gore-Tex graft. The patients are essentially allowed weight bearing and range of motion as tolerated. No cast or brace is used postoperatively. Most patients are off all walking aids by 2 to 3 weeks. Athletic endeavors are postponed for a minimum of 4 to 6 months, to allow complete bony ingrowth into the tunnels of the Gore-Tex.

Arthroscopic Reconstruction of the Posterior Cruciate Ligament

Prior to reconstruction of the posterior cruciate ligament (PCL), arthroscopy is performed with correction of any meniscal pathology. With the arthroscope positioned in the anterolateral portal, the femoral origin of the posterior cruciate ligament is visualized. Using the shaver through the anteromedial portal, soft tissue is removed as needed to allow visualization of the femoral attachment site. The femoral attachment is determined with the knee in 90° of

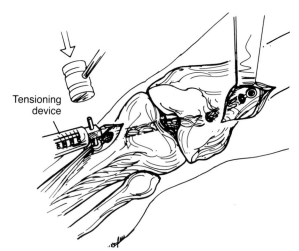

Figure 10–26

With the knee in complete extension, the tensioning device is held at the appropriate tension and used to create a hole in the tibial cortex at the corresponding position. (Reprinted from Friedman MJ: Gore-Tex anterior cruciate ligament reconstruction. Techniques in Orthopaedics 2(4):36–43, with permission of Aspen Publishers, Inc. © January, 1988.)[16]

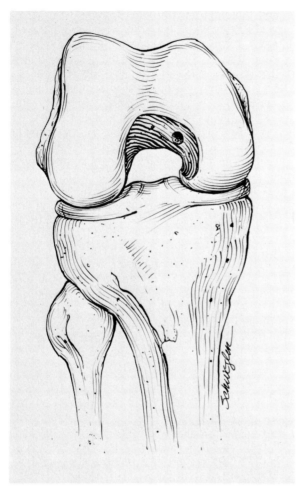

Figure 10–27
The attachment site for the PCL on the femur.

is at the level of the upper third of the patella with the knee in 90° of flexion (Fig. 10–28). The guidewire is then passed through the drill guide into the intercondylar notch (Fig. 10–29).

Attention is then directed to the tibial tunnel. The knee is placed in a figure 4 position and a posteromedial arthrotomy is made (Fig. 10–30). The normal PCL attachment site is onto the shelf, which is posterior to the articular surface of the tibia. The stylus of the drill guide is positioned, under direct visualization, through the arthrotomy over the area of the PCL insertion. The outrigger guide is positioned to create a tunnel beginning approximately 2 cm below the tibial tubercle. The direction of the tibial tunnel, therefore, is more vertical than that for the ACL reconstruction (Fig. 10–31). This results in minimal divergence from the femoral tunnel. The guide pin is then drilled through the drill guide from the tibia up to the insertion site. A periosteal elevator is placed behind the capsule to prevent damage to the neurovascular structures as the guide pin is advanced. After the guide pin has been properly positioned, the tibial tunnel is overdrilled with the appropriate-sized drill bit. This will generally be approximately 1 mm larger than the size of the graft used. The femoral hole is then also overdrilled to the appropriate size. The bony tunnels are beveled with chamfering rasps

flexion. The position is located approximately 8 mm proximal to the margin of the articular surface of the medial femoral condyle. This corresponds to the 2 o'clock position in the right knee or the 10 o'clock position in the left knee. The attachment site is situated posteriorly in the intercondylar notch, although the position is slightly more anterior than the position of attachment of the ACL (Fig. 10–27). With the arthroscope in the anterolateral portal, the femoral guide is passed through the anteromedial portal. The stylus is positioned in the center of the desired femoral attachment site. The outrigger is positioned along the medial aspect of the distal thigh. A small incision is made in the skin at the site of outrigger contact. Beneath the skin, the vastus medialis obliquus muscle is identified and retracted superiorly to expose the medial femoral condyle. The stylus of the femoral guide is again placed on the previously determined origin site for the PCL graft. The outrigger is positioned appropriately on the distal femur. With the knee flexed 90°, the site on the femur is midway between the medial femoral epicondyle and the margin of the medial articular surface of the femur. This hole

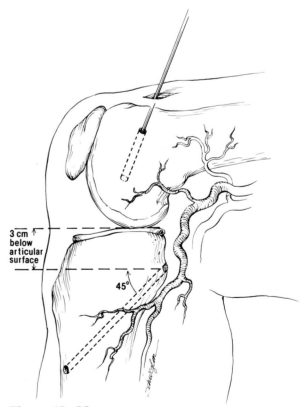

Figure 10–28
Schematic illustration of the femoral and tibial tunnels for PCL reconstruction. Note the proximity of the neurovascular structures to the tibial tunnel.

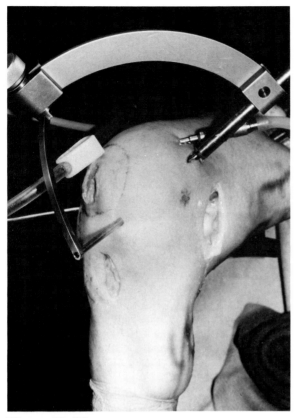

Figure 10–29
Guide in place for drilling a femoral tunnel.

through the tunnels. The knee is moved through a range of motion while the graft is observed arthroscopically. If impingement is noted in the intercondylar area, further resection can be performed. Depending on the graft material used, the femoral site is then fixed using either a screw or plastic button. The knee is placed in approximately 20° of flexion, and an anterior drawer force is applied to the tibia. The graft is placed under tension and fixed to the tibia, again using either screw or button fixation. The posterior drawer sign should be eliminated after proper graft positioning, and the knee should be able to pass through a full range of motion.

Several methods of fixing the femur and tibia during healing of the PCL have been advocated. A transfixion pin has been used, but problems with pin breakage or migration increase the morbidity of this procedure, and we have not used this technique for many years. If the knee is otherwise stable, it may be sufficient simply to immobilize the knee at approximately 0° of extension. This "tightens" the posterior capsule and pulls the tibia anteriorly.

The joint can also be fixed in position by fixing the patella to the tibia, a process termed *olecranoniza-*

or curettes. The graft is passed anterior to posterior through the tibia.

With the scope in the anteromedial portal, the leading sutures from the graft material are first passed through the tibial tunnel into the knee joint, using a straight pituitary. The upbiting pituitary is then inserted through the anterolateral portal to grasp the graft sutures. The sutures are pulled out through the anterolateral portal. A Red Robinson catheter is passed down the femoral tunnel from outside into the joint. This is grasped with the pituitary and also pulled out through the anterolateral portal. The sutures are passed through the Red Robinson catheter (Fig. 10–32). They are then pulled back with the Red Robinson catheter into the knee joint and out through the femoral tunnel. The graft is carefully advanced through the tibial tunnel into the knee joint and then out through the femoral tunnel.

Passing the graft out of the tibial tunnel and into the femoral tunnel can be difficult. Easier passage can often be obtained if the knee is flexed to 90° as the substitute is pulled through the notch. The knee can then be extended to approximately 30° to allow the graft to be pulled through the femoral tunnel. Manipulation of the graft through the posteromedial arthrotomy may then aid in passage.

The graft is held under tension after passage

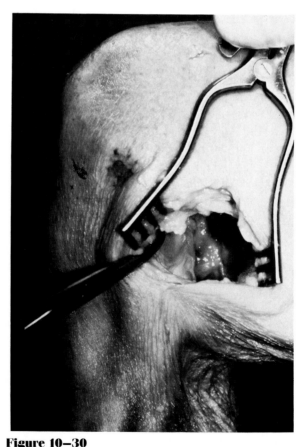

Figure 10–30
A posteromedial arthrotomy is made to allow visualization of the posterior tibia.

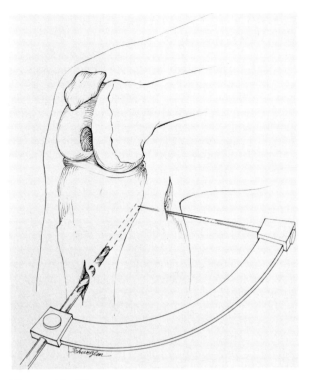

Figure 10–31
The drill hole guide stylus is positioned over the PCL attachment site on the tibia through the posteromedial arthrotomy, and the hole is drilled under direct vision.

tion. Under image intensification, a guidewire is first drilled through the patella in a longitudinal direction. The patella is then tipped forward and the guidewire is passed down into the tibia, fixing the patella to the tibia. After an appropriate position has been obtained, a Schanz screw can be passed through the patella to secure fixation to the tibia in approximately 30° of flexion (Fig. 10–33). Range of motion from 30° to 60° is possible. The screw is removed at 6 weeks, and full range of motion is allowed. Although this method is effective, it can also be associated with patellofemoral morbidity if careful attention is not paid to placement of the screw.

Specific rehabilitation depends on the type of graft material used. Substitution with patellar tendon, pes tendons, allograft, and synthetic ligaments has all been tried. A patellar tendon allograft may be especially useful in this situation. Use of the allograft prevents the associated patellofemoral morbidity of taking the autogenous patellar tendon graft. This may be especially important to patients with posterior cruciate ligament rupture who often have an increased incidence of preoperative patellofemoral problems. Use of an allograft also allows a larger and thus potentially stronger graft to be used than when an autogenous graft is used. Finally, using the bony plugs in the patellofemoral graft allows for stronger screw fixation and earlier mobilization. However, as noted for the ACL, the allograft may present problems of disease transmission and less complete incorporation.

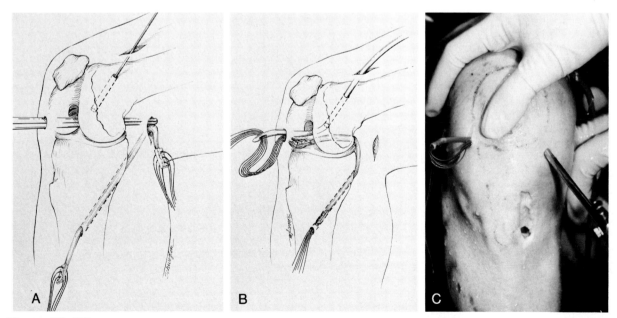

Figure 10–32
A, The graft has been passed through the tibial tunnel and brought out through the posteromedial arthrotomy. A straight Takahashi clamp has been passed through the anterolateral portal, through the notch, and out the arthrotomy. *B* and *C,* The graft has been pulled back and out through the anterolateral portal, and the sutures are passed through the Red Robinson catheter. The catheter is then pulled back through the femoral tunnel with the graft.

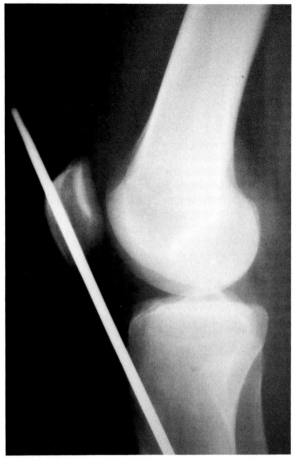

Figure 10–33
A Schanz screw is passed through the patella into the tibia to limit range of motion after PCL reconstruction, a process termed *olecranonization*.

RESULTS OF LIGAMENT RECONSTRUCTION

Recent studies have documented improvement in knee function following ACL reconstruction using open techniques.[17,22,23,38,41] Since arthroscopic reconstruction is a relatively new technique, there have been no published long-term studies of its efficacy. It remains to be seen whether the reported good results following open reconstruction will be achieved or even bettered arthroscopically.

DIRECTIONS FOR THE FUTURE

Understanding the principles of ligament reconstruction, including isometric placement of the graft, adequate notchplasty, and graft tensioning, has resulted in improved results from ACL reconstruction. It is hoped and expected that new developments will continue to improve these results. These advances probably will be in the form of new instrumentation and guide systems, allowing more precise graft placement with smaller incisions. A second area of improvement likely will involve artificial graft substitutes.

Devices currently being tested allow arthroscopic placement of a suture on the presumed femoral attachment site without creation of a drill hole (Fig. 10–34). A small drill hole is created appropriately on the tibia. The suture is passed through this hole by means of the special device and attached to the femoral origin of the ACL (Fig. 10–35). The sutures are then tensioned and moved through a range of motion attached to an isometry device. If the position of the attachment is found to be isometric, a guide pin is passed into this area and a drill hole is created as previously detailed. If placement of the femoral hole

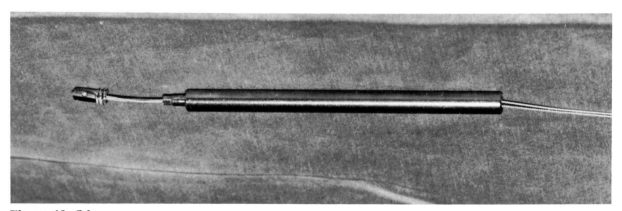

Figure 10–34
A device in development that allows a suture to be placed in the presumed isometric point on the femur to check isometry prior to drilling a femoral tunnel.

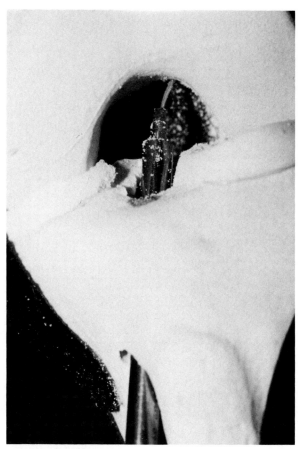

Figure 10–35
The suture has been imbedded in the femoral isometric position by passing the device up through the tibial tunnel.

attachment is not isometric, the device can be moved to the appropriate isometric position prior to creation of the drill hole. Another new development is the creation of the femoral drill hole from within the notch and fixation of the graft within the femur intraarticularly. This eliminates the need for an incision along the lateral aspect of the femur with its associated morbidity. This tunnel is created by drilling a straight line through the tibial tunnel through the knee joint and then into the femur. This tunnel is relatively convergent and therefore minimizes stress on the graft and allows easy graft passage.

The second area of important future developments will be in the area of prosthetic ligaments. Efforts are underway to develop prosthetic ligaments that more closely mimic the biomechanical characteristics of the natural ACL and have acceptable compatibility and strength. Work on ligament augmentation devices may improve their structural properties. The ideal ligament augmentation device would provide initial strengthening of the graft to allow rapid rehabilitation and return to activity. The device then would gradually be reabsorbed at a rate that allows gradual transfer of the stresses to the autogenous tissue.

While it is interesting to speculate on the future developments in ligament reconstruction, it is clear that the techniques emphasized in this chapter will continue to be important. Careful attention to the technical aspects noted here should give good results from anterior cruciate ligament reconstruction with a minimal amount of morbidity and a rapid rehabilitation.

References

1. Andrews JR, Sanders RA, Morin B: Surgical treatment of anterolateral rotatory instability. Am J Sports Med 13:112–119, 1985.
2. Arnoczky SP: Anatomy of the anterior cruciate ligament. Clin Orthop 172:19–25, 1983.
3. Baker CL Jr, Norwood LA, Hughston JC: Acute combined posterior cruciate and posterolateral instability of the knee. Am J Sports Med 12:204–208, 1984.
4. Clancy WG: Intra-articular reconstruction of the anterior cruciate ligament. Orthop Clin North Am 16(2):181–184, 1985.
5. Clancy WG, Nelson DA, Reider B, et al: Anterior cruciate ligament reconstruction using one-third of the patellar ligament, augmented by extra-articular tendon transfers. J Bone Joint Surg 64A:352–359, 1982.
6. Clancy WG Jr, Shelbourne KD, Zoellner GB, et al: Treatment of knee joint instability secondary to rupture of the posterior cruciate ligament. J Bone Joint Surg 65A: 310–322, 1983.
7. Cross MJ, Powell JF: Long-term followup of posterior cruciate ligament rupture: A study of 116 cases. Am J Sports Med 12:292–297, 1984.
8. DeHaven KE: Diagnosis of acute knee injuries with hemarthrosis. Am J Sports Med 9:209–214, 1981.
9. DeHaven KE: Arthroscopy in the diagnosis and management of the anterior cruciate ligament–deficient knee. Clin Orthop 172:52–56, 1983.
10. Eriksson E: Sports injuries of the knee ligaments; Their diagnosis, treatment, rehabilitation and prevention. Med Sci Sports 8:133–144, 1976.
11. Eriksson E: Rehabilitation of muscle function after sport injury. Major problems in sports medicine. Int J Sports Med 2:1–6, 1981.
12. Feagin JA, Curl WW: Isolated tears of the anterior cruciate ligament: 5 year follow-up study. Am J Sports Med 4:95, 1976.
13. Fowler P: Presentation at AAOS Summer Institute Instructional Course, San Diego, Sept. 9, 1988.

14. Fox JM, Sherman OH, Markolf K: Arthroscopic anterior cruciate ligament repair: Preliminary results and instrumented testing for anterior stability. Arthroscopy 1:175–181, 1985.
15. Friedman MJ: Arthroscopic semitendinosus (gracilis) reconstruction for anterior cruciate ligament deficiency. Tech Orthop 2(4):74–80, 1988.
16. Friedman MJ: Gore-Tex anterior cruciate ligament reconstruction. Tech Orthop 2(4):36–43, 1988.
17. Friedman MJ, Sherman OK, Fox JM, et al: Autogenic anterior cruciate ligament (ACL) reconstruction of the knee: A review. Clin Orthop 196:9–14, 1985.
18. Furman W, Marshall JL, Girgis FG: The anterior cruciate ligament. A functional analysis based on post-mortem studies. J Bone Joint Surg 58A:179–185, 1976.
19. Gillquist J, Hagberg G, Oretarp N: Arthroscopy in acute injuries of the knee joint. Acta Orthop Scand 48:190–106, 1977.
20. Gillquist J, Odensten M: Arthroscopic reconstruction of the anterior cruciate ligament. Arthroscopy 4(1):5–9, 1988.
21. Glousman R, Shields C, Kerlan R, et al: Gore-Tex prosthetic ligament in anterior cruciate deficient knees. Am J Sports Med 16(4):321–326, 1988.
22. Jensen JE, Slocum DB, Larson RL, et al: Reconstruction procedures for anterior cruciate ligament insufficiency: A computer analysis of clinical results. Am J Sports Med 11:240–248, 1983.
23. Johnson RJ, Eriksson E, Haggmark T, et al: Five-to-ten-year follow-up evaluation after reconstruction of the anterior cruciate ligament. Clin Orthop 183:122–140, 1984.
24. Kochum A, Markolf KL, Marei RC: Anterior-posterior stiffness and laxity of the knee after major ligament reconstruction. J Bone Joint Surg 66A:1460–1465, 1984.
25. Kohn D: Arthroscopy in acute injuries of the anterior cruciate–deficient knee: Fresh and old intraarticular lesions. Arthroscopy 2(2):98–102, 1986.
26. Kurosaka M, Yoshiya S, Andrish JT: A biomechanical comparison of different surgical techniques of graft fixation in anterior cruciate ligament reconstruction. Am J Sports Med 15(3):225–229, 1987.
27. Leland R, Burks RT: Determination of graft tension prior to fixation in anterior cruciate ligament reconstruction. Presented at 7th Annual Meeting, Arthroscopy Association of America, Washington, DC, March 26, 1988.
28. Lipscomb AB, Johnston RK, Snyder RB, et al: Evaluation of hamstring strength following use of semitendinosus and gracilis tendons to reconstruct the anterior cruciate ligament. Am J Sports Med 10(6):340–342, 1982.
29. Noyes FR, Bassett RW, Grood ES, Butler DL: Arthroscopy in acute traumatic hemarthrosis of the knee. Incidence of anterior cruciate tears and other injuries. J Bone Joint Surg 62A:687–695, 1980.
30. Noyes FR, Butler DL, Grood ES, et al: Biomechanical analysis of human ligament grafts used in knee ligament repairs and reconstructions. J Bone Joint Surg 66A:344–352, 1984.
31. Noyes FR, Butler DL, Paulos LE, Grood ES: Intra-articular cruciate reconstructions. I: Perspectives on graft strength, vascularization and immediate motion after replacement. Clin Orthop 172:71–77, 1983.
32. Odensten M, Gillquist J: Functional anatomy of the anterior cruciate ligament and a rationale for reconstruction. J Bone Joint Surg 67A:257–262, 1985.
33. Odensten M, Lysholm J, Gillquist J: Suture of fresh ruptures of the anterior cruciate ligament: A 5 year follow-up. Acta Orthop Scand 55:270–272, 1984.
34. Parolie JM, Bergfeld JA: Long-term results of nonoperative treatment of isolated posterior cruciate ligament injuries in the athlete. Am J Sports Med 14:35, 1986.
35. Paulos L, Drawbert JP, Rosenberg TD: Knee and leg soft tissue trauma. *In* Orthopaedic Knowledge Update 2. Park Ridge, IL, American Academy of Orthopedic Surgeons, 1987, p 412.
36. Penner DA, Daniel DM, Wood P, et al: An in vivo study of anterior cruciate ligament graft placement and isometry. Am J Sports Med 16:238–243, 1988.
37. Roth JM, Kennedy JC, Lockstadt M, et al: Intra-articular reconstruction of the anterior cruciate ligament with and without extra-articular supplementation by transfer of the biceps femoris. J Bone Joint Surg 69A(2):275–278, 1987.
38. Sandberg P, Ballefors B: The durability of anterior cruciate ligament reconstruction with the patellar tendon. Am J Sports Med 16:341–343, 1988.
39. Schinichi Y, Andrish JT, Manley MT, Bauer TW: Graft tension in anterior cruciate ligament reconstruction. An in vivo study in dogs. Am J Sports Med 15(5):464–470, 1987.
40. Shelbourne KD, Baele JR: Treatment of combined anterior cruciate ligament and medial collateral ligament injuries. Am J Knee Surg 1(1):56–58, 1988.
41. Tibone JE, Antioch TJ: A biomechanical analysis of anterior cruciate ligament reconstruction with the patellar tendon. A two-year followup. Am J Sports Med 16:332–335, 1988.
42. Wilcox PG, Jackson DW: Arthroscopic anterior cruciate ligament reconstruction. Clin Sports Med 6:513–524, 1987.

11

Stephen J. Lombardo
James P. Bradley
Arthroscopic Diagnosis and Treatment of Patellofemoral Disorders

A complete understanding of the anatomy, biomechanics, and radiographic and pathologic findings of the patellofemoral joint will permit the orthopedic surgeon to arrive at the best possible solution for the conservative and operative management of disorders of this joint. This chapter discusses these factors, plus the common arthroscopic procedures performed.

FUNCTIONAL ANATOMY AND BIOMECHANICS

The patella is a sesamoid bone, roughly triangular in shape, with its base proximal and apex distal. The quadriceps tendon envelops the patella, terminating distally at the tibial tubercle as the patella tendon. The primary tendinous-ligamentous attachments are located at the superior and inferior poles. On the anterior middle surface of the patella, the primary blood supply enters by way of an anatomic ring of vessels, as described by Scapinelli.[51] The posterior surface is oval; the articular surface is the thickest in the body (7 mm).[45] The architecture of the articular surface is divided into five facets: superior, inferior, medial, lateral, and odd (Fig. 11–1). Normally, they articulate fastidiously with the femoral trochlear groove. This congruence with the femoral surface permits transmission of a deceleration force at any knee flexion posture.[28] A longitudinal ridge separates the lateral from the medial facet, and a second ridge subdivides the medial half into medial and odd facets.[45]

The distal end of the femur articulates with the

patella by means of a lateral and medial facet; these make up the trochlea. The lateral facet is taller—it averages 5 mm, as described by Casscells.[7] The lateral patellar facet is longer with a greater slope,

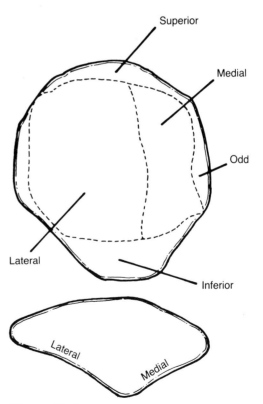

Figure 11–1
Patellar facets.

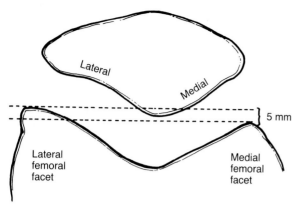

Figure 11–2
A tangential view of the patellofemoral articulation. Note the broad lateral femoral facet and the 5-mm difference in femoral facet height.

matching the higher and wider lateral femoral facet, thereby producing a broad surface for the excess forces attempting to displace the patella laterally (Fig. 11–2). The lateral femoral condyle is 1 cm higher than the medial femoral condyle on a tangential view at the functional position of 45 degrees of flexion, thus enhancing the patella's functional stability.[28]

The configuration of the patella is such that some portion of the articular surface is in contact with the femur throughout knee flexion almost to full extension. Goodfellow and associates, employing a dye method, demonstrated that initial patellar femoral engagement occurs at approximately 20 degrees of flexion, beginning along a narrow band at the inferior pole of the patella and involving both the medial and lateral facets.[23] As the knee is flexed, the patellofemoral contact area progressively moves upward, involving both the medial and lateral facets. As flexion increases, not only does the band move up, but it also becomes steadily broader. At 90 degrees of flexion, this band of contact engages the upper pole of the patella. The patella exclusively articulates with the trochlea until 90 degrees of flexion, then the broad quadriceps tendon begins to make contact with the trochlear groove. The odd facet does not articulate with the lateral margin of the medial femoral condyle until about 135 degrees of knee flexion. The marked change in the patellofemoral contact area, which occurs at 135 degrees of flexion, is secondary to the patella sliding off the true patellar facets of the trochlea and engaging the femoral condyles.

The load increases throughout flexion as the contact band of the patellofemoral articulation enlarges; however, the load increases at a greater degree than the contact area, thereby increasing the force per unit area on the patella (Fig. 11–3).

The patella provides six functions as described by Scott:[56]

1. It increases the moment arm of the quadriceps mechanism.
2. It provides a cartilage-on-cartilage articulation with a relatively low coefficient of friction to increase the efficiency of the quadriceps.
3. It centralizes the force of the quadriceps.
4. It is a sesamoid bone that, interposed between the quadriceps and the patellar tendons, protects them from attritional wear.
5. It shields the normal or prosthetic joint from direct trauma.
6. It serves a cosmetic function; its unilateral absence is sometimes quite apparent, especially when the knee is flexed.

Patellofemoral joint stability is influenced by a variety of factors, including (1) patellofemoral congruency, (2) static ligamentous stabilizers, and (3) dynamic quadriceps and hamstring muscle stabilizers.[10] The static ligamentous stabilizers include the patellotibial and patellofemoral medial and lateral ligaments, which assist in maintenance of proper patellar tracking (Fig. 11–4). The lateral patellofemoral ligament sometimes become excessively tight and may contribute to increased compressive forces to the patella with knee flexion.

The primary muscle group involved is the quadriceps, composed of four "heads": vastus lateralis, vastus intermedius, vastus medialis, and rectus femoris. It acts as the main decelerator force at any specific knee posture. Often overlooked is the function of the vastus medialis obliquus (VMO), which is an essential component of medial patellofemoral stability and proper tracking. In addition, the articular muscle of the knee, though small in size, enables the suprapatellar pouch to be retracted, thus maintaining proper position during knee flexion and extension.[28]

The angle of insertion of the muscles of the quadriceps is salient to the dynamic stability provided. The rectus femoris, arising from the pelvis, inserts at 0 degrees along the superior pole of the patella; Hughston and colleagues postulate that it acts as a

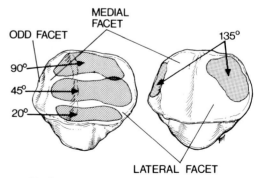

Figure 11–3
Patellar contact areas by the dye method. The contact area migrates superiorly as knee flexion increases.

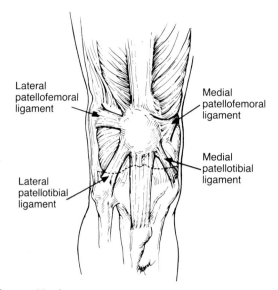

Figure 11–4
The static ligamentous stabilizers of the patellofemoral joint.

"command post" for coordinating various actions of the other components.[28] The other three members take origin from almost the entire circumference of the proximal three quarters of the femoral shaft, then blend to form the quadriceps tendon. The vastus intermedius has a virtually straight insertion into the quadriceps tendon, in relation to the long axis of the thigh. The vastus medialis longus inserts at an angle of approximately 50 degrees, whereas the distal third or VMO normally has a 65-degree orientation, which not only inserts into the quadriceps tendon but also the proximal third of the medial patellar border. The vastus lateralis fibers insert between 30 and 40 degrees into the lateral quadriceps tendon, terminating in an extremely strong, well-developed tendinous attachment at the superolateral pole of the patella (Fig. 11–5).[28,45] Aberrations in any of the insertion angles (especially the VMO), osseous anomalies (femoral anteversion, externally rotated tibia, increased Q angle, valgus knee), muscle imbalance, or ligamentous laxity of the extensor mechanism has the potential to create an abnormal condition. Also, failure of any of the other stabilizing mechanisms permits disruption of the patellofemoral articulation and increases loading on the articular surfaces.

Biomechanical force studies have indicated that the force across the patellofemoral joint during level gait is between one half and one times body weight. The reactive force increases three to four times the body weight in going up and down stairs and sometimes may climb as high as seven times body weight in squatting.[56] Obviously, any abnormality in patellofemoral contact area or tracking will produce a condition of localized pathologic forces that may cause attrition of the articular cartilage of the patella.

Anatomically, a synovial fold or plica is occasionally present in close proximity to the patella. It represents a normal embryologic synovial septum that persists into adulthood.[49] Three major types of plica exist: (1) the infrapatellar plica (ligamentous mucosum), (2) the suprapatellar plica partially separating the knee joint proper from the suprapatellar pouch, and (3) the medial patellar plica that originates along the anteromedial side of the joint, extending from the synovium above the medial patella to the synovium investing the fat pad. It is generally accepted that the medial patellar plica can produce symptoms that may mimic patellar pathology when it becomes inflamed, thickened, or fibrotic. However, concomitant aberrant patellofemoral mechanics may be an associated problem.

ROENTGENOGRAPHIC ANATOMY AND EVALUATION

Anteroposterior Film

The film should be taken with the patient standing with the feet straight ahead and the quadriceps relaxed. The patella normally rests in the center of the femoral sulcus and the inferior pole just proximal to

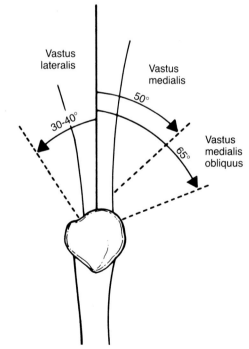

Figure 11–5
Angles of insertion of the components of the quadriceps on the patella. Note that the vastus medialis obliquus inserts at 65 degrees, thus enhancing the medial support of the patella.

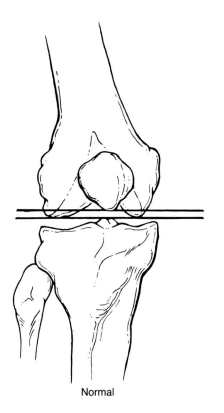

Normal

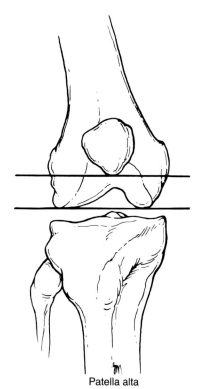

Patella alta

Figure 11–6
The patella normally rests in the center of the femoral sulcus and the inferior pole, just proximal to a line drawn across the distal margin of the femoral condyles. Patella alta is suspected if the tip of the inferior pole is more than 20 mm above this line.

a line drawn across the distal margin of the femoral condyles.[6] Patella alta is suspected if the tip of the inferior pole is more than 20 mm above this line[33] (Fig. 11–6). Evaluation of fractures and the bipartite configuration, usually at the superolateral margin, should be evident. Asymmetry of the femoral condyles is a clue to femoral anteversion, which is associated with patellofemoral malalignment.[23]

Lateral Film

The film is centered on the knee joint with the knee flexed 30 degrees. Blumensaat[3a] described the normal relationship of the patella to a line drawn along the intercondylar condensation. This line should touch the distal pole of the patella. If the distal pole is elevated above this line, patella alta should be suspected[8] (Fig. 11–7A). Inconsistency of knee flexion propagated inaccuracy in this technique. Insall and Salvati proposed a more accurate measurement.[31] They noted the distance from the superior patellar pole to the inferior patella pole approximately equals the distance from the inferior pole to the tibial tuberosity. The ratio of patellar tendon distance to the length of the patella with the knee flexed between 20 and 70 degrees should be approximately equal (1.0 ± 0.5). Variation of more than 20 percent of the length of the patellar tendon suggests patella alta[6,10,30] (Fig. 11–7B). An alternate method was proposed by Labelle and Laurin.[32] With the knee flexed

90 degrees, a line drawn down the anterior femoral cortex passes over the superior pole of the patella in 97 percent of normal knees. If the line bisects the superior pole, patella alta should be suspected, and if the superior pole lies below this line, patella baja is a possibility[6,10,19] (Fig. 11–7C).

Tangential Film

The most useful information concerning the patellofemoral articulation usually is ascertained from tangential films. Most popular are the Hughston,[6,26] Merchant,[40] and Laurin[35] techniques. In the Hughston view, the knee is flexed 50 to 60 degrees with the patient in the prone position. The cassette is placed under the flexed knee with the x-ray beam directed cephalad and inferiorly, approximately 45 degrees from the vertical. Hughston states that at this angle the height of the lateral femoral condyle is the greatest and its relation to the patella is evaluated.[28] Also, at 55 degrees of flexion, the extensor mechanism produces the greatest amount of lateral force on the patella as the quadriceps contracts; therefore, subluxation/dislocation could become evident.[6] The sulcus angle, which is the angle formed by placing lines from the center of the sulcus to the peaks of the femoral condyles, should be assessed. As the sulcus angle increases, the femoral groove becomes flatter and the buttress effect of the lateral femoral condyle is lost. This produces a propensity

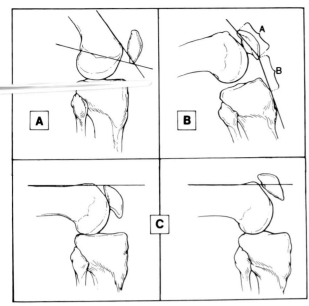

Figure 11-7

A, Blumensaat's line. A line drawn along the intercondylar condensation should touch the distal pole of the patella at 30 degrees of knee flexion. Patella alta should be suspected if the distal pole is elevated above this line. B, Insall's ratio of patellar tendon distance (B) to length of the patella (A), 1.0 ± 0.2 normal. Variation of more than 20 per cent of the length of the patellar tendon suggests patella alta. C, Labelle and Laurin line. A line drawn down the anterior femoral cortex passes over the superior pole of the patella in 97 per cent of normal knees with the knee flexed to 90 degrees. If the line bisects the superior pole, patella alta should be suspected and if the superior pole lies below this line, patella baja is suspected.

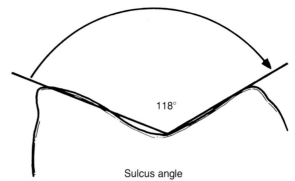

Sulcus angle

Figure 11-8

Hughston's sulcus angle. The sulcus angle is formed by placing lines from the center of the sulcus to the peaks of the femoral condyles. The normal angle is approximately 118 per cent.

for lateral tilt, subluxation, or dislocation of the patella[6,10] (Fig. 11-8). The normal sulcus angle has been determined to be 118 degrees.[33]

The patellar index is also obtained from Hughston's view. First described by Cross and Waldrop, it is expressed as the ratio of the width of the patella to the difference between the lateral and medial facet.[13] The number provides a radiographic index of the lateral position of the patella relative to the lateral femoral condyle. Applying the patellar index in an analysis of 1004 radiographs, Cross delineated that the medial patellar facet is significantly smaller in patients who have patellofemoral instability (Fig. 11-9).

Merchant and Mercer cited many problems with the Hughston view and described a view in which the patient is supine with the knee flexed 45 degrees, and the x-ray tube is directed caudad and inferiorly approximately 30 degrees from the horizontal[40] (Fig. 11-10). The congruence angle is delineated by bisecting the sulcus angle, thus establishing a reference line, then drawing a second line originating at the apex of the sulcus to the lowest point on the articular ridge of the patella. If the apex of the patella lies

lateral to the reference line (Fig. 11-11), a positive value is designated; conversely, if the apex lies medial, a negative value is designated.[6,10] Merchant and colleagues noted that in 200 normal knees the average congruence angle was −6 degrees ± 11 degrees. Any angle greater than +16 degrees was in the 95th percentile and associated with patellofemoral disorders.[41]

Laurin and associates proposed another tangential view with the knee flexed 20 degrees, noting that most subluxations and dislocations occur in the 0- to 20-degree range of motion.[35,36] For this view, the patient is in the sitting position, with the knee flexed 20 degrees; the cassette is held 12 cm proximal to the patella. The x-ray tube is directed cephalad and superiorly at approximately 160 degrees from the vertical. Salient measurements include the lateral patellofemoral angle and the patellofemoral index. Patellar tilt-

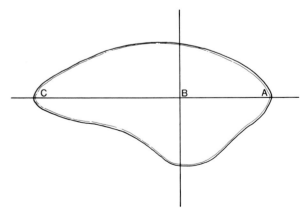

Figure 11-9

Diagram of the patella, demonstrating the measurements needed to calculate the patellar index. Perpendicular lines are drawn through the maximum height and width of the patella. The patellar index is the ratio of the sum of CB + AB, or AC to the difference BC − AB.

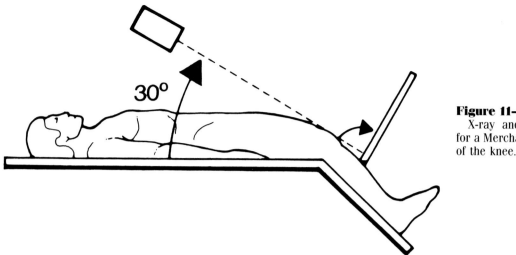

Figure 11–10
X-ray and patient position for a Merchant tangential view of the knee.

ing is determined by the lateral patellofemoral angle, which is constructed by drawing a line across the femoral condyles and drawing a second line along the lateral facet of the patella. Normally the two lines diverge laterally; however, if the lines are parallel or converge laterally, patellar subluxation or dislocation may be indicated (Fig. 11–12). "Mini-tilt" of the patella and possibly chondromalacia may be detected by the patellofemoral index. Laurin felt that it was a functional imbalance of the patella, yet not as severe as subluxation or dislocation.

The patellofemoral index is a ratio between the thickness of the medial patellofemoral interspace and that of the lateral patellofemoral interspace. The lateral patellar interspace is delineated by measuring the shortest distance between the lateral patellar facet and the surface of the lateral femoral condyle. The medial patellofemoral interspace is delineated by measuring the shortest distance between the lateral limit of the medial patellar facet and the medial femoral condyle[35] (Fig. 11–13). In 100 normal knees, the patellofemoral index is found to be 1.6 or less;

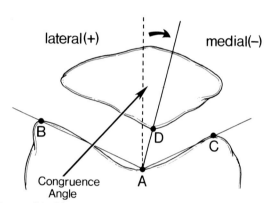

Figure 11–11
Congruence angle. The congruence angle is determined by bisecting the sulcus angle to establish a reference line, then drawing a second line originating at the apex of the sulcus to the lowest point on the articular ridge of the patella. If the apex of the patella lies lateral to the reference line, a positive value is designated; conversely, if the apex lies medial, a negative value is designated. The average angle is −6 degrees ±11 degrees; any angle greater than +16 degrees is associated with patellofemoral disorders.

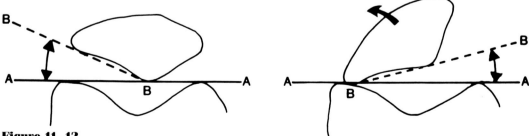

Figure 11–12
The patellofemoral angle is constructed by drawing a line across the femoral condyles and drawing a second line along the lateral facet of the patella. Normally, the two lines diverge laterally; however, if lines are parallel or converge laterally, patellar subluxation or dislocation is indicated.

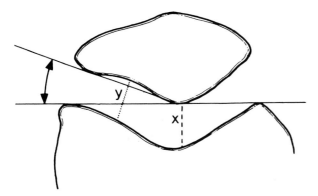

Figure 11-13
The patellofemoral index is the ratio between the thickness of the medial patellofemoral interspace (x) and that of the lateral patellofemoral interspace (y).

however, 93 percent of patients with chondromalacia patellae had an index greater than 1.6.

Aside from the specific calculations just discussed, patellar configuration was classified from the tangential films. Wiberg[60] and Baumgartl[1] described six types of patella. Type I has equal, yet slightly concave, patellar facets. Type II has a smaller medial facet that is slightly concave. Type III has a smaller medial facet that is convex. Type II/III has a smaller medial facet. Type IV has a very small, steeply sloped facet with the medial ridge still present. Type V (Jagerhut) has no central ridge or medial facet[60] (Fig. 11-14). Types I and II are considered the most stable configurations, with Type II the most common. The other types are subject to unbalanced forces and are prone to lateral subluxations.

COMPUTED TOMOGRAPHY (CT) OF THE PATELLOFEMORAL JOINT

CT scanning of the patellofemoral joint was first reported by Delgado-Martins in 1979, using normal patients to define patellar centering.[17] Subsequently, Martinez and associates in 1983 further defined patellar centralization at 0, 20, and 45 degrees of flexion in normal subjects.[38] Schutzer and colleagues in 1986 redefined centralization by noting that in asymptomatic normal knees some mild degree of lateralization of the patella between extension and 5 degrees of flexion is compatible with normal patellofemoral mechanics.[55] However, by 10 degrees of flexion, the congruence angle should be neutral or in the minus range. Using these criteria, they studied 20 patients with persistent patellofemoral pain and divided them into three types of malalignment by evaluating CT scans between 0 degrees and 30 to 40 degrees of flexion: (1) lateralized, nontilted, (2) lateralized, tilted, and (3) tilted, nonlateralized (Fig. 11-15). They emphasized, as did others, the

prime importance of scrutinizing the first 20° of flexion (the unstable range).[19,35,36,55] Most significantly, they defined three groups of malalignment, including a group of lateralized patellas, most of which became congruent by 20 to 30 degrees of flexion and therefore would not be detectable by traditional radiographs.

Fulkerson and colleagues further refined their technique and in 1987 reviewed 62 CT scans, including 21 patients before and after lateral release or anterior tibial tubercle transfer.[22] Again, it became apparent that three types of malalignment were present. They reported that types 1 (subluxed without tilt) and 2 (subluxed with tilt) (Fig. 11-16) may not respond as well to lateral release as did those patients with type 3 (tilt, not subluxed). In addition, when there is more advanced patellar degeneration, lateral release seems to be less effective both in restoring normal tracking (on CT) and in giving a good clinical result. Overall, they felt that CT scans provided an accurate diagnostic tool for defining tilt and subluxation of the patella.

In clinical studies at Kerlan-Jobe Sports Medicine Clinic, we and our colleagues concur that CT scans are helpful in delineating malalignment, especially in early flexion when tangential radiographs often fail to provide diagnostic information.

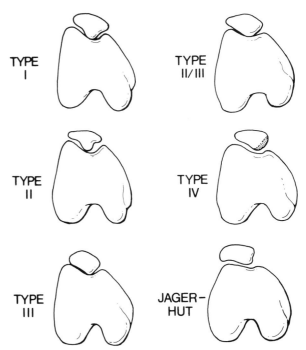

Figure 11-14
Wiberg and Baumgartal's patellar types. The medial facet is to the right. Type I has equal, slightly concave patellar facets. Type II, a smaller medial facet that is slightly concave. Type III, a smaller medial facet that is convex. Type II/III, a smaller medial facet. Type IV, a very small, steeply sloped facet with the medial ridge still present. Type V (Jagerhut) has no central ridge or medial facet.

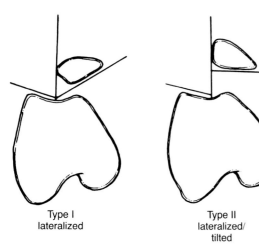
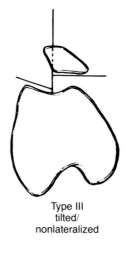

Type I
lateralized

Type II
lateralized/
tilted

Type III
tilted/
nonlateralized

Figure 11–15
Relationships of the patello-femoral joint by CT scan. Schutzer noted that most patients with patellofemoral pain could be divided into three types of malalignment: (1) lateralized, nontilted; (2) lateralized, tilted; and (3) tilted, nonlateralized.

Arthroscopic Determination of Patellofemoral Tracking

Arthroscopic evaluation of patellar tracking is equally as important as inspection of the cartilage surfaces. Employing an anteromedial portal, the patellofemoral alignment is determined according to the degree of knee flexion at which the lateral facet, patellar ridge, and medial facet of the patella initiate contact with the femur. Malalignment, according to Casscells[7] and Metcalf,[42] is failure of the midpatellar ridge to seat in the femoral groove during the first 45 degrees of knee flexion. In normal patellofemoral joints, the lateral facet aligns at a mean knee flexion of 20 degrees, the patellar ridge at 35 degrees, and the medial facet at 50 degrees of knee flexion.[58] In 1987, Søjbjerg and associates, using a constant intra-articular pressure and local anesthesia, noted that in 12 patients with patellar subluxation, contact of the lateral facet was equal to that in normal subjects; however, the alignment of both the patellar ridge and the medial facet was significantly different (55 and 85 degrees of knee flexion versus 35 and 50 degrees in normal subjects).[58] Also, the medial measurements in 20 patients with idiopathic anterior knee pain did not deviate significantly from normal measurements, in contrast to the patients with patellar subluxation.

CHONDROMALACIA

Classification

Chondromalacia means "soft cartilage." First described by Aleman in 1928, it is associated with specific patellar cartilage degeneration. This entity exists most often as a clinical asymptomatic condition.

The etiology of this condition often is not clear. Compression, lack of compression, instability, and malalignment may be predisposing factors to this disease process. Chondromalacia is identifiable by both gross anatomic and histologic characteristics of the patellar cartilage. This term should not be used indiscriminately to describe pain syndromes about the anterior knee and patella. Arthroscopy has proved very valuable in delineating this pathologic and anatomic diagnosis. Many investigators have reported its efficacy about the patellofemoral joint.[7,10,11,15,37,52,58,61]

The classification of chondromalacia employed in our clinic is a modification of the Outerbridge system described in 1961.[48]

Grade 0: Normal
Grade I: Light brownish-yellow discoloration; the cartilage yields to the touch of the arthroscope or to a blunt instrument, usually to a depth of 1 mm. A blister lesion is sometimes present. No fragmentation or fissuring.
Grade II: Fissuring within the soft areas, usually to a depth of 1 to 2 mm.
Grade III: Fissuring with fasciculation, not involving subchondral bone. It often has the appearance of "crabmeat," involving a depth of greater than one half the articular thickness.
Grade IV: Erosion of the articular cartilage down to subchondral bone. This grade cannot be distinguished from patellofemoral arthrosis.

In addition to the grade, the anatomic location of the lesion and its percentage of involvement in relation to the patellar facets is recorded (Figs. 11–17 through 11–20). The same grading system is applied to the facets of the femoral trochlea.

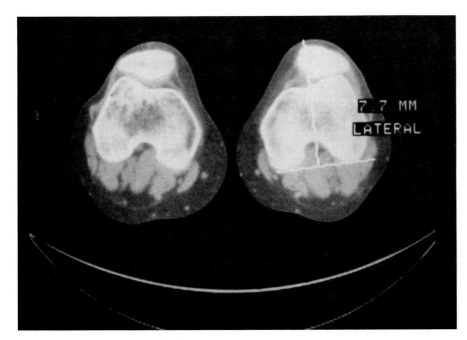

Figure 11–16
CT scan of Type 2, subluxed and tilted patella.

Treatment

CONSERVATIVE

Initially, the diagnosis of chondromalacia is established on the basis of history, physical examination, and radiographic findings. The examiner must rule out prepatellar bursitis, retropatellar tendon bursitis, pes anserinus bursitis, fat pad syndrome, generalized synovitis, meniscal lesions, ligamentous instability, hemophilia, rheumatoid arthritis, villonodular synovitis, osteochondritis dissecans, infectious arthritis, and foreign bodies.[12,24] The patients are then divided into one of the following five groups, as described by DeHaven and associates: (1) idiopathic, (2) post-traumatic, (3) recurrent subluxation, (4) recurrent dislocation, and (5) those that develop during rehabilitation after knee surgery for nonpatellar lesions.[16] The most prevalent is recurrent subluxation (51 percent), followed by idiopathic (30 percent), post-traumatic (10 percent), recurrent dislocation (4 percent), and rehabilitation-induced (5 percent).

All groups are then placed into the Kerlan-Jobe chondromalacia knee rehabilitation protocol with no regard to the etiology of the chondromalacia. The protocol consists of three phases;

Phase I—symptomatic control and isometric exercises, including electrical stimulation to VMO, quadriceps sets, isometric exercises (adduction hamstring sets), straight leg raises, achilles stretching, ice, compression, and nonsteroidal anti-inflammatory drugs.

Phase II—discontinue electrical stimulation. Continue with Phase I exercises with the addition of short arc quadriceps, active hop adduction, hamstring curls, Fitron bike (low resistance), Cybex (200 degrees), and, lastly, eccentric quadriceps exercises.

Phase III—Active quadriceps strengthening exercises, Fitron bike (increasing resistance), and light jogging. When the patient is able to jog 1.5 to 2 miles without pain or discomfort, progressive agility drills are added. Ice is continued after the termination of exercises.

Many workers have reiterated the need for a su-

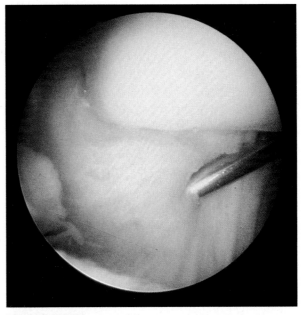

Figure 11–17
Chondromalacia, Grade I.

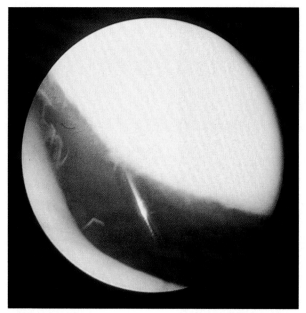

Figure 11–18
Chondromalacia, Grade II.

pervised rehabilitation program as the initial treatment of chondromalacia.[2,16,24,29,39] The duration of the rehabilitation regimen is variable; however, at least a 3- to 5-month supervised program is indicated. If the patient remains symptomatic, surgical intervention may be necessary. The natural history of patellar disease has not been well studied. Therefore, definitive data on this salient point are lacking. Insall noted anecdotally that in most patients the pain does

not become progressively worse and, in time, a certain level becomes acceptable in their daily lives.[29]

Overall restraint and careful evaluation beforehand are required before performing an operative procedure.

Surgical Indications for Chondromalacia and Malalignment

Surgical indications are hard to delineate and are varied in nature. However, the following indications may be helpful:

1) Failure of a supervised rehabilitation program to improve symptoms within 6 to 12 months.
2) Progressive, unremitting pain localized to the patella.
3) Inability to perform normal daily activities.
4) Expected associated pathology (i.e., osteochondral fracture, chondral fracture, or meniscal derangement).
5) Recurrent instability.

Generally, surgical intervention for malalignment is successful, with patellar instability having by far the best results. The results are not nearly as impressive when patellar pain is due to other causes. Surgery is contraindicated for sympathetic dystrophy and overuse syndromes.[31] General treatment guidelines for evaluating the patient with patellar or peripatellar pain are illustrated in Figure 11–21.

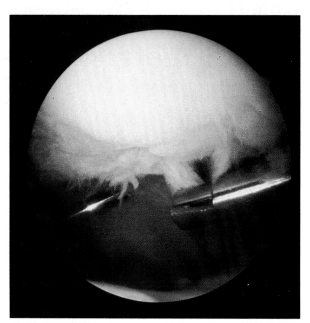

Figure 11–19
Chondromalacia, Grade III.

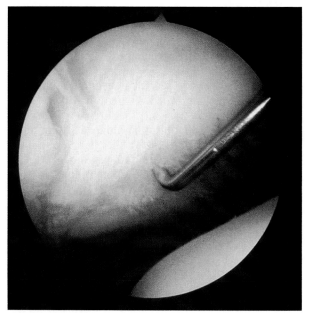

Figure 11–20
Chondromalacia, Grade IV.

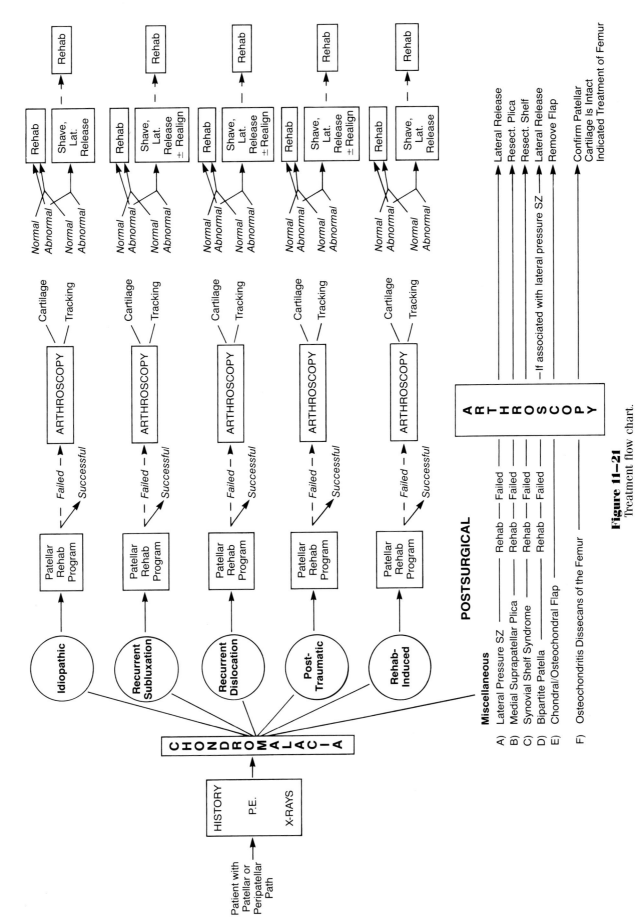

Figure 11-21
Treatment flow chart.

165

Arthroscopic Treatment of Chondromalacia

PATELLAR AND FEMORAL GROOVE SHAVINGS AND DEBRIDEMENT

This remains a controversial topic. Renewed interest in shaving has surfaced following new advances in arthroscopic instrumentation. Many investigators have found that removal of fibrillated and damaged areas of cartilage is advantageous to the patient's recovery.[29,46,52] Wissinger noted excellent results with removal of intra-articular debris in a prospective study of 100 patients.[61] Ogilvie-Harris and Jackson described the efficacy of patellar shavings, especially in post-traumatic chondromalacia with no evidence of malalignment. The technique of patellar shaving involves excision of damaged and fibrillated cartilage with the use of an arthroscopic shaver. Care must be taken to avoid accidental removal of normal articular cartilage. At completion, a relatively smooth cartilage surface that does not violate the subchondral bone is desirable, and copious lavage to remove debris is recommended. Besides removal of destructive collagenases, one of the main, and probably most important, benefits of patellar shaving is the elimination of articular cartilage flaps as mechanical factors that may aggravate the problem. The question arises, "Which grade of chondromalacia is most amenable to shaving and debridement?" Grade I should be left alone. Grade II, when it occurs in the area of the central ridge, and Grade IV, when there is irregular diseased articular cartilage remaining, may require debridement if clinical judgment so indicates. In most cases, Grade III with fissuring and flap formation falls into the category of the treatable group. The healing potential of the different histologic zones of articular cartilage is reviewed in other segments of this book. Overall, results of our debridements have been unpredictable.

LOCAL EXCISION OF THE DEFECT

This arthroscopic technique involves removal of the cartilage defect to the level of the subchondral plate and drilling of the subchondral plate to expose the cancellous portion of the patella. Care must be taken to lavage the joint copiously to remove all debris from drilling. Childers and Ellwood, using an open technique, reported that good-to-excellent results were recorded in patients under 30 years old, but less favorable results were noted in patients over 30 years of age.[8] This method is specifically useful in the treatment of isolated grade IV chondromalacia not secondary to malalignment. Our overall surgical experience with this stage of the disease is limited and not very favorable. We have had no experience with nor have plans for the use of abrasion chondroplasty.

ARTHROSCOPIC LATERAL RETINACULAR RELEASE (ALRR)

Principal indications for ALRR include malalignment with recurrent subluxation and dislocation of the patella not responding to a structured rest and rehabilitative program. Congenital dislocation, lateral facet pressure syndrome,[34] and bipartite patella associated with lateral pressure syndrome are relative indications.

The diagnosis of patellar instability is made by a positive history of dislocation laterally with manual or spontaneous relocation. Subluxation is a more subtle entity. A precise history with the description of a "catching" sensation, "giving way," or anteromedial knee pain is usually given. Physical findings of apprehension, medial retinacular discomfort, or abnormal tracking through a range of motion may be present. This may or may not be accompanied by abnormal radiologic findings previously described.

Excessive lateral facet compression syndrome, as described by Ficat and Hungerford[19] and Larson and associates,[34] results in increased pressure on the lateral facet and decreased pressure on the medial facet. This may be caused by shortening or fibrosis of the lateral structures or abnormal insertion of the iliotibial band. The rationale of the ALRR is to release the tight, tethering lateral retinacular structures to improve seating and tracking of the patella in the femoral trochlea. Accurate evaluation, diagnosis, and operative technique will yield the best results.

The technique of arthroscopic lateral release discussed and illustrated is a modification of the techniques described by Fox and Ferkel.[20] A comprehensive understanding of the equipment and technique is necessary before the procedure is undertaken. The procedure is performed without a leg holder to facilitate evaluation of patellofemoral relationships through a complete range of motion. General anesthesia is preferred due to the use of electrosurgical instrumentation. A pneumatic tourniquet is secured on the upper thigh but not inflated. Standard prepping and draping is completed per routine. Through a superomedial portal, a large in-flow cannula (4 mm) is inserted; the diagnostic arthroscope is inserted through the standard anterolateral portal. A thorough arthroscopic examination is completed, with special consideration given to patellofemoral tracking, lateral facet compression, and areas of chondromalacia. Usually, the nature of the patellofemoral disorder has been documented preoperatively and arthroscopy assumes a confirmatory or qualitative role.

After confirmation of the germane pathology, the arthroscope is transferred to the anteromedial portal and a spinal needle is inserted approximately 2 cm proximal to the superolateral margin of the patella. This needle helps orient the surgeon during the re-

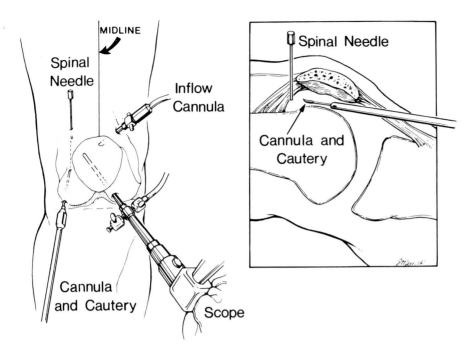

Figure 11–22
The portal and instrument locations with the Fox technique of arthroscopic lateral release.

lease. A surgical cannula is inserted into the anterolateral portal (it is sometimes necessary to enlarge this portal to improve mobility), and the electrolytic irrigation solution is changed to nonconductive sterile water (Fig. 11–22). The joint is suctioned free of electrolytic solution and irrigated with sterile water. The electrocautery unit is dialed to the appropriate setting, preferably the lowest cutting and coagulation setting to minimize tissue damage. The lateral release is begun at the musculotendinous junction of the vastus lateralis, usually at the superolateral border of the patella. The synovium and lateral capsule ligaments are sequentially transected. The release progresses distally approximately 1 cm from the bony patellar edge.

During this proximal release, the superolateral geniculate artery is often encountered; however, visualization and coagulation are usually attainable. Other vessels are visualized and coagulated to enhance visualization. If voluminous bleeding is encountered, inflate the tourniquet, use coagulation, and sequentially obtain hemostasis. Once hemostasis is maintained, deflate the tourniquet.

As the release proceeds externally, subcutaneous fat is encountered. It is very important to maintain this layer because of its insulating properties. As the release is carried distally, it is paramount to release the bands of capsular or ligamentous structures running from the inferolateral pole of the patella to the lateral tibial plateau (Fig. 11–23). Adequate release is verified by digitally everting the patella to 90 degrees, that is, the lateral border of the patella points straight up from the femoral notch (Fig. 11–24). Occasionally it is necessary to perform a small arthrot-

omy through the anterolateral portal to complete the distal portion of the release.

An alternative method was described by Schreiber, in which a proximal superomedial portal was used so

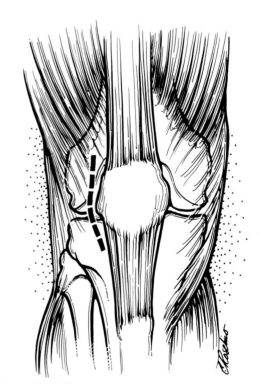

Figure 11–23
The lateral release extends approximately from the superolateral border of the patella distally to the lateral aspect of the patellar tendon.

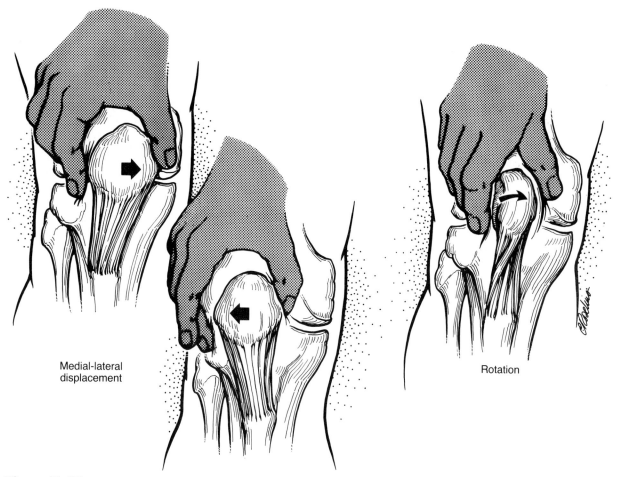

Medial-lateral displacement

Rotation

Figure 11–24
The lateral release is complete when the lateral aspect of the patella can be rotated 90 degrees to a point anterior with the medial facet in contact with the intercondylar notch.

that the arthroscope would approximate the midline at the 25-degree angle, and the tip of the arthroscope would center 1 cm proximal to the femoral groove.[54] The skin entry point is estimated by using a sterile goniometer to measure the angle; the point is usually 6 cm (2.5 inches) proximal to and in line with the medial edge of the patella (Fig. 11–25). The supero-medial portal is initially used for inflow, and the standard anteromedial and anterolateral portals are used to examine the knee. The arthroscope is then switched to the superomedial portal while sterile water is introduced for inflow through the antero-medial portal. The anterolateral portal is used for the electrosurgical arthroscopy electrode. The remainder of the procedure is similar to the previously described modified technique of Fox and Friedman.[20] The theoretical advantages of this approach are a better estimation of patellar tracking and improved visualization to ensure completion of the distal portion of the lateral release.

Arthroscopic lateral release has gained popularity in parallel with the improvement in arthroscopic technique and instrumentation. Diagnostic arthroscopy, evaluating the patellar articular cartilage and patellofemoral tracking in association with an arthroscopic lateral release, has been described by many investigators.[2,4,21,25,39,42,44,46]

Recently, Sherman and colleagues reviewed electrosurgical ALRR in 39 patients (45 knees) with recurrent patellar subluxation or dislocation (average follow-up, 28 months).[57] They state that this technique yields results comparable with those of open extensive realignment and avoids the complications inherent to lateral release, particularly hematoma and hemarthrosis. This series did show significant quadriceps weakness by isokinetic testing in two thirds of the patients. Three patients had marked weakness and were unable to generate sufficient torque to make a reliable comparison. Schonholtz and associates, in a retrospective study of 22 patients (average age, 22 years) after ALRR, concluded that ALRR is a reasonable initial step in the surgical treatment of patellar dislocation or subluxation resistant to conservative treatment.[53] It is interesting

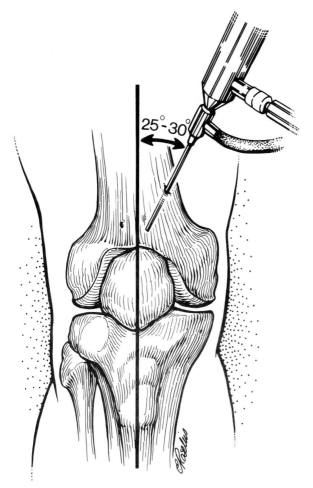

Figure 11–25
The Schreiber technique of arthroscopic lateral release, with the arthroscope in a superior medial patellar position.

that satisfactory results were obtained in 11 of 22 knees (50 per cent). Six of eight (75 per cent) dislocators and four of seven (56 per cent) subluxators were improved. On the other hand, only one of seven patients (14 per cent) with pain without instability was improved. Micheli and Stanitski, assessing functional and anatomic criteria, noted an overall excellent or good result in 76.7 per cent following open release in 33 young patients (average age, 18 years) for symptomatic patellalgia not responsive to conservative measures.[43] Also, benefits of the procedure long-term tended to remain at the same level without decline as noted 3 months postoperatively. Henry and associates, contrasting arthroscopic lateral release with open patellofemoral reconstruction in 100 patients (average age, 28 years), reported that the ALRR involves less surgery and that the patient's improvement parallels that of patellofemoral reconstruction.[25] They recommend that if the patient does not improve after ALRR, patellofemoral reconstruction should be considered. Henry's arthroscopic series, performed without electrosurgery, had a complication rate of 13 per cent. There were nine

hematomas and four cases of sympathetic dystrophy. Additionally, this series showed no correlation between surgical results and degree of chondromalacia. Metcalf[42] and McGinty and McCarthy[39] reported 86 per cent and 82 per cent good-to-excellent results using an ALRR technique in similar groups of patients (average age, 18 years). They conjointly emphasized the importance of an aggressive postoperative rehabilitation program.

Complications during and after ALRR, although rare, sometimes are debilitating. Intraoperative complications include:

(1) Too-high power setting, causing skin burns, especially if digital pressure is applied over the skin.[20]

(2) Poor electrocautery insulation, located at the hub of the contact point; this will produce sparking external to the joint and skin blistering.[20]

(3) Compartment syndrome due to extravasation of subcutaneous fluid.[57]

The most common postoperative complication of ALRR is hematoma/hemarthrosis.[25,42,44,46] Other complications occasionally reported are deep venous thrombosis,[4,39] pulmonary emboli,[39] reflex sympathetic dystrophy,[39] rupture of the quadriceps tendon,[3] and adhesions.[57] Recently, Hughston and Deese studied the status of 54 patients post-ALRR for failure to improve or worsening of their preoperative symptoms.[27] With surprise, they noted 30 patients with medial subluxation after ALRR (Fig. 11–26). This complication was previously unreported. CT scan evaluation demonstrated severe atrophy and retraction of the vastus lateralis muscle, with loss of this dynamic lateral stabilizer contributing to the medial subluxation. Teitge likewise has reported on a series of patients with medial patellar instability, both as a primary disorder and secondary to surgery.[59]

We strongly concur with Hughston and Teitge that ALRR be preceded by a documented cause of injury, a diagnosis, and a trial of supervised conservative treatment. This regimen should be specifically rendered by the orthopedist who is anticipating surgery on the knee.

Postoperative Program for ALRR

The institution of an aggressive rehabilitation program is linked to the achievement of a good result. Therefore, active range of motion and exercise programs are started immediately. The knee is held in 30° of flexion when not being exercised for the first few weeks. Most patients use crutches for 1 to 3 weeks. Approximately 75 per cent of the patients achieve an active arc of 0 to 90 degrees of flexion 1 week postoperatively; a few patients require aspiration for recalcitrant hemarthrosis. Continued therapy

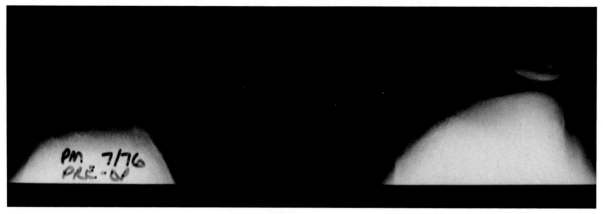

Figure 11–26
Medial subluxation of the patella in a postoperative patient with a lateral release.

is a necessity to re-establish the dynamic equilibrium of the hamstrings and quadriceps and to ensure range of motion, power, and endurance.

Many investigators have reported a high percentage of good-to-excellent results with ALRR for a variety of pathologic lesions associated with the patellofemoral joint, especially malalignment syndromes.[4,25,39,42–44,46,47,53,57] However, none have reported specifically on the results of a population with high-demand activities after ALRR in their studies. We concur that, for activities of daily living, ALRR will produce these percentages of good-to-excellent results. However, we think from our clinical experience that high-demand, elite athletes and individuals involved with physically demanding activities do not fare as well as other populations. Therefore, we recommend that any enthusiasm for similar results concerning ALRR in this latter group be dampened till shown otherwise. The question arises as to whether there is a long-term strength loss of the extensor mechanism from the incision into and diminished vector component of the vastus lateralis muscle tendon retinaculum unit. Additionally, we do not recommend the procedure for anterior knee pain syndrome.

In summary, ALRR is an effective procedure when appropriately performed, but it is only one of a spectrum of approaches to the complex issue of extensor mechanism problems and malalignment. No surgical treatment or an open surgical approach often may be the only reasonable alternatives to a given problem in a patient.

ARTHROSCOPIC REPAIR OF MEDIAL RETINACULUM AND ALRR

Controversy surrounds treatment of acute dislocations of the patella. Studies by Cofield and Bryan[9] and Power[50] on the natural history of acute patellar

dislocation revealed a 52 to 56 per cent recurrence rate.

Dainer and colleagues, in 1988, reviewed 29 cases undergoing arthroscopy after acute traumatic patellar dislocation.[14] Twenty-five of twenty-nine patients were noted to have significant osteochondral free fragments in the joint. Additional treatment consisted of 15 lateral releases. The lateral release group had 73 per cent good-to-excellent results with four recurrences, compared with 93 per cent with no recurrence in the group without release. The conclusion of the authors was that realignment and lateral release procedures are not warranted in acute traumatic dislocations. Our experience with arthroscopy in this group is limited and, overall, most patients have done well with closed treatment without significant clinical problems from loose fragments.

Detrisac and associates recently reported on 77 patients with arthroscopic patellar realignments consisting of arthroscopic lateral release and arthroscopic medial capsular imbrication; 80 per cent had no recurrence at a minimum of 1 year of follow-up.[18] They feel that the procedure allows monitoring of the surgical correction and patellar tracking intraoperatively.

Yamamoto described an arthroscopic medial capsular-retinacular repair and lateral retinacular release on 30 cases of documented lateral dislocation without prior patellar instability.[62] Follow-up was from 1 to 7 years with "gratifying" results in all instances with the exception of one traumatic redislocation. Although Yamamoto proposes that this technique provides early accurate diagnosis and early restoration of normal anatomy, we have no experience in its application or efficacy. We have continued to perform appropriate open proximal and distal realignment procedures when indicated.

PLICA SYNDROME

The medial synovial plica, as alluded to earlier, is a rare but accepted source of peripatellar pain, snapping, giving way, or pseudolocking. These symptoms may lead the clinician to suspect meniscal, anterior cruciate ligament, or patellar pathology. Trauma is commonly associated with this syndrome; however, strenuous athletics (i.e., basketball) also play a role by converting a normal elastic plica into an inflamed, thickened, nonelastic pathologic plica.[49] If the plica is large enough, it will impinge on the medial femoral condyle during flexion and sometimes, over a long period of time, produce a notch in the medial femoral condyle (Fig. 11–27). The plica does not have to contact the medial femoral condyle to produce symptoms. The tethering effect of the fibrotic plica may interfere with normal quadriceps function and place excessive traction on its synovial insertions, which are rich in nerve endings.[5] The treatment is arthroscopic excision. Some debate exists over simple excision that is sometimes followed by recurrence of symptoms, or radical excision down to the subcutaneous fat, which may cause a tight, fibrous cicatrix.[15] Removal of a 1-cm segment down to but not including the synovial wall, as advocated by Dandy,[15] is probably sufficient. This is probably an overdone operative procedure.

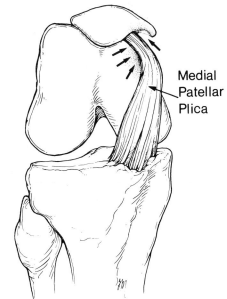

Medial Patellar Plica

Figure 11–27
The medial fibrotic plica can impinge on the medial femoral condyle and create symptoms as well as alter patellofemoral tracking.

Summary

It is obvious that an abundance of anomalies exists to explain peripatellar and patellar pathology. Careful history, physical examination, and radiologic review will usually allow an accurate diagnosis. The arthroscope has become an important adjunct not only in the diagnosis but also in the surgical treatment of patellofemoral problems. It is hoped that this chapter will provide a basic foundation for the clinician to understand the arthroscopic diagnosis and possible management alternatives of patellofemoral disorders and to administer treatment wisely.

References

1. Baumgartl F: Das Krieglenk. Berlin, Springer-Verlag, 1944.
2. Bently G: The surgical treatment of chondromalacia patellae. J Bone Joint Surg 60B:74, 1978.
3. Blasier RB, Ciullo JV: Rupture of the quadriceps tendon after arthroscopic lateral release. J Arthros Rel Surg 4:262, 1986.
3a. Blumensaat C: Die Lageabweichungen und Verrenkungen der Kniescheibe. Ergebn d Chir u Orthop 31:149–223, 1938.
4. Bray RC, et al: Arthroscopic lateral release for anterior knee pain: A study comparing patients who are claiming Worker's Compensation with those who are not. J Arthros Rel Surg 3(4):237, 1987.
5. Broom MJ, Fulkerson JP: The plica syndrome: A new perspective. Orthop Clin North Am 17:2, 1986.
6. Carson WG, et al: Patellofemoral disorders: Physical and radiographic evaluation. Clin Orthop 185:178, 1984.
7. Casscells SW: The arthroscope in the diagnosis of disorders of the patellofemoral joint. Clin Orthop 144:45, 1979.
8. Childers JC, Ellwood SC: Partial chondrectomy and subchondral bone drilling for chondromalacia. Clin Orthop 144:114, 1979.

9. Cofield RH, Bryan RS: Acute dislocation of the patella: Results of treatment. J Trauma 17(7):526, 1977.
10. Cox JJ: Chondromalacia of the patella: A review and update. Part I. Contemp Orthop 6:6, 1983.
11. Cox JJ: Chondromalacia of the patella: A review and update, Part II. Contemp Orthop 7:1, 1983.
12. Crenshaw AH: Campbell's Operative Orthopaedics. 7th ed. St. Louis, CV Mosby, 1987.
13. Cross MC, Waldrop J: The patella index as a guide to the understanding and diagnosis of patellofemoral instability. Clin Orthop 110:174, 1976.
14. Dainer RD, Barrack RL, Alexander AH, Buckley SL: Arthroscopy in acute patellar dislocations. Presentation at Annual Meeting of the Arthroscopy Association of North America, Washington, DC, March, 1988.
15. Dandy DJ: Arthroscopy in the treatment of young patients with anterior knee pain. Orthop Clin North Am 17(2):221, 1986.
16. DeHaven KE, Dolan WA, Mayer PJ: Chondromalacia patellae in athletes: Clinical presentation and conservative management. Am J Sports Med 7:5, 1979.
17. Delgado-Martins H: A study of the position of the patellae using computerized tomography. J Bone Joint Surg 61B:443, 1979.
18. Detrisac DA, Austin MD, Johnson LL: Arthroscopic patellar realignment. Presentation at Annual Meeting of the Arthroscopy Association of North America, Washington, DC, March, 1988.
19. Ficat RP, Hungerford DS: Disorders of the Patellofemoral Joint. Baltimore, Williams & Wilkins, 1977.
20. Fox JM, Ferkel RD: Use of electrosurgery and arthroscopic surgery. *In* Parisien J (ed): Arthroscopic Surgery. New York, McGraw-Hill, 1988, pp 315–330.
21. Fulkerson JP, Schutzer SF: After failure of conservative treatment for painful patellofemoral malalignment: Lateral release or realignment? Orthop Clin North Am 17:283, 1986.
22. Fulkerson JP, Schutzer SF, Ramsby GR, Bernstein RA: Computerized tomography of the patellofemoral joint before and after lateral release or realignment. J Arthros Rel Surg 3:19, 1987.
23. Goodfellow J, Hungerford DS, Woods C: Patellofemoral joint mechanics and pathology. J Bone Joint Surg 58B:921, 1976.
24. Gruber MA: The conservative treatment of chondromalacia patella. Orthop Clin North Am 10:105, 1979.
25. Henry JH, Goletz TH, Williamson B: Lateral retinacular release in patellofemoral subluxation. Am J Sports Med 14:121, 1986.
26. Hughston JC: Subluxation of the patella. J Bone Joint Surg 50A:1103, 1968.
27. Hughston JC, Deese M: Medial subluxation of the patella as a complication of lateral retinacular release. Am J Sports Med 16: 383–388, 1988.
28. Hughston JC, Walsh WM, Puddu G: Patellar Subluxation and Dislocation. Philadelphia, WB Saunders, 1984.
29. Insall J: Patellar pain: Current concept review. J Bone Joint Surg 64A:147, 1983.
30. Insall J, Goldberg V, Salvati E: Recurrent dislocation and the high riding patella. Clin Orthop 88:67, 1972.
31. Insall J, Salvati E: Patella position in the normal knee joint. Radiology 101:101, 1974.
32. Labelle H, Laurin CA: Radiological investigation of normal and abnormal patellae. J Bone Joint Surg 57B:530, 1976.
33. Larson RL: Subluxation and dislocation of the patella. *In* Kennedy JC (ed): The Injured Adolescent Knee. Baltimore, Williams & Wilkins, 1979, pp 161–204.
34. Larson RL, et al: The patellar compression syndrome. Clin Orthop 134:158, 1978.
35. Laurin CA, Dussault R, Levesque HP: The tangential x-ray investigation of the patellofemoral joint: X-ray technique, diagnostic criteria and their interpretation. Clin Orthop 144:16, 1979.
36. Laurin CA, Levesque HP, Dussault R, Labelle H, Peides JP: The abnormal lateral patellofemoral angle. J Bone Joint Surg 60A:55, 1978.
37. Lund F, Nilsson B: Arthroscopy of the patellofemoral joint. Acta Orthop Scand 51:297, 1980.
38. Martinez S, Korobkin M, Fondren F, Hedlund L, Goldner JL: Computed tomography of a normal patellofemoral joint. Invest Radiol 18:249, 1983.
39. McGinty JB, McCarthy JC: Endoscopic lateral retinacular release: A preliminary report. Clin Orthop 158:120, 1981.
40. Merchant AC, Mercer RL: Lateral release of the patella. Clin Orthop 103:40, 1974.
41. Merchant AC, Mercer RL, Jacobsen RH, Coal CR: Roentgenographic analysis of patellofemoral congruence. J Bone Joint Surg 56A:1391, 1974.
42. Metcalf RW: An arthroscopic method of lateral release of the subluxating or dislocating patella. Clin Orthop 167:9, 1983.
43. Micheli LJ, Stanitski CL: Lateral patellar retinacular release. Am J Sports Med 9:30, 1981.
44. Miller K, et al: The use of electrosurgery for arthroscopic subcutaneous lateral release. Orthopaedics 5:309, 1982.
45. Nicholas JA, Hershman EB: The Lower Extremity and Spine in Sports Medicine. St. Louis, CV Mosby, 1986.
46. Ogilvie-Harris DS, Jackson RW: Arthroscopic treatment of chondromalacia patellae. J Bone Joint Surg 66B:660, 1984.
47. Osborne AH, Fulford PC: Lateral release for chondromalacia patellae. J Bone Joint Surg 64B:202, 1982.
48. Outerbridge RE: The etiology of chondromalacia patellae. J Bone Joint Surg 43B:752, 1961.

49. Pipkin G: Knee injuries. The role of suprapatellar plica and suprapatellar bursa in simulating internal derangements. Clin Orthop 74:161, 1971.
50. Power MA: Natural history of recurring dislocation of the patella. J Bone Joint Surg 59B:107, 1977.
51. Scapinelli R: Blood supply of the human patella. J Bone Joint Surg 49B:563, 1967.
52. Schonholtz GJ, Ling B: Arthroscopic chondroplasty of the patella. J Arthros Rel Surg 1:92, 1985.
53. Schonholtz GJ, et al: Lateral retinacular release of the patella. J Arthros Rel Surg 3:269, 1987.
54. Schreiber SN: Arthroscopic lateral retinacular release using a modified superomedial portal, electrosurgery, and postoperative positioning in flexion. Orthop Rev 17:375, 1988.
55. Schutzer SF, Ramsby GR, Fulkerson JP: The evaluation of patellofemoral pain using computerized tomography. Clin Orthop 204:286, 1986.
56. Scott RD: Prosthetic replacement of the patellofemoral joint. Orthop Clin North Am 10:129, 1979.
57. Sherman OH, et al: Patellar instability: Treatment by arthroscopic electrosurgical lateral release. J Arthros Rel Surg 3:152, 1978.
58. Søjbjerg JO, Lauritzen J, Hvid I, Boe S et al: Arthroscopic determination of patellofemoral malalignment. Clin Orthop 215:243, 1987.
59. Teitge RA: Personal communication. June, 1988.
60. Wiberg G: Roentgenographic and anatomic studies of the patellofemoral joint. Acta Orthop Scand 12:319, 1941.
61. Wissinger HA: Chondromalacia patellae: A non-operative program. Orthopaedics 5:315, 1982.
62. Yamamoto RK: Arthroscopic repair of the medial retinaculum and capsule in acute patellar dislocations. J Arthros Rel Surg 2:125, 1986.

12

Kelly G. Vince

Osteochondritis Dissecans of the Knee

Osteochondritis dissecans is a condition of disputed etiology that involves the development of a focal area of radiolucent subchondral bone adjacent to but not always extending up to the articular margin. In some cases this piece of bone may detach from the surrounding osseous tissue and form a loose body together with the overlying cartilage. The cartilage remains normal until it detaches or deforms, at which time degeneration may occur. The condition is not primarily a disorder of articular cartilage.

The term *osteochondritis dissecans* is attributed to Konig who, in 1887, described "corpora mobile" of the knee.[61] He hypothesized that trauma produced osseous necrosis followed by "dissecting inflammation" that produced a loose body. Other writers have taken exception to the older term, preferring instead *osteochondrosis dissecans*.[79,92,100] *Osteochondritis* is regarded by some as a misnomer since the pathology is that of a "reparative rather than an inflammatory process."[73] Throughout the literature both names are used to describe the same clinical entity.

Sir James Paget described the condition in 1870 as the result of "quiet necrosis of bone."[98] Paget acknowledged that the idea of localized osteonecrosis causing intra-articular loose bodies had already been suggested by Broca, Lebert, and Klein.[73] The origins of loose bodies in the knee and other joints was debated exhaustively in the German literature during the early part of this century. Nagura has published a scholarly chronicle of this debate with a detailed bibliography.[88] Numerous etiologies for this disorder have been proposed and can be grouped into four categories: direct trauma, indirect trauma, ischemia, and constitutional. Before they can be discussed meaningfully, however, osteochondritis dissecans should be distinguished from other similar conditions.

Although some similarities in anatomic location of occurrence, theories of etiology, and clinical presen-

tation may exist between osteochondritis dissecans and osteonecrosis, the differences are of greater significance. Ischemia has been proposed as a cause common to both, but Aichroth points out that when loose bodies result from both conditions, the craters that are left behind are quite different.[4] Gross dissection at the time of arthrotomy shows that osteochondritis leaves a defect of vascularized bone in relatively close proximity to the fragments[4] even if separation occurs through a thin layer of ischemic bone.[44] By comparison, large amounts of surrounding bone are avascular in osteonecrosis[4] (Fig. 12–1).

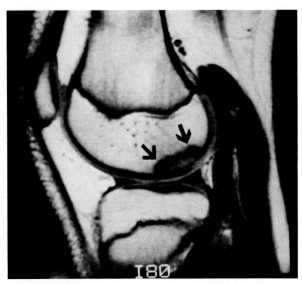

Figure 12–1

Magnetic resonance imaging (MRI) of the knee of a 24 year old man with insidious onset of knee pain and stiffness due to osteochondritis dissecans. A relatively large lesion of the posterior femoral condyles is apparent (arrows). The affected area, however, is circumscribed, unlike the case with osteonecrosis. Note the excellent depiction of articular cartilage with MRI.

Osteochondritis dissecans tends to occur in younger, more active individuals,[3,4] whereas osteonecrosis occurs either in specific risk groups (patients on steroid therapy, caisson workers, diabetics) or spontaneously in older patients as an "idiopathic" disorder (Fig. 12–2).[1,2,111]

Osteochondritis dissecans should be distinguished from fresh osteochondral[3,59,76,94] or chondral fractures,[41] such as occur in conjunction with patellar dislocation[53] and ruptures of the anterior cruciate ligament.[26,93] These lesions are definite sequelae of trauma; this cannot be stated conclusively of osteochondritis dissecans. The osteochondral-fracture fragments separate immediately at the time of trauma, whereas formation of loose bodies in osteochondritis dissecans occurs gradually.[44]

A relationship between osteochondritis dissecans and radiographic irregularities of ossification of the distal femoral epiphysis has not been completely determined. Clearly, however, irregularities of ossification of the distal femoral epiphysis, which are said to be extremely common in people under the age of 10 years, should not be confused with or treated like symptomatic osteochondritis dissecans.[15,87,112,128,135] This distinction is explored further in the discussion of etiology.

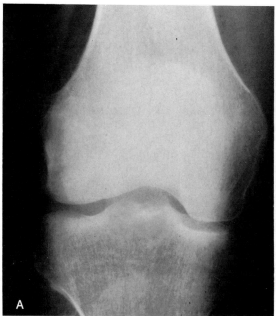

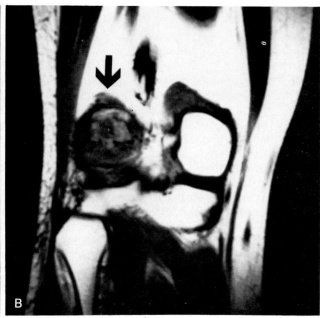

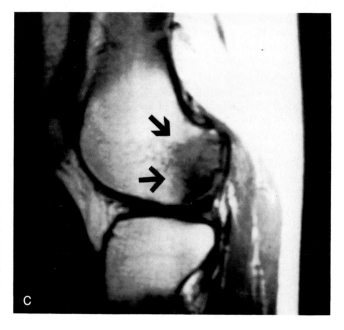

Figure 12–2

A, Anteroposterior radiograph of 39 year old woman with diabetes and spontaneous onset of knee pain. The diagnosis of osteonecrosis is not apparent. B, Anteroposterior section of MRI of the same patient, showing extensive involvement of the lateral femoral condyle with osteonecrosis. C, Sagittal MRI showing extensive involvement of bone by osteonecrosis. Compare this with Figure 12–1, an example of osteochondritis dissecans.

Table 12–1
Physical Finding in Osteochondritis Dissecans[56]*

	PER CENT
Joint line tenderness	46
Effusion	44
Palpable loose body	22
Grating	21
Locked knee	11
Decreased motion	5

*Patients past age of epiphyseal closure predominate.

DIAGNOSIS

Osteochondritis dissecans occurs most commonly in the knee but can affect other joints. It usually occurs during the first half of the second decade of life but may also affect young adults. The incidence of osteochondritis dissecans in individuals under the age of 30 years is probably at least twice that in the over-30 age group.[117] Most clinical studies identify a higher proportion of males than females affected with the disorder.[3,4,44,56,87] Pain, sometimes accompanied by an effusion, develops insidiously and is aggravated by physical activity. It is generally low grade. If irregularities of the articular surface overlying the lesion develop, or if an osteochondral fragment breaks off and becomes a loose body, then mechanical symptoms of joint locking, painful buckling, instability, and articular degeneration may ensue.[13]

Physical examination may confirm stiffness in association with the other findings of a knee effusion. The most consistent physical finding among juveniles is thigh muscle atrophy.[45,87] Physical findings are more frequent in study groups that have a majority of patients past the age of epiphyseal closure[56,113] (Table 12–1).

There can be localized tenderness to palpation of the flexed knee directly over the site of the lesion, if accessible, on the distal femoral condyle. Sometimes, to avoid painful impingement of a lesion situated on the lateral aspect of the medial femoral condyle against the tibial eminence, a patient may walk with the tibia externally rotated.[21,114] Wilson has described a sign in which pain is produced in a flexed knee when it is internally rotated and then extended slowly, if osteochondritis is present in the most common location—the lateral aspect of the medial femoral condyle. A positive sign is confirmed if the pain is relieved by external tibial rotation.[6] The diagnosis is apparent on radiographs that demonstrate the typical crescent radiolucency in the subchondral area. Radiologic investigation should include anteroposterior, lateral, tunnel, and merchant[80] views of the knee,[101] to evaluate the locations where osteochondritis and other potential causes of symptoms may be found.

The classic location of osteochondritis dissecans is the intercondylar area of the medial femoral condyle: the incidence is 47 to 75 per cent of cases[3,4,44,56,66–68,87] (Table 12–2). Outerbridge described 14 patients (16 knees) with osteochondritis dissecans affecting the posterior femoral condyle.[96] These lesions tended to be large and occurred equally on the posterior aspects of the medial and lateral condyles. The age at onset was typical of osteochondritis dissecans in other locations. Hughston and associates also distinguished between lesions on the most distal, weight-bearing part of the femoral condyle and those that occurred posteriorly. They found that the great majority of defects on the medial femoral condyle occurred distally (67 of 69), whereas lesions of the lateral condyle were equally distributed between posterior and distal locations. A minority of defects on both condyles was large and extended from the distal surface to the posterior condyle.[56]

Osteochondritis dissecans also has been observed on the patella[4,28,122] and the lateral femoral trochlea.[8,85] Some care should be taken in calling lesions of the patello-femoral joint true osteochondritis dissecans, because of the possibility that they may be osteochondral fractures resulting from patellar instability. Osteochondritis dissecans also has been reported to occur on the tibial plateau.[127]

Imaging techniques other than plain radiographs

Table 12.2
Location of Osteochondritis Dissecans of the Knee

	MUBAREK[87] (1981) (%)	AICHROTH[3] (1971) (%)	HUGHSTON[56] (1984) (%)	GREEN[44] (1966) (%)	(1977) (%)	LINDEN[67] (ADULT)	(CHILD)
Medial Femoral Condyle							
Intercondylar area	62	75	47	74	59	59	57
Weight-bearing area	Nil	10	33	12	17	17	30
Lateral Femoral Condyle							
Intercondylar area	0	0	1	0	11	11	9
Weight-bearing area	22	10	17	14	13	13	4
Patella	16	5	0	0	0	0	0

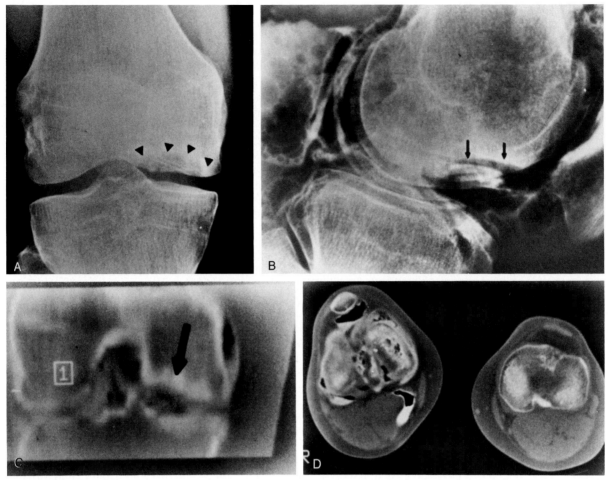

Figure 12–3

A, Anteroposterior radiograph of 19 year old boy with a large, well circumscribed defect of the medial femoral condyle caused by osteochondritis dissecans (arrows). Mechanical symptoms of locking and buckling have developed. *B*, Double-contrast arthrogram demonstrating the articular cartilage defect (arrows) in this patient. *C*, Computed tomography (CT) reconstruction shows the articular defect, but with resolution inferior to MRI. CT arthrogram cross-section demonstrating extensive involvement of the right femoral condyle in the same patient. (Courtesy of Dr. John Insall, The Hospital for Special Surgery.)

have been used to diagnose, stage, or distinguish osteochondritis dissecans from other lesions. Arthrography can be very helpful in assessing the integrity of cartilage overlying the lesion[133] (Fig. 12–3). Conventional scintigraphy is sensitive but does not readily discriminate between osteochondritis dissecans and other lesions in the differential diagnosis. Cahill and Berg have used scintigraphy to stage lesions, evaluate healing, and plan surgery. They also feel it discriminates true osteochondritis dissecans from ossification defects.[16] Litchman and colleagues used a computerized refinement of scintigraphy (computerized blood flow analysis) to provide a quantitative analysis of regional blood flow. This technique gave information about the healing potential of osteochondritis dissecans.[73]

To date, literature on the application of magnetic resonance imaging (MRI) to osteochondritis dis-

secans has been limited.[9,81,84] It provides a highly satisfactory depiction of articular cartilage overlying specific lesions,[9] usually with adequate resolution to determine the extent of cartilage disruption.[81] Because MRI gives excellent information regarding medullary bone, it is extremely useful in differentiating osteochondritis dissecans from osteonecrosis. Osteonecrosis typically produces very extensive, diffuse areas of decreased signal over an entire condyle, whereas osteochondritis dissecans creates more focal involvement (see Figs. 12–1 and 12–2). No literature exists as yet that clearly distinguishes osteochondritis dissecans from osteochondral fractures on MRI.

Arthroscopy has been used in the diagnosis of osteochondritis dissecans. Some investigators described it as useful in avoiding arthrotomy[124,138] and identifying concomitant pathology.[33] Arthroscopy has been used to evaluate the healing of lesions treated surgically[12,33] and in this respect may assist in planning rehabilitation postsurgery. Generally speaking, however, the role of simple diagnostic arthroscopy has been contracted, if not eliminated, while the capability of treating osteochondritis dissecans by arthroscopy has expanded.

PATHOLOGY AND STAGING

Whatever its etiology, osteochondritis dissecans appears to be a progressive phenomenon that may eventually produce an intra-articular loose body. As such, staging is useful to understand the natural history of the disorder, to evaluate the effectiveness of treatment, and to establish prognosis. The most basic type of staging divides patients according to age. Some writers have appropriately defined their study groups as including only children, or "juvenile osteochondritis dissecans."[11,16,45,87] With or without treatment, the natural history of osteochondritis dissecans is worse in a postadolescent or adult population than in a younger group.[56,67] In a study of 40 knees with osteochondritis dissecans that developed in adulthood, Linden found that signs and symptoms of osteoarthritis developed in every knee.[67]

Pappas described three treatment categories based on the patient's age, because of the correlation with healing capacity.[100] Category I comprises children up to skeletal age 11 years for girls and 13 years for boys, who usually present with mild symptoms related to activity. Lesions may be incidental findings and are more frequently bilateral in this group. The capacity for healing is excellent. Category II includes girls of skeletal age 12 years and boys of skeletal age 14 years to about age 20 years for both sexes. The integrity of the fragment and the condition of the cartilage may be in question; treatment depends on these variables. Category III includes patients aged 20 years and older who are likely to have more severely disrupted lesions and a poor prognosis.

Osteochondritis dissecans may be staged anatomically according to the progression of the lesion. In the literature antedating arthroscopy, three stages were described.[22] Stage I is a lesion that is well formed in bone and apparent on radiographs. The overlying articular cartilage remains intact. Visualization of the joint surface would reveal little or no abnormality at this stage, but direct digital palpation would locate spongy areas that compress more easily than adjacent cartilage, with solid bone underneath (Fig. 12–4A).

Stage II lesions have some articular surface defect. The lesion, though held in place by a band of tissue, may be capable of significant rotational and translational motion. Symptoms of buckling or locking may occur. This stage was subdivided by Guhl (Fig. 12–4B) based on the degree of separation observed at arthroscopy.[47–51] Subsequent investigators have

adopted the new system.[33] Guhl's Stage II is characterized by *early separation,* with a break in the articular cartilage from which fibrous tissue protrudes. His Stage III is a *partially detached* lesion usually held only by a hinge of articular cartilage. The fragment may be completely displaced from the crater despite the hinge. Lesions that Guhl calls Stage IV are identical to what Conway originally called Stage III: completely detached from their osseous bed with completely loose bodies (Fig. 12–4C). A crater filled with fibrous tissue is left. A further stage has been used by some to depict the development of degenerative changes on the opposite joint surface[8] (Fig. 12–4D).

Outerbridge combined the concepts of age and morphology to establish guidelines for treatment of osteochondritis dissecans affecting the posterior condyles. He felt that Group I included patients from the time of onset of symptoms until age 15 years, that Group II included patients from that age until the fragment separated, and that Group III, with the worst prognosis, included all patients with separated fragments.[96]

Chiroff and Cooke made the point that the microscopic pathology of osteochondritis dissecans differs depending upon the stage of the lesion.[20] This is useful to bear in mind when assessing pathologic studies that are used in support of a specific theory of etiology. Chiroff and Cooke examined Conway's Stage II (Fig. 12–4B) osteochondritis lesions from six patients aged 13 to 29 years. The hyaline cartilage and underlying bone were viable in all cases. Repair and resorption were apparent in the osseous nucleus, with bone and cartilage formation predominating in the deeper portions adjacent to the osseous beds. The beds were composed of mesenchymal tissue in varying stages of differentiation, from very primitive, spindling fibrous tissues to histologically normal fibrocartilage. The appearance suggested an ongoing maturation process. At least part of the bone in the base of the lesion had resulted from endochondral ossification. Chiroff and Cooke felt that at least some of the bone of the ossific nucleus was newly formed and not merely separated from the femoral condyle by trauma. No evidence of osteonecrosis was seen in any lesion. One large, informative review article erroneously cited Chiroff and Cooke's work in support of the statement that "the underlying bone pathology presents findings consistent with focal avascular osteonecrosis followed by repair or nonunion with occasional separation of the fragment."[100] Although this is consistent with the findings of Linden,[67] as well as those of Green and Banks,[45] it is not supported by Chiroff and Cooke who, in fact, reported no osteonecrosis. Milgram, in a study of 50 specimens, noted avascular necrosis of bone inconsistently and did not feel that bone death was responsible for the lesions.[83]

Nagura described the histology from one case in which he removed a (Conway Stage III) lesion from

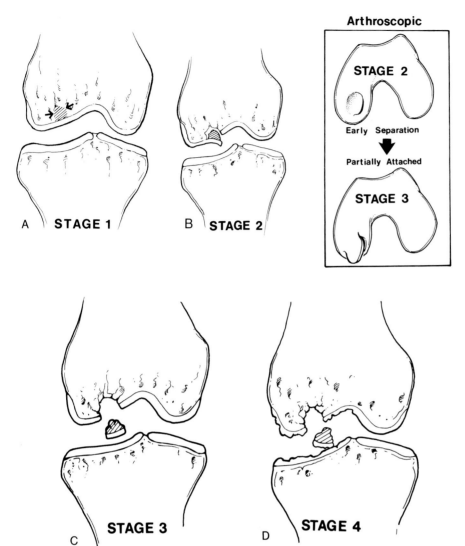

Figure 12–4

A, A Stage I (Conway and Guhl) lesion is well formed in bone and apparent on radiographs. The overlying articular cartilage is intact. *B*, A Stage II (Conway) articular surface defect is present, but no loose body has formed. Conway did not distinguish degrees of separation. The lesion, though held in place by at least a band of tissue, may rotate and cause locking. (*Inset*) Stages II and III (Guhl). The advent of arthroscopy enabled the original Conway Stage II to be divided by degree of separation. *C*, A Stage III (Conway) and Stage IV (Guhl) loose body broken off in the joint, leaving a crater. *D*, Stage IV (Bayne) degenerative joint disease developed on the adjacent articular surface. These stages depict the natural history of osteochondritis dissecans. Although Stage I lesions may sometimes heal, once progression to Stage II occurs degenerative joint disease is almost inevitable.

the distal humerus of a 23-year-old laborer. Bone and cartilage in the detached piece were "markedly changed," giving the appearance of regressive changes including "fissures, bruising, and bone death." Tissue from the bed was quite different, characterized by Nagura as a reparative response to an interruption in the continuity of subchondral bone, i.e., fracture healing.[88] Most investigators consider that the tissue in loose bodies is viable to some degree. Whereas the bone may sometimes, but not invariably, die,[21] the cartilage can proliferate because of synovial nutrition.[21,36,82,103]

The pathologic appearance of Stage I osteochondritis dissecans has not been reported. The aforementioned different histology may have resulted from examining different stages, including some that have already suffered degenerative joint disease. The later stages of the disorder have been better characterized than the early phases; unfortunately, it is the early phases that would probably contain the most useful information regarding the etiology of the disorder.

Caffey and associates were impressed with the frequency of marginal irregular ossification of the distal femoral epiphyses in healthy children,[15] a finding also noted by others.[29,119] They conducted a radiographic study to document normal patterns of ossification and found that "the margins of the ossification centers were more commonly irregular than smooth." They divided these irregularities into three groups. Group I had varying degrees of roughening of the margins, occasionally with small separate foci of calcification just beyond the roughened edge of the main center. Group II had larger, localized marginal irregularities in the form of indentations. Group III had irregularities of the same kind as Group II except that there was an independent island of bone in the marginal crater. They felt that the uneven marginal ossification in the femoral condyle was a feature of healthy endochondral bone formation. At what point, if any, these lesions may progress to a symptomatic osteochondritis dissecans is the subject of controversy.

ETIOLOGY

The etiology of osteochondritis dissecans has been debated, at a sophisticated level, for well over a century in the literature of several languages.[88] This debate originated prior to roentgenograms and safe surgical treatments. Early medical thinkers tried to explain the origins of loose intra-articular bodies and had never visualized what we now recognize as the classic radiographic appearance of osteochondritis dissecans. The commonly considered theories of etiology are direct trauma, indirect trauma, ischemia, and constitutional factors.

Direct or Exogenous Trauma

The evidence that has been frequently cited in favor of direct trauma as the etiology of osteochondritis dissecans is the frequency with which patients report accidents[64] or chronic injury[13] in association with this diagnosis. One of the strongest contemporary proponents of a traumatic etiology is Aichroth, who presents supporting clinical and laboratory evidence.[3,4]

However, lesions that are undeniably of traumatic origin, such as a Colle's fracture, universally have a history of trauma. In many studies of osteochondritis dissecans, patients give a history of trauma inconsistently and sometimes report injuries that occurred up to 18 months prior to the development of symptoms. This kind of loose association is reminiscent of patients with musculoskeletal malignancy who may attribute the first appearance of a mass or pain to some recent injury.

Trauma does not easily explain multiple lesions that have been found in as many as 47 per cent of patients (Fig. 12–5).[87] Some reports claim that more patients, especially children, with osteochondritis dissecans participated in organized sports, as an indication of exogenous knee trauma.[3,4,71] Outerbridge, in a series of patients with osteochondritis dissecans of the posterior femoral condyles, found that most were of "outstanding athletic ability."[96] Mubarak and Carroll, who found that many of their patients with osteochondritis dissecans reported some recent trauma, also established a control group to determine the incidence of sports participation in the general adolescent population. They found that 48 per cent of patients and 44 per cent of controls participated in some form of organized sports and discounted the effect of athletic trauma.[87]

Interesting laboratory experiments have been done to test the theory of a traumatic etiology, but a satisfactory animal model has never really been created. Clanton and Delee[21] cited the experimental studies of Rehbein,[105] who subjected the anterior aspect of the knees of dogs to repeated minor trauma. Rehbein produced lesions resembling osteochondritis dis-

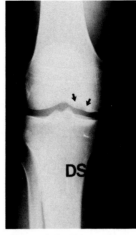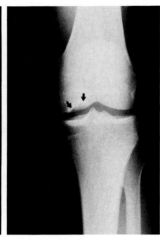

Figure 12–5

Symmetric lesions of osteochondritis dissecans in an adolescent. Vague aching pain, worse in the left knee, was associated with activity. The pains resolved with nonsurgical treatment. (Courtesy of Dr. James Tibone.)

secans by histology and radiography. No loose bodies resulted, however. Using mathematical models and energy estimates led to the conclusion that the force necessary to produce lesions resembling osteochondritis dissecans exceeded that which was likely to occur clinically.[14] Lesions resembling osteochondritis dissecans have been produced by cutting segments of articular cartilage in young rabbits, leaving the cartilage attached to synovium in the joint and then replacing the piece into its bed.[3,4,55,62,125] Theoretically, neglected chondral injuries in early childhood may produce ossification defects and, eventually, osteochondritis dissecans.[55]

Osteochondritis dissecans tends to occur in the same parts of the knee. This consistency is not easily explained by random exogenous trauma. The fact that in the early stages the articular cartilage overlying the lesion remains intact is also unlikely to happen as the result of trauma.[20] Two groups of investigators were unable to produce a fracture of the subchondral bone experimentally without also fracturing the overlying articular cartilage.[9,18]

Indirect or Endogenous Trauma

Some manifestations of osteochondritis dissecans become more plausible when a mechanism of endogenous or internal trauma is postulated.

Fairbanks first suggested that the typical lesion might result from impingement of the tibial spine on the lateral aspect of the medial femoral condyle during internal rotation of the tibia.[34] This mechanism (the basis for Wilson's sign[136]) was supported by Smillie[117] but disputed by Green, who showed cases of incomplete fragment separation, noting that the *intact* cartilage lay on the side of the fragment *clos-*

est to the tibial spine.[44] The medial tibial spine is larger than the lateral spine around age 12 years and can abut on the lateral or intercondylar aspect of the medial femoral condyle—the classic location.[34,38,117] By grading the prominence of tibial spines,[42] Mubarek and Carroll found that a minority of their juvenile patients with osteochondritis dissecans had prominent spines, but half of these patients did not have the osteochondritis defect in the predicted, classic spot. Instead, it was on the patella or the lateral condyle.[87]

Other supporters of the theory of endogenous trauma indicate that the medial facet of the patella articulates only with the posterolateral aspect of the medial femoral condyle at 135 degrees of flexion.[3,43] Presumably, repeated trauma between patella and femur might produce the lesion of osteochondritis dissecans: a type of fatigue failure. Factors such as patellar instability, meniscal tears, knee ligament laxity, and genu recurvatum have been implicated in the causation of osteochondritis by contributing to a mechanism of endogenous trauma.[3,4,117]

It should be remembered in this discussion that a distinction between osteochondritis dissecans and osteochondral fracture has been assumed. Trauma, endogenously or exogenously applied, can result in damage to the articular cartilage and underlying bone. It may be that osteochondritis results from the nonunion of undisplaced osteochondral fractures,[110] a view that has also been suggested by others.[55,62,88,125]

Ischemia

One of the strongest contemporary proponents of ischemia as the major factor leading to osteochondritis dissecans is Enneking.[30,31] Comparing the blood supply of subchondral bone to that of the bowel mesentery with its end arterial arcade and poorly developed anastomoses, he concluded that embolic obstruction creates wedge-shaped areas of bone necrosis immediately below the articular cartilage. The lesion may heal spontaneously, or, if the overlying cartilage is disrupted traumatically, a loose body may be produced.

Ischemia has been proposed as the etiology of osteochondritis dissecans for many years. Nagura details the long history of this debate from Broca, who proposed "spontaneous necrosis of part of the protective cartilage of the joint surface" in 1854.[88] Blockage of end-arteries by tubercle bacilli,[7] fat emboli,[107] and thrombosis[132] all have been suggested. Watson-Jones, proposing thrombosis, sought an explanation for the many cases he saw with either multiple site involvement or no history of antecedent trauma.[132]

The work of Rogers and Gladstone, demonstrating abundant blood supply to subchondral bone, has cast doubt upon ischemia as a cause of osteochondritis

dissecans.[109] It is well recognized that osteonecrosis results from ischemia. Whether of the spontaneous, idiopathic type[2] or in association with caisson, Gaucher's, or sickle cell disease, osteonecrosis can cause lesions of bone that later result in degenerative joint disease. As indicated earlier, these diseases are different from osteochondritis dissecans. Ficat and colleagues illustrated this distinction by demonstrating increased marrow pressure and circulatory obstruction in patients with osteonecrosis—findings that were absent with osteochondritis dissecans.[35] Lesions caused by ischemia are more extensive and lead to osseous collapse rather than to production of loose bodies.

Constitutional Factors

Mubarak and Carroll, in a thoughtful clinical review of children with osteochondritis dissecans, favored what they called a "constitutional" theory of etiology. They concluded that four factors might be involved in a constitutional etiology: familial occurrence, endocrine abnormalities, generalized tissue laxity, and epiphyseal abnormality.[87] The implication of this hypothesis is that the epiphyseal bone is already abnormal and that trauma plays a minor role, if any, in causation.

Familial occurrence has been noted frequently[6,10,37,39,52,86,89,92,97,104,118,120,121,126,131] in studies that are generally case reports of individual patients or pedigrees.

However, Petrie, who studied first-degree relatives of 34 patients with osteochondritis dissecans, found only one relative with the disorder.[102] Although this does not eliminate genetic influence or etiology, it does suggest that variable penetrance may occur and that clinically apparent disease may be a multifactorial event.

In a study of osteochondritis affecting the capitulum, Nielson found that 17 per cent of nearest male relatives of 80 patients with osteochondritis dissecans were also affected.[90] The true familial incidence, of course, cannot really be known unless radiographs are performed on all asymptomatic relatives. Mubarak and Carroll identified two pedigrees with autosomal dominant inheritance and associated abnormalities, such as short stature, osteochondritis dissecans of the capitellum, and patellar instability.[86]

Osteochondritis dissecans has been reported in association with other disorders such as tibia vara[126,135] and Legg-Perthes disease.[137] While one may infer a constitutional disorder in cases such as these, it is not clear that a direct genetic etiology is implied.

Mubarak and Carroll noted endocrine abnormalities in 19 per cent of the patients with osteochondritis dissecans in their review. These took the form of minor alterations in thyroid or sex hormone levels, or

Fröhlich-type body habitus.[87] Smillie also noted the association between Fröhlich syndrome and osteochondritis dissecans.[117]

Mubarak and Carroll investigated "tissue laxity" as an indication of some generalized collagen disorder. In their own study, modestly increased laxity was present occasionally.[87] Patellar instability, also observed by others in association with osteochondritis, has been used alternatively to support theories of traumatic[3,4,117] and constitutional etiologies.[87]

The collagen disorder hypothesis has been alluded to by authors who observed osteochondritis dissecans in association with Osgood-Schlatter disease[18,45,117] and nonossifying fibroma.[18] The incidence of these disorders in patients with osteochondritis dissecans, however, may not be appreciably different from that in the general population.[87]

The fourth constitutional factor is that of epiphyseal abnormalities, such as may be manifested by mild dwarfism. The association with mild dwarfism has been noted by others,[6,79,87,104,117,121,126,134] and the theory that osteochondritis dissecans may be a constitutional disorder of the epiphysis was suggested by Mau, who used the term *enchondral dysostoses.*[79] Multiple epiphyseal dysplasia (MED) should be considered in patients with osteochondritis dissecans.[21,106] Mubarak and Carroll, citing their own experience of short stature in 30 per cent of individuals affected by osteochondritis dissecans and a 47 per cent incidence of multiple lesions, feel that osteochondritis dissecans may actually be a forme fruste of epiphyseal dysplasia.[87] Others have observed a high incidence of bilateral disease in juvenile patients,[57,63] as well as multiple sites of involvement.[57] Langer and Percy support the idea that osteochondritis dissecans may be related to anomalies in the centers of ossification.[63] This idea relates to the aforementioned irregularities of ossification of the distal femoral epiphysis described by Caffey and associates.[15] Hypothetically, these irregularities may be the precursor of osteochondritis dissecans,[87,91,106,119,131] with either endogenous or exogenous trauma playing some note in the development of symptoms and loose bodies.

TREATMENT

The prognosis for any case of osteochondritis dissecans depends on the stage of the lesion, the extent of articular surface involvement,[56] and the age of the patient.[45,66,67,116,128,135] These variables have not been strictly controlled in any of the many studies of the treatment of osteochondritis dissecans. As such, it is difficult to critically evaluate different treatments that have been recommended over the last several decades.

What constitutes healing of osteochondritis dissecans? "Spontaneous resolution" may mean dissipation of symptoms with the radiographic image of osteochondritis remaining static, or dissolution of the lesion by fusion of the bone fragment to adjacent bone without trace of the previous process.[135] The former may occur relatively quickly; the latter may take years or never occur at all. Resolution of lesions has been reported,[27,74,128,135] although some confusion exists as to which cases may simply have been the normal maturation of ossification irregularities.[31,123] This decision will remain unanswered until the relationship between symptomatic osteochondritis dissecans and these irregularities is clarified. There is general agreement that younger patients are more likely to have spontaneous healing, and Van Demark aptly drew a parallel with the natural history of Legg-Perthe's disease in that respect.[128]

Stage I

Nonoperative therapy has included observation with avoidance of athletics,[135] no weight-bearing with braces or crutches, immobilization in a plaster cast, quadriceps strengthening,[45,128,135] and even complete bed rest for up to 6 months.[25] Smillie reported 32 patients, aged 10 to 28 years, in whom he found no cases of true spontaneous healing. He contended that observation alone may be dangerous by allowing progression of the lesion, and that early cases should be treated at least with immobilization.[116] This is based on the belief that osteochondritis dissecans is the result of trauma and should be treated like an osteochondral fracture. Green and Banks felt that some form of protection of the joint was necessary, based on their view that osteochondritis dissecans results from osteonecrosis and that bone collapse will lead to cartilage destruction.[45] Clearly, while the surgeon's belief about etiology will influence the choice of therapy, there seems to be progressive acceptance of conservative (or nonsurgical) treatment of early lesions in the young patient.[114]

Hughston, in a relatively large series, divided patients into conservative and surgical groups. For the conservative group, quadriceps exercises and slight modification of sports activities were prescribed. Sports were permitted if there was no discomfort or swelling in the knee joint.[56] Some activity was generally preferred because of the deleterious effects of immobilization, such as stiffness, atrophy, and possibly cartilage degeneration.[32] Surgery was recommended eventually if a bone fragment failed to heal in a crater after closure of the distal femoral epiphysis. The conservatively treated group comprised 18 patients with a mean age of 16.7 years (range, 10 to 44). Three of these patients had incidental findings on comparison radiographs made for contralateral injury. The results in this group were generally very good, due to the younger age and lesser involvement.[56] The key to good results without surgery is correct patient selection.

By contrast, once mechanical symptoms have developed (especially if disruption of the articular surface can be confirmed by magnetic resonance imaging or arthrogram), then a poor outcome is likely, and surgical intervention is generally recommended.[56,100] The types of surgical treatment, antedating arthroscopy, are drilling of lesions to promote new blood supply and healing, excision of loose bodies, curettage of the base of lesions with or without bone graft followed by fixation of fragments, and osteochondral graft reconstruction. Most but not all of these techniques have now been adapted for use with arthroscopy.[24,47–51]

Smillie was an early proponent of the efficacy of drilling through the fragment and beyond the sclerotic zone of the femoral condyle to reach a satisfactory blood supply.[115,116] This blood then fills up the space between the fragment and bone to promote healing. He felt strongly that osteochondritis dissecans represented nonunion of a fracture, and his ideas of treatment were based on established methods of treating nonunions.

Some experts recommend drilling across the cartilage, through sclerotic bone of osteochondritis dissecans, and into healthy bone even for Stage I lesions with an intact cartilage surface.[3,4,47–49,115,116] Guhl describes using this treatment under arthroscopic visualization when the knee is symptomatic, the patient is of musculoskeletal age over 12 years, and the lesion is larger than 1 centimeter over a weight-bearing surface.[49] He uses a 0.062 smooth Kirschner wire, admitted into the knee through a cannula with standard triangulation technique. The arthroscope and wire are alternated between inferolateral and inferomedial approaches to maintain drilling perpendicular to the surface of the defect. About six to eight drill holes are placed with care to avoid the weight-

bearing surfaces. The small, smooth wire is not felt to be injurious to the joint surface. These intact lesions are then maintained for 3 to 6 weeks with a nonweight-bearing cast, followed by a period of restricted activity.[49]

In 1980, Lee and Mercurio described a method of bone grafting Stage I lesions by drilling through the femoral condyle from outside the knee joint while visualizing the lesion through an arthrotomy.[65] The goal of the technique is to promote union of the fragment to the host bone without disturbing the intact articular cartilage. They recommend introducing a guide pin from the flare of the condyle across normal bone to the affected subchondral area under fluoroscopic control. A bone biopsy needle or coring device of about 50 per cent of the diameter of the lesion is introduced over the guide wire and through the lucent area of fibrocartilage. Firm, gentle counterpressure is applied to the articular surface with a finger, to prevent iatrogenic detachment of the fragment. The core of bone is removed and reversed in the drill hole such that its cancellous end bridges the fibrocartilaginous layer of the osteochondritis dissecans, and the distal end may be sent for pathology. Additional autogenous cancellous bone may be curetted from the surrounding condyle if necessary. Immobilization in plaster is required. Limited follow-up, less than 1 year's duration in each case, was provided for three patients.[65] Satisfactory results were described, without complication. A similar method has been used by others to reconstruct defects.[58]

Guhl has described another method of retrograde bone grafting, or "grafting from above" under direct arthroscopic control (Fig. 12–6).[49] In his technique, a Kirschner wire is passed from inside the knee, across the articular surface and lesion, and out through the femoral condyle. A 5-millimeter, cannu-

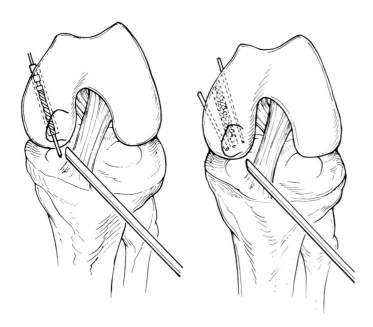

Figure 12–6

Left, Retrograde drilling of osteochondritis dissecans under arthroscopic visualization. A Kirschner guide wire is introduced across the lesion under arthroscopic control. A reamer is advanced over the guide wire and up to the lesion but not across the articular surface. Precise measurement of wire lengths or radiographic control is necessary to avoid damage to the joint surface. *Right,* The original bone core and/or cancellous chips are packed in. Kirschner wires may be required for fixation. This technique has been used (without fixation) for completely intact lesions or (with fixation) for partially detached lesions.

lated, calibrated reamer is introduced superiorly from outside the knee, over the guide wire, and down through the condyle to the articular cartilage, without broaching it.[49]

Detached Lesions

Once the articular surface has been partially or completely disrupted, the indications for surgical treatment, if not the preferred technique, become clearer. The objectives of treatment that most investigators agree on are re-establishing a fresh blood supply to the lesion by drilling or curetting the base, using bone graft to support articular fragments at a level where they are flush with adjacent cartilage, and then securely fixing the reconstruction.[72]

Fixation

Smillie popularized methods of securing partly or completely separated osteochondral fragments.[115,116] Previously, it was relatively common practice to sim-

ply excise fragments,[22] and some success has been described recently by treating even partially detached lesions in adults by arthroscopic excision.[33]

Smillie felt he could successfully replace fragments if they could be fixed solidly.[116] He had observed viable cartilage, even in completely separated loose bodies, and believed that the bone could become revascularized and heal. He worked initially with screw fixation, later abandoned because of the difficulty of insertion in favor of slender stainless steel nails measuring about 1 to 1.25 inches in length (Fig. 12–7). He designed instruments to drive and countersink these nails, which had grooves about their ends near the articular surface to facilitate removal. He advocated fixation of partially attached lesions by preserving soft tissue hinges. Access to the crater to create a vascular bed by drilling was important. Immobilization for 12 to 16 weeks with no weight bearing followed. Migration of these devices into the knee joint has been reported.[77]

Smillie-type nails and other similar forms of fixation require additional surgery for removal. Consequently, other techniques of fixation have been developed. Experimental work was reported with porous,

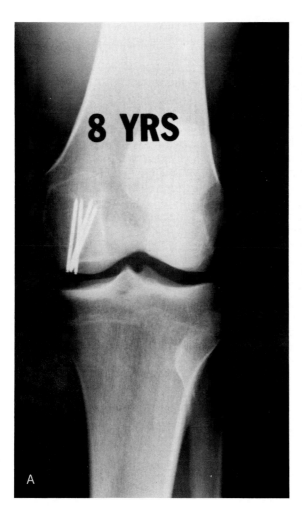

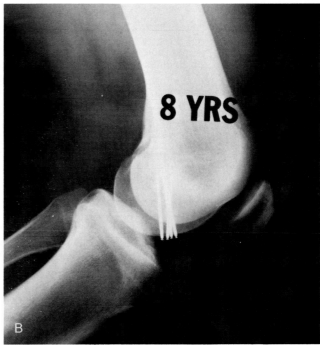

Figure 12–7

Anteroposterior (A) and lateral (B) radiographs of a 17 year old male with left knee pain, first noted after a football injury. The diagnosis was confirmed by arthroscopy and the osteochondritis dissecans was treated with arthrotomy, bone grafting, and fixation with Smillie pins as seen here. Full activities were resumed after 3 months of protected weight bearing. Eight years later, the patient had been running marathons and experienced some posterior knee pain without effusion, which resolved with decreased activity. (Courtesy of Dr. Frank Jobe.)

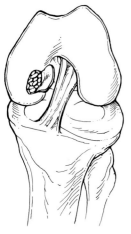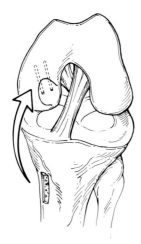

Figure 12–8

Cancellous bone grafting (left) and bone peg fixation (right) of partially detached osteochondritis dissecans. Arthrotomy was performed, with harvesting of cortical matchstick grafts from proximal tibia.

coated nails that were expected not to migrate because of bone ingrowth and so be left in situ.[17] No clinical experience with these devices was published.

It is possible to remove necrotic bone from a lesion by gaining access from the intercondyloid fossa at the time of arthrotomy. The weight-bearing surface is left intact, graft may be packed under the cartilage, and the flap can then be sutured into position.[129] Scott and Stevenson described the use of bone pegs and buried Kirschner wires for fixation, neither of which necessarily required removal.[113]

The idea of using bone pegs was mentioned in 1955 by Osborne in the discussion of a paper by Smillie.[115] Greville, in 1964, described the technique of shaping cortical strips from the proximal tibia to resemble match sticks and using them to pin fragments[46] (Fig. 12–8). This method has since been used successfully by others.[11,40,57,69,70] One of the largest series is reported by Gillespie and Day, who used the bone peg fixation technique to treat 18 defects in 17 patients.[40] They reported union in all cases with good results in 16. Their technique, endorsed by other experts,[48,49] has the advantages that second arthrotomy for removal is not necessary, pegs are easily harvested from the proximal tibial bone, and, at least theoretically, the pegs stimulate healing of the subchondral bone.

The problem of fixation that requires repeat arthrotomy for retrieval can also be solved by the use of Kirschner wires that can be pulled back out through the femoral condyle once union is achieved. Lipscomb, Jr., and colleagues acknowledged that Kirschner wires that are placed subcutaneously for easy removal had long been used to fix osteocartilaginous fractures, and they adapted the technique to osteochondritis.[72] They described the technique in six pa-

tients with follow-up of from 5 to 15 years. All fragments were loose at the time of surgery. The lesions were exposed with an arthrotomy, bleeding subchondral bone was exposed in the crater by drilling multiple small holes, and fragments were denuded of fibrous tissue on the undersurface. Cancellous bone was obtained locally for grafting when necessary. The fragment was held in place with 0.045 or 0.062 Kirschner wire drilled through the fragment and condyle until it protruded through the side of the femur. The distal ends were cut off flush with the articular surface. The wires were left in place for 3 to 16 weeks; immobilization originally was enforced for an average of 3 months. With later patients, motion and weight bearing were resumed within 3 weeks. They reported that three patients had no symptoms, physical findings, or radiographic incongruities. Three had a minimum of symptoms or signs with normal radiographs. One patient had both clinical and radiographic abnormalities, with clinical improvement as a result of treatment.

Hughston and associates used a similar technique of Kirschner wire fixation for fragments that were *partially attached*.[56] (Loose fragments were removed.) They bent the tip of the wire to 45 degrees at the end where it engaged the fragment, which could then be compressed in its crater. Wires were generally left for 6 to 8 weeks and then removed through the skin. In a detailed paper that reviews several important variables, they concluded that knees did better when the fragment was reduced than when it was excised. Generally, however, the latter group had more advanced disease at the time of treatment.

Unstable lesions (Guhl Stages II and III) may be pinned during arthroscopy. Guhl emphasizes removal of fibrous tissue from the periphery of the lesion with basket forceps or dental drill and favors the use of 9-inch long, smooth, 0.062 diameter Kirschner wires that have a raised thread over the distal 3 inches.[49] A jig or guide is useful for placement of the wires, which are eventually withdrawn in a retrograde direction through the femoral condyle until the threads disappear under the articular surface. This technique is well suited to lesions of the medial femoral condyle, but similar treatment on the lateral condyle may not be practicable (Fig. 12–9).

Following the aforementioned principles of revascularization, grafting, and fixation, Guhl reported 43 cases treated entirely via the arthroscope.[49] Some were drilled, some drilled and pinned, and others curetted and/or grafted. Thirty-four healed, eight showed evidence of healing at last follow-up, nine lacked long follow-up, and one was clearly a failure.

Restoration of a normal articular surface, where a crater is present with a loose body in the joint, is difficult. Replacing the fragment often is not feasible. Most commonly, the base of the crater is curetted to expose bleeding bone, hoping that fibrocartilage will proliferate in the defect. If fibrous healing has al-

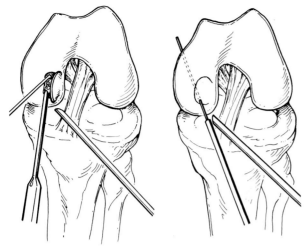

Figure 12–9

Arthroscopic curettage and drilling of partially detached osteochondritis dissecans (left). Kirschner wires for fixation are introduced across the articular surface and out through the femoral condyle to permit retrograde removal (right).

ready occurred, the lesion is left. Several writers have reported the results of curetting empty craters, usually remarking that the results in these patients are inferior to those patients in whom fragments can and have been successfully replaced.[56,96] Aichroth dissents, saying that "the results of simple excision were the same as those of internal fixation when the lesion was on the weight-bearing surface."[3]

Ewing and Voto reported a series of patients, all of whom were treated arthroscopically by excision of fragments and drilling or abrasion of the crater.[33] All the 29 patients reported on were skeletally mature. By the classification of Guhl, 3 were Stage II (early separation), 7 were Stage III (partially attached), and 19 were Grade IV (loose body with empty craters). Patients were followed on an average of 35 months (range, 11 to 75 months), and results were graded by the Lysholm/Gillquist knee rating scale.[75] Accordingly, 10 patients were excellent, 11 were good, 7 were fair, and 1 was poor. This represents a somewhat more aggressive, though simpler, technique for dealing with osteochondritis dissecans. The long-term results are unavailable.

Faced with a loose body and large crater, several clinicians have reported methods of reconstructing the defect and at times the articular surface. Guhl describes a technique, using arthroscopy, of bone grafting "from below."[49] This involves placement of a Kirschner wire into the lesion from inside the knee. A reamer is introduced over this wire and passed through the previous articular surface to a depth of about 3 centimeters. A 5-millimeter cannula is then inserted into the knee through the reamer portal and aligned with the channel that has been reamed. Can-

cellous graft, preferably from the iliac crest, is passed through the cannula into the channel and countersunk just below the level of the surrounding articular cartilage. The goal is to decrease the size of the crater and allow fibrocartilage to fill in over it, as a substitute for hyaline cartilage.

Rinaldi has described a surgical technique and set of instruments for harvesting a bone plug from the nonweight-bearing lateral femoral trochlea, with its articular cartilage intact, and then transferring it by means of a solid press fit into a cylindrical hole drilled in the crater.[108] No other fixation is used, and surgery is performed via arthrotomy. He treated patients between the ages of 17 and 35 years, reconstructing defects from 9 to 19 millimeters in diameter. Eleven of the fifteen cases were due to osteochondritis dissecans, the others due to osteochondral fracture. Patients were followed from 6 months to 2 years, and good radiographic incorporation was observed. Two patients had persistent pain and giving way at 6 months. Long-term results are not available.[108] Rinaldi cited earlier autograft reconstruction methods, using cartilage autografts from the nonweight-bearing surfaces of the femoral condyles[99,130] and from the patella.[23] Disadvantages with these procedures included the need for repeat arthrotomy to retrieve hardware.

In a paper devoted mainly to describing reconstruction of osteochondral defects resulting from osteonecrosis, Bayne and colleagues report techniques that they also used in six adult patients with osteochondritis dissecans.[8] Fresh osteochondral allografts were used in the majority of cases: four on the femur and one on the patella. All cases were Bayne Stage III: empty craters, without degenerative changes on the tibial surface. Necrotic bone was excised down to an even bed of bleeding bone and the allograft was shaped to allow a snug press fit that was secured on the femoral side with two cancellous AO screws. Of all diagnostic groups treated, those with osteochondritis dissecans and traumatic arthritis had the best results, at a mean follow-up of 4.8 years (range, 2 to 10 years).

Animal work on the reconstitution of experimental defects has included filling them with a mechanically minced preparation of autologous hyaline cartilage moistened by thrombin solution and then mixed with a fibrin adhesive. A plug of this material is compressed into the defect until it solidifies. In a rabbit model, some restitution of a quasi-"juvenile" status of new cartilage has been reported.[5] Other investigators have used periosteal grafts in animals, along with continuous passive motion, in an effort to restore articular surface defects.[95]

When osteochondritis dissecans progresses to significant degenerative joint disease, then treatment is similar to other forms of arthritis. In the appropriate circumstances, osteotomy, arthroplasty, and arthrodesis will be useful.

References

1. Aglietti P, Insall JN, Buzzi R, et al: Idiopathic osteonecrosis of the knee: Aetiology, prognosis and treatment. J Bone Joint Surg 65B:588, 1983.
2. Ahlback S, Bauer GCH, Bohne WH: Spontaneous osteonecrosis of the knee. Arthritis Rheum 11:705, 1968.
3. Aichroth PM: Osteochondritis dissecans of the knee. J Bone Joint Surg 53B:440, 1971.
4. Aichroth PM: Osteochondritis dissecans. In Insall JN (ed): Surgery of the Knee. London, Churchill Livingstone, 1984, pp 167–190.
5. Albrecht R, Roesner A, Zimmerman E: Closure of osteochondral lesions using chondral fragments and fibrin adhesive. Arch Orthop Traum Surg 101:213, 1983.
6. Andrew T, et al: Familial osteochondritis dissecans and dwarfism. Acta Orthop Scand 52:519, 1981.
7. Axhausen G: Die Aetiologie der kohlerschen Erkrankung der Metatarsalkopfchen. Beit Z Klin Chir 126:451, 1922.
8. Bayne O, Langer F, Pritzker KPH, Houpt J, Gross AE: Osteochondral allograft in the treatment of osteonecrosis of the knee. Orthop Clin North Am 16:727, 1985.
9. Berndt A, Harty M: Transchondral fractures (osteochondritis dissecans) of talus. J Bone Joint Surg 41A:988, 1959.
10. Bernstein MA: Osteochondritis dissecans. J Bone Joint Surg 7:319, 1925.
11. Bigelow DR: Juvenile osteochondritis dissecans. J Bone Joint Surg 57B:530, 1975.
12. Bots RA, Slooff TT: Arthroscopy in the evaluation of operative treatment in osteochondritis dissecans. Orthop Clin North Am 10:685, 1979.
13. Brackett EG, Hall CL: Osteochondritis dissecans. Am J Orthop Surg 15:79, 1917.
14. Buchner L, Rieger H: Können freie Gelenkkörper durch Trauma entstehen? Arch Klin Chir 116:460, 1921.
15. Caffey J, Maddell SH, Roger C, Morales P: Ossification of the distal femoral epiphysis. J Bone Joint Surg 40A:647, 1958.
16. Cahill BR, Berg BC: 99m-Technetium phosphate compound joint scintigraphy in the management of juvenile osteochondritis dissecans of the femoral condyles. Am J Sports Med 11:329, 1983.
17. Cameron HU, Pilar RM, MacNab I: Fixation of loose bodies in joints. Clin Orthop 100:309, 1974.
18. Campbell CJ, Ranawat C: Osteochondritis dissecans. The question of etiology. J Trauma 6:201, 1966.
19. Cayea PD, Pavlov H, Sherman MF, Goldman AB: Lucent articular lesion in the lateral femoral condyle: Source of patellar femoral pain in the athletic adolescent. Am J Radiol 137:1145, 1981.
20. Chiroff RT, Cooke CP III: Osteochondritis dissecans: A histologic and microradiographic analysis of surgically excised lesions. J Trauma 15:689, 1975.
21. Clanton TO, DeLee JC: Osteochondritis dissecans: History, pathophysiology and current treatment concepts. Clin Orthop 167:50, 1982.
22. Conway FM: Osteochondritis dissecans: Description of the stages of the condition and its probable traumatic etiology. Am J Surg 38:691, 1937.
23. Crova M, Gallinaro P, Lorenzi GL: Il trapianto osteocondrale di rotula nel tratamento chirurgico della osteocondrosi di ginocchio. G Ital Orthop Traumatol 3:273, 1977.
24. Debacker A, Casteleyn PP, Opdecam P: Osteochondritis dissecans of the knee: Present state: The role of arthroscopy and arthroscopic surgery. Acta Orthop Belg 49:468, 1983.
25. Decker P: Guerison d'une osteo-chondrite dissequante bilateralke du genou. Schweiz Med Wochenschr 19:221, 1938.
26. Dehaven KE: Diagnosis of acute knee injuries with hemarthrosis. Am J Sports Med 8:9, 1980.
27. Edelstein JM: Osteochondritis dissecans with spontaneous resolution. J Bone Joint Surg 36B:343, 1977.
28. Edwards DH, Bentley G: Osteochondritis dissecans patellae. J Bone Joint Surg 59B:58, 1977.
29. Elliot HC: Studies on articular cartilage. Am J Anat 58:127, 1936.
30. Enneking WF: Principles of Musculoskeletal Pathology. Gainesville, FL, Storter Printing Company, 1970, p 140.
31. Enneking WF: Clinical Musculoskeletal Pathology. Gainesville, FL, Storter Printing Company, 1977, p 147.
32. Enneking WF, Horowitz M: The intra-articular effects of immobilization on the human knee. J Bone Joint Surg 54A:973, 1972.
33. Ewing JW, Voto SJ: Arthroscopic surgical management of juvenile osteochondritis dissecans of the femoral condyles. Am J Sports Med 11:329, 1983.
34. Fairbanks HAT: Osteochondritis dissecans. Br J Surg 21:67, 1937.
35. Ficat P, Arlet J, Mazieres B: Osteochondritis and osteonecrosis of the lower end of the femur: Interest of functional investigation of the marrow. Sem Hôp Paris 51:1907, 1975.
36. Fisher AGT: A study of loose bodies composed of cartilage and bone occurring in joints. With special reference to their pathology and etiology. Br J Surg 8:493, 1921.
37. Fraser WNC: Familial osteochondritis dissecans. J Bone Joint Surg 48B:598, 1966.
38. Freiberg AH: Osteochondritis dissecans. J Bone Joint Surg 5:13, 1923.

39. Gardiner TB: Osteochondritis dissecans in three members of one family. J Bone Joint Surg 37B:139, 1955.

40. Gillespie HS, Day B: Bone peg fixation in the treatment of osteochondritis dissecans of the knee joint. Clin Orthop 143:125, 1979.

41. Gilley JS, Gelman MI, Edson DM, et al: Chondral fractures of the knee. Radiology 138:51, 1981.

42. Giorgi B: Morphological variations of the intercondylar eminence of the knee. Clin Orthop 8:209, 1956.

43. Goodfellow J, Hungerford DS, Zindel M: Patello-femoral joint mechanics and pathology. Functional anatomy of the patello-femoral joint. J Bone Joint Surg 58B:287, 1976.

44. Green JP: Osteochondritis dissecans of the knee. J Bone Joint Surg 48B:82, 1966.

45. Green W, Banks HH: Osteochondritis dissecans in children. J Bone Joint Surg 35A:26, 1953.

46. Greville NR: Osteochondritis dissecans treatment by bone peg bone grafting. South Med J 57:886, 1964.

47. Guhl J: Arthroscopic treatment of osteochondritis dissecans; Preliminary report. Orthop Clin North Am 10:671, 1979.

48. Guhl J: Arthroscopic treatment of osteochondritis dissecans. Clin Orthop 167:65, 1982.

49. Guhl J: Update in the treatment of osteochondritis dissecans. Orthopaedics 7:1744, 1984.

50. Guhl J: Osteochondritis dissecans. *In* Shahriaree H. (ed): O'Connor's Textbook of Arthroscopic Surgery. Philadelphia, JB Lippincott, 1984, p 211.

51. Guhl J: Osteochondritis dissecans. *In* Cassells SW (ed): Arthroscopy—Diagnostic and Surgical Practice. Philadelphia, Lea and Febiger, 1984, p 113.

52. Hanley WB, McKusick VA, Barranco FT: Osteochondritis dissecans with associated malformation in two brothers. A review of familial aspects. J Bone Joint Surg 49A:925, 1967.

53. Harilainen A, Myllynen P: Operative treatment in acute patellar dislocation: Radiological predisposing factors, diagnosis and results. Am J Knee Surg 1:178, 1988.

54. Hartzman S, Reicher MA, Bassett LW, Gold RH: Magnetic resonance imaging of the knee. Part II. Chronic disorders. Radiology 162:553, 1987.

55. Hidaka S, Sigioka Y, Kameyama H: Pathogenesis and treatment of osteochondritis dissecans: An experimental study on chondral and osteochondral fractures in adult and young rabbits. Nippon Seikeigeka Gakkai Zasshi 57:81, 1983.

56. Hughston JC, Hergenroeder PT, Courtenay BG: Osteochondritis dissecans of the femoral condyles. J Bone Joint Surg 66A:1340, 1984.

57. Johnson EW, McLeod TL: Osteochondral fragments of the distal end of the femur fixed with bone pegs. J Bone Joint Surg 59A:677, 1977.

58. Johnson RP, Aaberg TM: Use of retrograde bone grafting in the treatment of osseous defects of the lateral condyle of the knee. Am J Knee Surg 1:89, 1988.

59. Kennedy JC, Grainger RW, McGraw RW: Osteochondral fractures of the femoral condyles. J Bone Joint Surg 48B:436, 1966.

60. Kingston S: Magnetic resonance imaging of the abnormal knee. Am J Knee Surg 1:153, 1988.

61. Konig F: Ueber freie Korper in den Gelenken. Dtsch Z Chir 27:90, 1887–1888.

62. Langenskiold A: Can osteochondritis dissecans arise as a sequel of cartilage fracture in early childhood? Acta Chir Scand 109:204, 1955.

63. Langer F, Percy EC: Osteochondritis dissecans and anomalous centers of ossification: A review of 80 lesions in 61 patients. Can J Surg 14:208, 1971.

64. Lavner G: Osteochondritis dissecans. Am J Roentgenol 57:56, 1947.

65. Lee CK, Mercurio C: Operative treatment in osteochondritis dissecans in situ by retrograde drilling and cancellous bone graft; A preliminary report. Clin Orthop 158:129, 1981.

66. Linden B: The incidence of osteochondritis dissecans in the condyles of the femur. Acta Orthop Scand 47:664, 1976.

67. Linden B: Osteochondritis dissecans of the femoral condyles. J Bone Joint Surg 59A:769, 1977.

68. Linden B, Telhaz H: Osteochondritis dissecans. Acta Orthop Scand 48:681, 1977.

69. Lindholm S, Pylkkanen P: Internal fixation of the fragment of osteochondritis dissecans in the knee by means of bone pins. Acta Chir Scand 140:626, 1974.

70. Lindholm S, Pylkkanen P, Osterman K: Fixation of osteochondral fragments in the knee joint. Clin Orthop 126:256, 1977.

71. Lindholm TS: Osteochondritis dissecans of the knee. A clinical study. Am Chir Gynaecol Fenn 63:69, 1974.

72. Lipscomb PR Jr, Lipscomb PR Sr, Bryan RS: Osteochondritis dissecans of the knee with loose fragments. J Bone Joint Surg 60A:235, 1978.

73. Litchman HM, McCullough RW, Gandsman EJ, Schatz SL: Computerized blood flow analysis for decision making in the treatment of osteochondritis dissecans. J Pediatr Orthop 8:208, 1988.

74. Lofgren L: Spontaneous healing of osteochondritis dissecans in children and adolescents. Acta Chir Scand 106:460, 1953.

75. Lysholm J, Gillquist J: Evaluation of knee ligament surgery results with special emphasis on use of a scoring scale. Am J Sports Med 10:150, 1982.

76. Makin M: Osteochondral fracture of the lateral femoral condyle. J Bone Joint Surg 33A:262, 1951.

77. Marcus RE, Albers WE, Thompson GH: Extruded osteochondral nail: An interesting cause of knee locking. Clin Orthop 157:161, 1981.

78. Matthewson MH, Dandy DJ: Osteochondral fractures of the lateral femoral condyle. J Bone Joint Surg 60B:199, 1978.
79. Mau H: Juvenile osteochondroses—enchondral dysostoses. Clin Orthop 11:154, 1958.
80. Merchant AC, Mercer RL, Jacobsen RH, Cool CR: Roentgenographic analysis of patello-femoral congruence. J Bone Joint Surg 56A:1391, 1974.
81. Mesgarzadeh M, Sapega AA, Bonakdarpour A, Maurer AH, Moyer RA, Alburger PD: Osteochondrosis dissecans: Analysis of mechanical stability with radiography, scintigraphy and magnetic resonance imaging. Radiology 165:775, 1987.
82. Milgram JW: The development of loose bodies in human joints. Clin Orthop 124:292, 1977.
83. Milgram JW: Radiological and pathological manifestations of the distal femur. Radiology 126:305, 1978.
84. Mink JH, Reicher MA, Crues JV III: Magnetic Resonance Imaging of the Knee. New York, Raven Press, 1987. p 113.
85. Mollan RAB: Osteochondritis dissecans of the knee: A case report of an unusual lesion on the lateral femoral condyle. Acta Orthop Scand 48:517, 1977.
86. Mubarak SJ, Carroll NC: Familial osteochondritis dissecans of the knee. Clin Orthop 140:131, 1979.
87. Mubarak SJ, Carroll NC: Juvenile osteochondritis dissecans of the knee: Etiology. Clin Orthop 157:200, 1981.
88. Nagura S: The so-called osteochondritis dissecans of Konig. Clin Orthop 18:100, 1960.
89. Nicholas JA: Injuries to knee ligaments. Relationship to looseness and tightness in football players. JAMA 212:2236, 1970.
90. Nielson NA: Osteochondritis dissecans capituli humeri. Acta Orthop Scand 4:307, 1933.
91. Novotny H: Osteochondritis dissecans in two brothers. The pre- and developed state. Acta Radiol 37:493, 1952.
92. Novotny H: Preventive and conservative treatment of osteochondritis dissecans. Acta Orthop Scand 21:40, 1951.
93. Noyes FR, Bassett RW, Grood ES, Butler DL: Arthroscopy in acute traumatic hemarthrosis of the knee. Incidence of anterior cruciate tear and other injuries. J Bone Joint Surg 62A:687, 1980.
94. O'Donoghue DH: Chondral and osteochondral fractures. J Trauma 6:469, 1966.
95. O'Driscoll S, Keeley F, Salter R: The chondrogenic potential of free autogenous periosteal grafts for biological resurfacing of major full-thickness defects in joint surfaces under the influence of continuous passive motion. An experimental investigation in the rabbit. J Bone Joint Surg 68A:1017, 1986.
96. Outerbridge RE: Osteochondritis dissecans of the posterior femoral condyle. Clin Orthop 175:121, 1983.
97. Paatsama S, Rokkanen P, Jussila J: Etiological factors in osteochondritis dissecans. Acta Orthop Scand 46:906, 1975.
98. Paget J: On the production of some of the loose bodies in joints. St. Bartholomew's Hosp Rep 6:1, 1870.
99. Palazzi CS, Palazzi CC, Palazzi DAS: Osteocartilaginous autograft of the knee. Int Orthop 1:48, 1977.
100. Pappas A: Osteochondrosis dissecans. Clin Orthop 158:59, 1981.
101. Pavlov H: Radiographic examination of the knee. In Insall JN (ed): Surgery of the Knee. New York, Churchill-Livingstone, 1984, p 73.
102. Petrie PWR: Aetiology of osteochondritis dissecans. J Bone Joint Surg 59B:366, 1977.
103. Phemister DB: The causes of and changes in loose bodies arising from the articular surface of the joint. J Bone Joint Surg 6:278, 1924.
104. Pick MP: Familial osteochondritis dissecans. J Bone Joint Surg 37B:142, 1955.
105. Rehbein F: Die Entschung der Osteochondritis dissecans. Arch Klin Chir 265:69, 1950.
106. Ribbing S: The hereditary multiple epiphyseal disturbance and its consequences for the aetiogenesis of local malacias—particularly the osteochondritis dissecans. Acta Orthop 24:286, 1954.
107. Rieger H: Zur Pathogenese von Gelenkmausen. Muenchener Med Wochensch 67:719, 1920.
108. Rinaldi E: Treatment of osteochondritis dissecans and cartilaginous fractures of the knee by osteo-cartilaginous autografts. Ital J Orthop Traumatol 8:17, 1982.
109. Rogers WM, Gladstone H: Vascular foramina and arterial supply of the distal end of the femur. J Bone Joint Surg 32A:867, 1950.
110. Rosenberg NJ: Osteochondral fractures of the lateral femoral condyle. J Bone Joint Surg 46A:1013, 1964.
111. Rozing PM, Insall JN, Bohne WH: Spontaneous osteonecrosis of the knee. J Bone Joint Surg 62A:2, 1980.
112. Scheller S: Roentgenographic studies on epiphyseal growth and ossification in the knee. Acta Radiol [Suppl] 195:1, 1960.
113. Scott DJ Jr, Stevenson CA: Osteochondritis dissecans of the knee in adults. Clin Orthop 76:82, 1971.
114. Sisk TD, Canale ST: Traumatic affections of joints. In Edmonson AS, Crenshaw AH (eds): Campbell's Operative Orthopaedics. 6th ed. St. Louis, CV Mosby, 1980, pp 873–1030.
115. Smillie IS: Treatment of osteochondritis dissecans. J Bone Joint Surg 37B:723, 1955.
116. Smillie IS: Treatment of osteochondritis dissecans. J Bone Joint Surg 39B:248, 1957.
117. Smillie IS: Osteochondritis Dissecans. Edinburgh and London, E & S Livingstone, 1960.

118. Smith AD: Osteochondritis of the knee joint. A report of three cases in one family and a discussion of the etiology and treatment. J Bone Joint Surg 42A:289, 1960.

119. Sontag LW, Pyle SI: Variations in the calcification pattern in epiphysis. Am J Roentgenol Radium Ther Nucl Med 45:50, 1941.

120. Stougaard J: The hereditary factor in osteochondritis dissecans. J Bone Joint Surg 43B:256, 1961.

121. Stougaard J: Familial occurrence of osteochondritis dissecans. J Bone Joint Surg 46B:542, 1964.

122. Stougaard J: Osteochondritis dissecans of the patella. Acta Orthop Scand 45:111, 1974.

123. Strange TB: Osteochondritis dissecans. Am J Surg 63:144, 1944.

124. Suman RK, Stother IG, Illingworth G: Diagnostic arthroscopy of the knee in children. J Bone Joint Surg 66B:535, 1984.

125. Tallqvist G: The reaction to mechanical trauma in growing articular cartilage. Acta Orthop Scand [Suppl] 53, 1962.

126. Tobin WJ: Familial osteochondritis dissecans with associated tibia vara. J Bone Joint Surg 39A:1091, 1957.

127. Towbin J, Towbin R, Crawford A: Osteochondritis dissecans of the tibial plateau: A case report. J Bone Joint Surg 64A:783, 1982.

128. Van Demark RE: Osteochondritis dissecans with spontaneous healing. J Bone Joint Surg 34A:143, 1952.

129. Van der Weyer FAA: Osteochondritis dissecans. J Bone Joint Surg 46B:574, 1964.

130. Wagner H: Traitement operatoire de l'osteochondrite dissequante, cause de l'arthrite deformante du genou. Rev Chir Orthop 50:335, 1964.

131. Wagoner G, Cohn BNE: Osteochondritis dissecans. A resume of the theories of etiology and the consideration of hereditary as an etiologic factor. Arch Surg 23:1, 1931.

132. Watson-Jones R: Fractures and Joint Injuries. 4th ed. Vol 1. London, E & S Livingstone, 1952, p 97.

133. Wershba M, Dalinka MK, Coren GS, Cotler J: Double contrast knee arthrography in the evaluation of osteochondritis dissecans. Clin Orthop 107:81, 1975.

134. White J: Osteochondritis dissecans in association with dwarfism. J Bone Joint Surg 39B:261, 1957.

135. Wiberg G: Spontaneous healing of osteochondritis dissecans in the knee joint. Acta Orthop Scand 14:270, 1940.

136. Wilson JN: A diagnostic sign in osteochondritis dissecans of the knee. J Bone Joint Surg 49A:477, 1967.

137. Woodward AH, Decker JS: Osteochondritis dissecans following Legg-Perthes disease. South Med J 69:943, 1976.

138. Ziv I, Carroll NC: The role of arthroscopy in children. J Pediatr Orthop 2:243, 1982.

13
Michael A. Kelly
Christopher M. Magee

The Arthroscopic Diagnosis and Treatment of Loose Bodies

Loose bodies may occur in all joints and frequently present in the knee. They may occur as a single entity or be multiple in origin. The etiology of loose bodies is varied; a detailed evaluation is required to identify any underlying associated pathologic processes.

Arthroscopic removal of loose bodies in the knee, when successful, is a very rewarding procedure. It often can be accomplished with minimal trauma to the patient's knee and may provide a rapid resolution of symptoms. Arthroscopic techniques have reduced the postoperative rehabilitation period and often facilitated the swift recovery to normal activity.[5] Despite this fact, an ill-conceived or poorly planned surgical procedure for removal of loose bodies may prove to be a frustrating excursion for the unwary arthroscopist.

ORIGIN OF LOOSE BODIES

A frequent cause of loose bodies in the knee is a traumatic injury, either direct or indirect in nature. The injury may involve only the chondral surface of the articular cartilage, or it may be an osteochondral fracture with resulting hemarthrosis.[10,11,13,14] Paget described the production of intra-articular loose bodies following a direct joint injury in 1870.[13] Kennedy and colleagues discussed the importance of recognizing osteochondral fractures of the femoral condyles in the symptomatic adolescent knee and proposed a classification system based on the mechanism of injury[10] (Fig. 13–1).

Patella malalignment may be a source of loose body formation, especially in the younger pa-

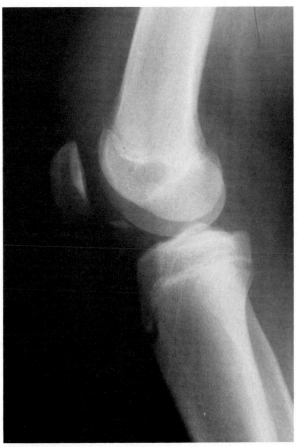

Figure 13–1
Lateral roentgenogram of a 13 year old girl with an osteochondral fracture of a lateral femoral condyle following patellar dislocation.

193

Figure 13–2
Merchant view of an acute, traumatic patellar dislocation. An osteochondral fracture of the medial patellar facet was noted at arthroscopy.

tient.[2,4,7,8] Patella subluxation or dislocation may produce either a chondral or an osteochondral fracture, commonly of the lateral femoral condyle or the medial patellar facet (Fig. 13–2).

Another cause of loose body production in the young patient is osteochondritis dissecans.[2] The etiology and arthroscopic treatment of this condition are well outlined in Chapter 12.

A common cause of loose bodies in the older patient is osteoarthritis. These particles may be numerous, and their size may vary. On occasion, the loose body may attain a very large size (Fig. 13–3).

Synovial disorders affecting the knee joint may be involved in the production of intra-articular loose bodies. Synovial chondromatosis with radiolucent loose bodies, as well as synovial osteochon-

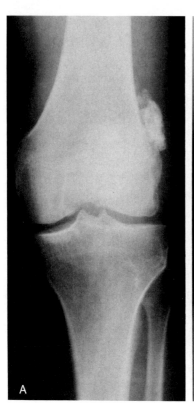
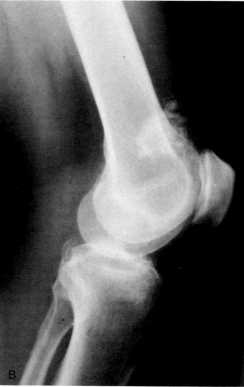

Figure 13–3
Anteroposterior (A) and lateral (B) roentgenograms of a large, osteoarthritic loose body located in the suprapatellar pouch of an elderly patient.

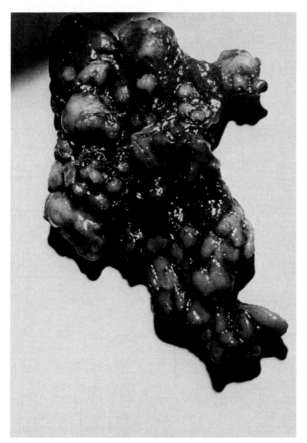

Figure 13—4
Synovial specimen of a knee with synovial chondromatosis.

dromatosis, may be a source of pathology. In synovial chondromatosis, metaplastic foci of cartilage arise de novo in the synovial membrane or subsynovial lining, and cartilaginous debris may be exuded into the joint (Fig. 13—4). Osteochondromatosis may present with multiple radiopaque loose bodies, which are occasionally located in intra-articular locations that may prove technically difficult for arthroscopic removal (Figs. 13—5 and 13—6). Rice bodies may be associated with disorders such as rheumatoid arthritis. These bodies may be multiple, radiolucent, and small. Rarely, endocrine disorders, such as gout, may be responsible for loose body formation.

Intra-articular loose bodies of meniscal origin may be produced with arthroscopic partial meniscectomy techniques. Despite advanced arthroscopic techniques, small loose meniscal fragments may persist in the joint following such procedures. The ultimate clinical outcome of such fragments is unclear. Recent experimental work on a canine model suggests a reduction in fragment size with time.[1]

A variety of foreign materials introduced into the knee may be encountered as loose bodies.[3,6,9,12] These may include pieces of glass, bullet fragments, and other metallic objects (Fig. 13—7). In addition,

arthroscopic instruments, such as knife blades, basket forceps, or even the arthroscope, may break during arthroscopic procedures and require arthroscopic removal (Fig. 13—8).

DIAGNOSIS OF A LOOSE BODY

A detailed patient history is the initial step in the diagnosis of a loose body. The history should be based on a sound understanding of the various factors involved in producing loose bodies. Frequent patient symptoms include pain and a catching or buckling sensation in the knee. These may be associated with intermittent knee effusions and the sensation of something "moving about" the knee with changing knee positions. If the loose body is of large dimensions, it may be palpable by the patient in the suprapatellar pouch. In our experience, sustained locking of the knee is uncommon.

The physical examination should include a routine, detailed inspection of the involved knee. One may palpate a large loose body, especially in the suprapatellar pouch, or localize an area of tenderness. The

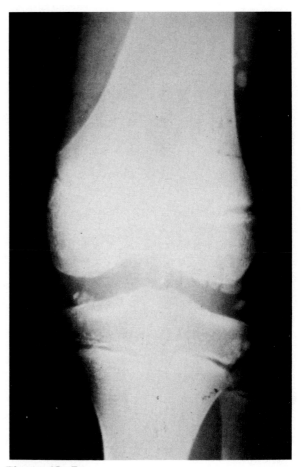

Figure 13—5
Anteroposterior roentgenogram of a knee demonstrating osteochondromatosis.

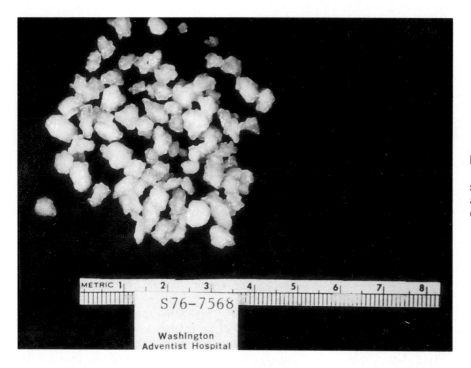

Figure 13–6
Multiple chondral and osseus fragments obtained from a knee with osteochondromatosis.

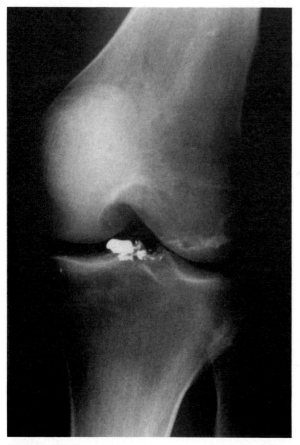

Figure 13–7
Anteroposterior roentgenogram of a knee following a gunshot wound and residual bullet fragments within the knee.

presence of an effusion or associated quadriceps atrophy should be noted. Particular attention should be paid to patellofemoral tracking in the younger patient. If the patient has any other joint complaints, a complete examination should be performed, especially if a synovial etiology is suspected. In addition, specific laboratory tests should be obtained as needed.

Routine radiographs are mandatory in the evaluation of patients. A suspected diagnosis of intra-articular loose bodies may be confirmed radiographically in approximately 70 per cent of cases.[5] Full views of the knee should be obtained, including standing anteroposterior (Fig. 13-9A), lateral (Fig. 13–9B), tunnel, and tangential patellar (Fig. 13–10) views. Oblique radiographs may be indicated in specific cases. Comparison views with previous radiographs, if available, may be helpful in evaluating any change in intra-articular location of the body. It should be remembered that a significant number of loose bodies may be radiolucent and later demonstrated at arthroscopy.

ARTHROSCOPIC REMOVAL OF LOOSE BODIES

Planning the Procedure

The initial step in the treatment of loose bodies is planning the procedure. A careful review of the preoperative radiographs is necessary. The fabella, if

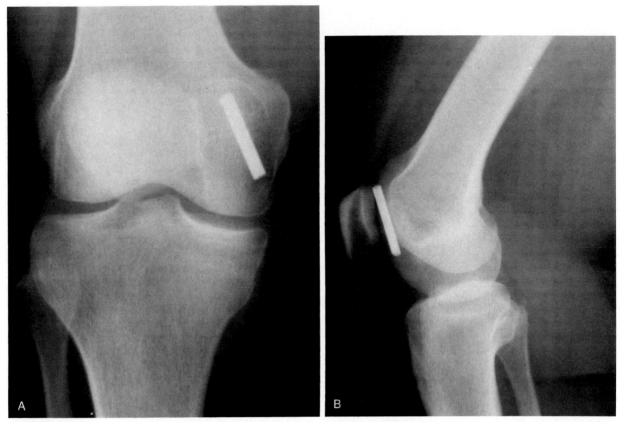

Figure 13—8
    Anteroposterior (*A*) and lateral (*B*) roentgenograms demonstrating the broken tip of an arthroscope located intra-articularly adjacent to the lateral femoral condyle. This was retrieved arthroscopically.

present, should be identified and distinguished from other calcified bodies in all views. Repeat radiographs may provide confirmation that the radiopaque bodies, if their positions have changed, are indeed floating freely within the knee joint. Single or multiple bodies also may exist within soft tissue or enclosed within bursae, making them inaccessible to arthroscopic retrieval (Fig. 13–11). At the time of arthroscopy, considerable time can be saved in the localization and retrieval of calcified loose bodies by having a C-arm x-ray or fluoroscopy machine available in the operating room. This is especially helpful when the loose bodies have migrated to an extra-articular location.

Intra-articular loose bodies have a tendency to localize to certain sites within the knee. The suprapatellar pouch, the lateral recess both above and below the lateral plica, and the posteromedial compartment are the most common locations. Gravitational pull may cause these bodies to migrate into the popliteal recess or posterior compartments of the knee. Additional sites of involvement include the interocondylar notch, beneath either meniscus, and occasionally within a popliteal or Baker's cyst (Fig. 13–12).

The arthroscopist should be familiar with the arthroscopic portals necessary to visualize the loose bodies in these various intra-articular locations be-

fore attempting the procedure. A clear understanding of the associated anatomy of the knee is quite helpful when establishing additional arthroscopic portals for loose body extraction.

Techniques of Loose Body Removal

The arthroscopic removal of loose bodies consists of three stages, as emphasized by Dandy:[3] (1) finding the loose body, (2) grasping it, and (3) extracting it. Arthroscopic visualization of the loose body is the initial step in its successful removal. This procedure may be performed under either local or general anesthesia. A tourniquet is not routinely inflated but is utilized if intraoperative visualization is compromised because of bleeding.

FINDING THE LOOSE BODY

A thorough arthroscopic examination is necessary. This often can be accomplished with the arthroscope in the standard anterolateral portal. The examination begins with the suprapatellar pouch. The pouch is examined in detail, with special attention given to the medial recess. A large loose body may be concealed in this area and difficult to visualize. The arthroscope

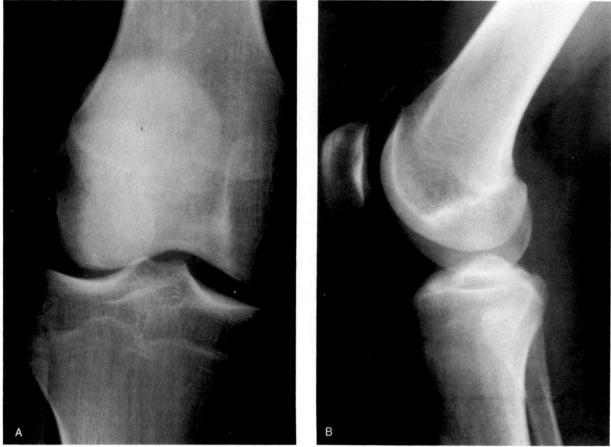

Figure 13—9
  Anteroposterior (*A*) and lateral (*B*) roentgenograms demonstrating a loose body within the suprapatellar pouch.

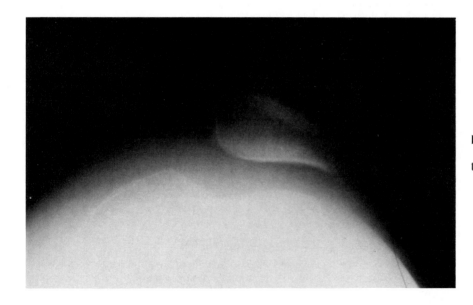

Figure 13—10
  Merchant patellar view of the knee.

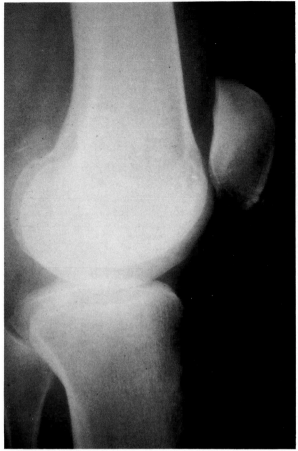

Figure 13–11
Lateral roentgenogram of a knee with multiple loose bodies in the prepatellar bursa.

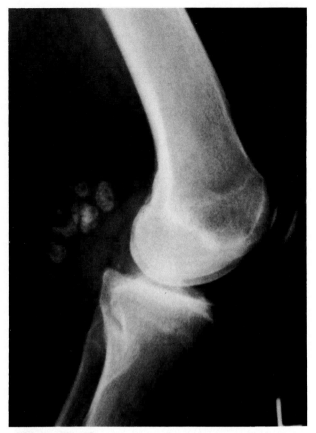

Figure 13–12
Multiple chondro-osseus loose bodies are visualized within a "Baker's" cyst on this lateral roentgenogram of the knee.

can be redirected through an anteromedial portal to search the medial recess further. The patellofemoral articulation is then examined and a careful search for evidence of possible chondral or osteochondral defects performed. This may be accomplished by rotating the 30-degree arthroscope to visualize the undersurface of the patella.

If no loose body is encountered at this stage, the examination proceeds with the lateral recess. One may "milk" the area of the popliteus tendon sheath at the time of visualization in an effort to manipulate any loose bodies into view (Fig. 13–13). Throughout this portion of the examination, care is taken to prevent any possible migration of the loose body into the posterior compartments of the knee. The medial recess is then examined.

If the loose body remains elusive at this point, the examination proceeds to the anteromedial compartment, the intercondylar notch, and the lateral compartment, in sequence (Fig. 13–14 and 13–15). The loose body may be "hiding" beneath the meniscus or entrapped within the tough ligamentous tissue or synovium within the intercondylar notch. A probe in-

serted through an anteromedial portal is essential to this portion of the examination. Visualization of a particularly stubborn loose body located in the extreme anterior aspects of the knee joint may be improved by means of a midpatellar arthroscopic portal, either medial or lateral.

The search for a loose body is not complete without examining posteromedial or posterolateral compartments (Fig. 13–16). This may be accomplished through an anterior arthroscopic portal, directing the arthroscope via the intercondylar notch into the posterior knee and using a 70-degree arthroscope to visualize the entire posterior compartment. A posteromedial portal may be best suited for localizing a loose body in this compartment if attempts from an anterior portal fail.

GRASPING THE LOOSE BODY

Grasping the fragment following localization may prove to be a frustrating task to even a seasoned arthroscopist. The removal of a large loose body from within the knee should be attempted as soon as the

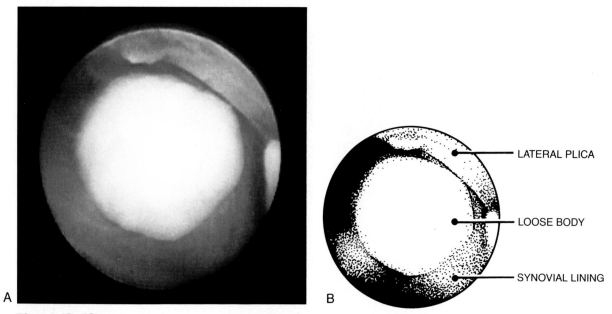

Figure 13–13
Arthroscopic view and sketch of a large, osseus loose body contained within the lateral recess of the knee.

body is encountered. This can be accomplished most easily with the outflow occluded and distention of the joint maintained with gentle inflow going through the arthroscope. Unnecessary motion of the knee should be avoided and immobilization of the loose body carried out with precise movements. When one encounters many large loose bodies, the smallest fragment should be removed first, if possible.

Loose bodies located within the suprapatellar pouch may be immobilized with external finger pressure or fixed stationary with a percutaneous needle. A locating needle is then inserted transcutaneously to mark the optimal location for placement of the suprapatellar portal. A generous portal is then established and an appropriately sized grasping instrument is inserted into the knee.

Because of the relative laxity of tissue in the suprapatellar pouch, loose bodies are most easily removed

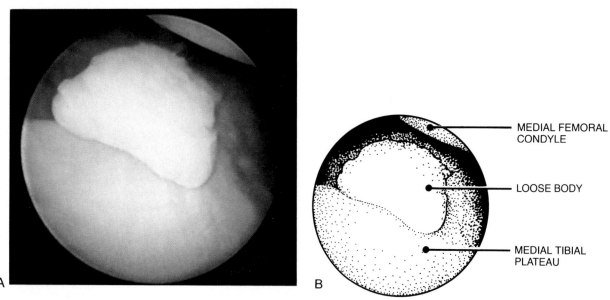

Figure 13–14
Chondro-osseus body floating within the medial compartment.

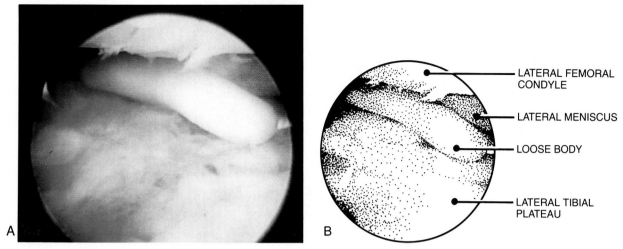

Figure 13–15
Chondral body in the lateral compartment of an arthritic knee.

through these portals. Therefore, it is most desirable if a loose body can be coaxed into the upper compartment with suction or probing. This is especially true of loose bodies within the recesses; transfixation with a percutaneous needle is especially helpful in immobilizing slippery loose bodies here.

Loose bodies in the intercondylar notch may be immobilized by the surrounding ligamentous structures. They may also be attached within the synovium and present greater difficulties during extraction. A firm hold on the fragment with the grasping instrument is essential here to avoid losing the body within the fat pad.

Loose bodies in the posterior compartments often can be visualized from an anterior portal and the grasping instruments introduced through a posterior portal. Rarely, posterior portals are required for both visualization of the loose body as well as introduction of the instruments.

A variety of arthroscopic grasping instruments is available for extrication of loose fragments from the joint. These include a 5-mm toothed loose body forceps, loose body forceps with suction, pituitary grasping forceps, and a tendon-passing forceps (Figs. 13–17, 13–18, and 13–19). A hemostat may be helpful in removing small loose bodies (Fig. 13–20). A standard motorized shaving system may be especially helpful in removing multiple small loose bodies.

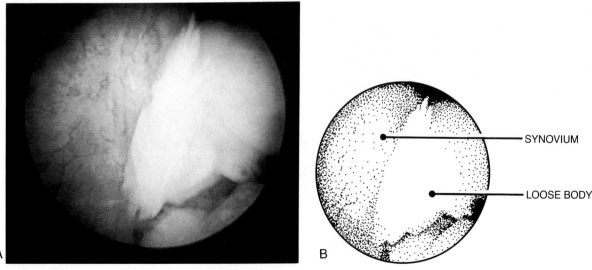

Figure 13–16
Arthroscopic view of multiple chondral fragments in the posterior compartment of the knee.

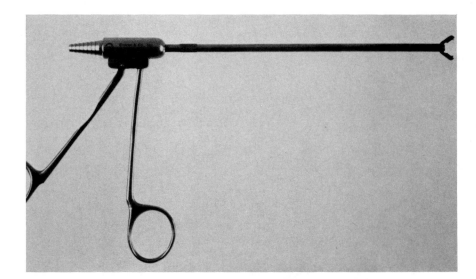

Figure 13–17
A toothed loose body forceps is available for rapid removal of loose bodies.

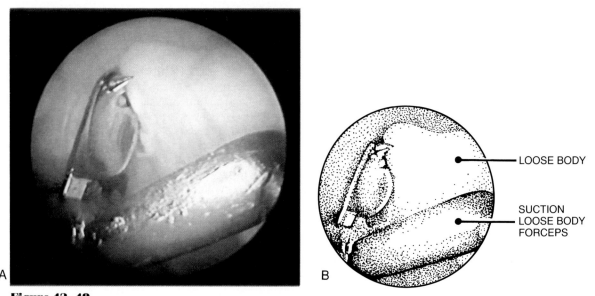

Figure 13–18
Suction loose body forceps provide for speedy localization and retrieval of a chondral loose body, as demonstrated here.

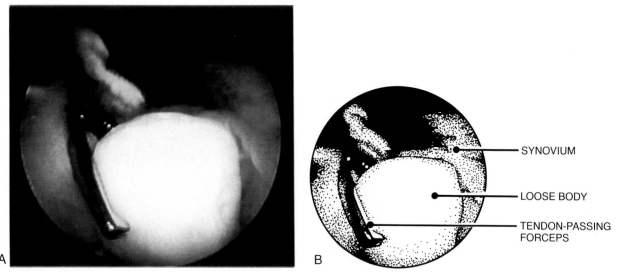

Figure 13–19
The use of a tendon-passing forceps to retrieve a single large loose body from the lateral recess of the knee.

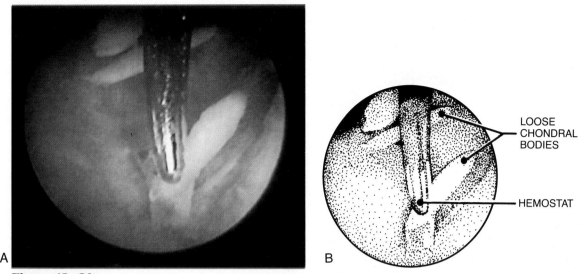

Figure 13–20
The use of a hemostat for removal of smaller chondral fragments.

REMOVING THE LOOSE BODY

The technique of loose body removal often varies with the size and location of the fragment in the knee.

Multiple small loose bodies may most easily be transported out of the knee with a flow of irrigant through a large cannula or sheath attached to suction. Similarly, a motorized shaver serves as an excellent vacuum device for extraction of multiple small bodies within the recesses of the joint (Fig. 13–21). A careful search beneath the menisci and in the popliteus sheath should always be part of this proce-dure. Additionally, the presence of multiple intra-articular loose bodies always necessitates a careful search of the posterior compartment via the inter-condylar notch of the posteromedial approach. A careful re-examination of the joint after repetitive flexion and extension may sometimes uncover some lingering fragments.

In cases of synovial osteochondromatosis, multiple loose bodies may be encountered (Fig. 13–22). Loose body removal should be accompanied by partial syno-vectomy in areas of involved synovium in which new chondral fragments appear to be developing.

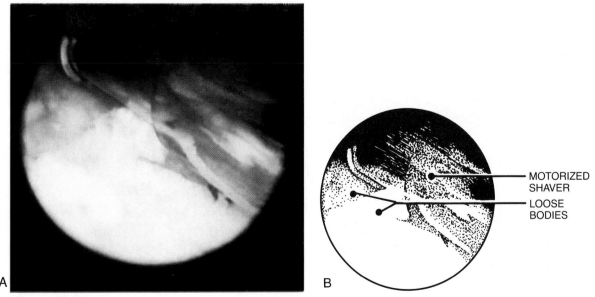

Figure 13–21
A motorized shaver is particularly useful in the rapid removal of multiple loose bodies in any compartment.

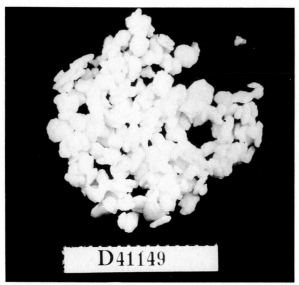

Figure 13–22
Multiple osseus bodies from synovial osteochondromatosis of the knee.

Larger loose bodies in the suprapatellar pouch or gutters are grasped firmly following immobilization. It may be necessary to enlarge the portal at the time of withdrawal of the grasping instrument (Fig. 13–23). This is best accomplished by running a scalpel along the shaft of the forceps and into the joint, being certain to incise the synovial lining. The grasper can then be withdrawn with the loose body in its jaws.

The removal of a particularly large or slippery loose body occasionally may be accomplished by "pushing" it rather than "pulling" it out of the joint.

The loose body is held firmly against the opposite wall of the knee and an exit portal of the appropriate size is established in this position to permit the fragment to be driven out of the joint. Very large loose bodies sometimes may require fragmentation and removal in piecemeal fashion.

Extraction of loose bodies from the posterior compartment presents a considerable challenge. These may be visualized with a 30-degree or a 70-degree arthroscope directed through the intercondylar notch from an anterior portal and retrieved transcutaneously through a posteromedial or posterolateral portal. Alternatively, it may be necessary to locate the fragment through a posteromedial portal and, after localization with a transcutaneous needle, make a separate posteromedial portal for grasper insertion. It is difficult to extract a loose fragment with the grasper directed through an anterior portal.

A loose body encountered in the intercondylar notch may be removed directly or by remanipulating the fragment into the suprapatellar pouch. Manipulating the fragment into the pouch facilitates its removal but does run the risk of allowing the body to escape into a less desirable location, such as the posterior compartment of the knee.

Visualization may prove difficult because of the overlying fat pad, but the loose fragment can be grasped from an anteromedial portal. Again, it is crucial to gain a firm grasp of the fragment to avoid losing it within the fat pad or subcutaneous tissues during removal.

Foreign Bodies

Foreign bodies may consist of a variety of materials, including arthroscopic instruments. A surgical

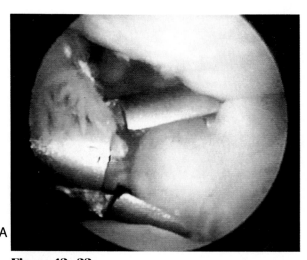

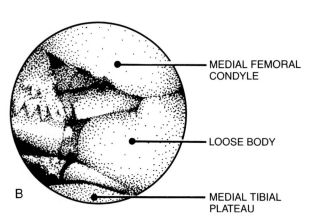

Figure 13–23
Removal of a large osseus body from the medial compartment. Extraction required enlargement of the portal, as described in the text.

instrument broken during an arthroscopic procedure is often visualized at the time of injury. The first step is to stop the irrigation inflow and outflow and maintain arthroscopic visualization. These metallic foreign bodies may be quite small and are difficult to relocate if they are lost from sight. They are most easily removed with the aid of a magnetized suction rod, such as the "golden retriever," introduced through the largest cannula available, with an associated grasper as needed.

Some foreign bodies are embedded in soft tissue and provoke a soft tissue reaction. This reactive tissue must be divided before arthroscopic removal of the object can be accomplished, which may require the introduction of additional instrumentation through a third portal.

Summary

The value of arthroscopy in the removal of loose bodies within the knee is clear. The arthroscopic procedure may be performed with minimal surgical trauma and may provide a rapid relief of symptoms. It is essential that a detailed preoperative evaluation of the patient be performed, including appropriate radiographs. The arthroscopic removal of a loose body may appear simple but can test the patience of even the experienced arthroscopist. The frustration of removing such a body often can be relieved with a careful surgical plan and a thorough understanding of arthroscopic techniques.

References

1. Agins HJ, Riddle JM, Sadasivan KK: The fate of intraarticular loose bodies of meniscus origin in canine species. Clin Orthop 209:298–312, 1986.
2. Aichroth P: Osteochondritis dissecans of the knee. *In* Insall JN (ed): Surgery of the Knee. New York, Churchill Livingstone, 1984, pp 181–188.
3. Dandy DJ: Loose bodies, foreign bodies, joint surfaces and ligaments. *In* Dandy DJ: Arthroscopic Surgery of the Knee. New York, Churchill Livingstone, 1981, pp 53–69.
4. Dandy DJ: The patellofemoral joint and loose bodies. *In* Dandy DJ: Arthroscopy of the Knee; A Diagnostic Color Atlas. Philadelphia, Lea & Febiger, 1984, pp 4.1–4.16.
5. Dandy DJ, O'Carroll PF: The removal of loose bodies from the knee under arthroscopic control. J Bone Joint Surg 64B:473–474, 1982.
6. Fergusson C, Burge P: An unusual loose body in the knee. Clin Orthop 206:233–235, 1986.
7. Johnson LL: Arthroscopic Surgery. Principles and Practice. St. Louis, Mosby, 1986, pp 704–712.
8. Joyce JJ: Surgery of loose bodies in the knee joint. *In* Casscells SW (ed): Arthroscopy; Diagnostic and Surgical Practice. Philadelphia, Lea & Febiger, 1984, pp 108–112.
9. Joyce JJ: Osteochondral loose bodies, foreign bodies, osteochondritis dissecans. *In* Parisien JS (ed): Arthroscopic Surgery. New York, McGraw-Hill, 1988, pp 173–188.
10. Kennedy JC, Grainger RW, McGraw RW: Osteochondral fractures of the femoral condyles. J Bone Joint Surg 48B:436–440, 1966.
11. Matthewson MH, Dandy DJ: Osteochondral fractures of the lateral femoral condyle. A result of indirect violence to the knee. J Bone Joint Surg 60B:199–202, 1978.
12. McGinty JB: Arthroscopic removal of loose bodies. Orthop Clin North Am 13(2):313–328, 1982.
13. Paget J: On the production of some of the loose bodies in joints. St Bartholomew's Hosp Reports 6:1, 1870.
14. Rosenberg NJ: Osteochondral fractures of the lateral femoral condyle. J Bone Joint Surg 46A:1013–1026, 1964.

Russell E. Windsor

Arthroscopic Diagnosis and Treatment of the Septic Knee

The septic knee is an orthopedic emergency that, if left untreated, poses dire consequences for its future function. Laboratory studies have shown that it is not the bacterial organism itself that causes cartilage destruction. Rather, it is the proteolytic lysosomal enzymes that are secreted by the synovial cells, polymorphonuclear leukocytes, and macrophages that migrate to the knee to combat the infection.[1-3,6,7,28,30] Thus, it is of utmost importance to treat this disorder as a true emergency so that both bacteria and these destructive enzymes may be expeditiously removed. The faster the diagnosis can be made, the quicker the treatments can commence and the best prognosis obtained for preservation of the articular cartilage and the future function of the infected knee.

The diagnosis of septic knee is made by obtaining a thorough history and performing a complete physical examination of the knee. Spontaneous sepsis of a knee more commonly occurs in the pediatric population because of the increased vascularity that is found in the physis of the proximal tibia and distal femur. In children, the knee is second only to the hip in frequency of infection. Hematogenous infection of the knee follows trauma in many cases.[4,5,9,11,21,22,24,25,29] An infected knee in this population generally presents with an acute onset of pain, swelling, and erythema; frequently the patient has a systemic feeling of malaise. The child will be irritable and have fever and chills. The erythrocyte sedimentation rate is usually elevated, but an elevated leukocyte count is not always present.[23,24,28]

In adults, on the other hand, sepsis may result from spontaneous hematogenous seeding of organisms from a remote anatomic site. Immunosuppressed patients (e.g., a steroid-dependent rheumatoid arthritic individual) are susceptible to this mode of infection. Sepsis may result from a laceration or a puncture wound that communicates with the skin. Adult joint infection most commonly affects the knee, which shows swelling, erythema, and pain. The patient may not always have fever and chills; the leukocyte count and sedimentation rate are unpredictable and are not necessarily elevated.[4,5,19,26,28] The clinician must have a high degree of suspicion that infection is present in the knee. Diagnosis is confirmed by aspiration of the joint fluid. The specimen should be sent for synovial fluid analysis, immediate Gram stain, and culture and sensitivity tests for aerobic and anaerobic bacteria, fungi, and acid-fast bacilli.

The principle of treatment of an infected knee is fast, effective decompression and drainage of all infected material, with intravenous antibiotic therapy that is specific for the organism(s) involved. A broad-spectrum antibiotic, based on the initial Gram stain, is administered immediately after the initial aspiration.[12,23] When the antibiotic sensitivities are known, the broad-spectrum agent is changed to one to which the bacteria are specifically sensitive.[12,23] Antibiotic combinations are sometimes used to obtain synergistic bactericidal effects.

The internal medicine and rheumatology literature supports repeated needle aspiration and intravenous antibiotic therapy as a method of adequately decompressing the septic knee.[10] The knee is initially immobilized; early motion begins when the symptoms improve. This method has been especially effective in gram-positive bacterial infections with high antibiotic sensitivity. The potential benefit of repeated needle aspirations and antibiotic therapy is early mobility of the knee without having to violate the extensor mechanism of the knee. However, the principal disadvantage of this procedure is that the clinician cannot be assured of complete debridement and decompression of the knee. Frequently, intra-articular fibrosis is severe, and numerous small abscesses make it impossible to decompress completely these abscess cavities by aspiration alone.

The surgical literature has supported open arthrotomy and formal debridement and irrigation of the septic joint as a means of removing bacteria and proteolytic enzymes that are present in the knee in order to preserve cartilage viability.[5–7,19] This procedure is coupled with concurrent intravenous antibiotic therapy. Postoperatively, the knee is drained for up to 72 hours until symptoms improve. Some reports favor the use of ingress/egress irrigation tubes through which antibiotic solution passes in order to sterilize the fluid within the knee.[8,19] However, this method of treatment has recently fallen out of favor since the tubes frequently became clogged and the risk was too great of infecting the knee with a more resistant organism that gained access to the knee by way of these tubes. In addition, continuous antibiotic irrigation has been shown to cause a chemical synovitis in the knee by this technique.[25]

The benefit of arthrotomy, open drainage, and irrigation of the knee is complete drainage of all infected material. However, the disadvantage of this method of treatment is that the extensor mechanism is surgically violated, which poses, postoperatively, a delay in complete return of knee motion.

Advances in the technique and instrumentation of arthroscopy over the last two decades have made it possible for the surgeon to visualize the entire knee joint.[15,16,18] Hence, arthroscopic debridement and drainage of the knee have gained considerable favor over the last few years.[8,15–18,29] This method potentially combines the benefit of early motion, which the repeated aspiration technique provides, with complete control of drainage of all abscess cavities, which formal arthrotomy ensures. The arthroscopic technique theoretically eliminates the disadvantages of those two procedures in that early motion may begin. In the laboratory, it has been shown that early motion of a septic knee is favorable, provided adequate incision and drainage of the septic knee are performed. Salter and associates showed in a rabbit model that septic knees responded favorably to early passive motion and that cartilage viability was preserved.[27]

Skyhar and Mubarak treated 15 children with arthroscopy lavage and suction drainage for several days, and all infections improved.[29] The knees demonstrated early functional recovery after a mean time of 10 days. The researchers felt that the arthroscopy caused little postoperative scarring, and they believed that motion returned quickly after the procedure. They believed, however, that the arthroscopic technique may have some limitation in knees that had severe joint loculation or fibrosis. Ivey and Clark treated 16 knees in 12 adult patients and saw the

infection eradicated in all patients, with an average of 34 months of follow-up.[14] The patients demonstrated no loss of motion or roentgenographic evidence of cartilage loss. In their series, the peripheral leukocyte count showed a mean of 9600 per cubic millimeter (range, 1300 to 20,600 per cubic millimeter). The mean sedimentation rate was 49 mm/hr (range, 18 to 78 mm/hr). The mean temperature was 38.4°C (range, 36.4 to 40.8°C).

Loss of ground substance and collagen matrix of articular cartilage through continued enzymatic activity can occur even in the absence of viable organisms. Thus, a loculated and inadequately drained joint fluid may continue to destroy the articular cartilage by enzymatic destruction. The arthroscope enables the surgeon to drain all loculated areas completely and allow for a large volume of saline irrigation to be used during the procedure.

The indication for arthroscopic decompression and irrigation lavage is an acute or chronic septic knee in an adult or pediatric population. Contraindications include a chronic infection in which a significant amount of scarring and fibrosis is suspected in a severely ankylosed knee joint.

An infected total knee replacement represents a unique challenge to the orthopedic surgeon. Early (i.e., within 3 months of implantation) and late (i.e., more than 3 months after implantation) infections of a total knee replacement cannot be readily irrigated by the arthroscopic technique for several reasons: first, it is quite difficult to maneuver the arthroscope in the knee without causing scratching of the implant, especially in a severely ankylosed knee; second, it is difficult to decompress the posterior aspect of the knee joint. On the Knee Service at The Hospital for Special Surgery, we have not had success in performing arthroscopic debridement of infected total knee replacements and have treated numerous infected total knee replacements that had failed arthroscopic debridement elsewhere.[13] In a review of 38 infected total knee replacements that underwent two-stage reimplantation, it was found that 12 knees had failed irrigation and drainage elsewhere without removal of the implant, and four of these were done by the arthroscopic technique.[13]

The best method of treating the infected total knee replacement is by formal arthrotomy, debridement, and removal of the prosthesis. However, there may be an occasion when irrigation and antibiotic suppression without removal of the implants may be done in a medically frail patient who might not be able to survive the two-stage reimplantation protocol.

TECHNIQUE

The technique of arthroscopic drainage and debridement of an infected knee is similar to the technique of arthroscopic synovectomy done for other

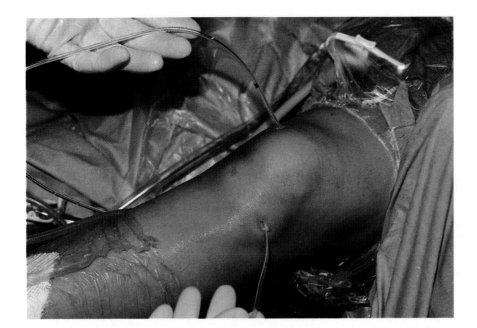

Figure 14–1
The knee is draped free to allow the use of all portals.

rheumatologic diseases. Usually, four portals are utilized, and sometimes as many as six portals may be necessary to adequately decompress all loculated areas. The leg is prepared and draped to allow exposure of the entire knee (Fig. 14–1). A superomedial portal is used for placement of the irrigation cannula, through which sterile saline solution passes through the knee and distends the joint. An inferolateral portal is used for the insertion of a 30-degree arthroscope, and an inferomedial portal is used for insertion of a probe and other rotary instruments.

The arthroscope is placed through the inferolateral portal and inserted into the suprapatellar pouch. Frequently fibrous adhesions are observed in this area, and the purulent material that is present in the knee is allowed to pass through the exit cannula that is present on the sheath of the arthroscope. If thick, fibrous adhesions are not easily decompressed with the arthroscope itself, then a basket punch or scissors can be used to excise dense, fibrous adhesions that may be present in the knee (Fig. 14–2). Alternatively, a rotary suction instrument can be placed through the inferomedial portal to excise the fibrous adhesions and remove debris by suction (Fig. 14–3*A*, *B*). Care should be taken to decompress the entire suprapatellar pouch fully. All infected synovium should be removed as well by means of a rotary suction instrument. If the suprapatellar pouch can not be completely debrided by way of the inferomedial portal, then a superolateral portal should be made to complete the debridement of this region.

After debridement of the suprapatellar pouch is completed, the arthroscope is then rotated to visualize the medial and lateral femoral gutters, and suction instruments are used, along with basket punches, to remove fibrous adhesions that may be

present in this area. The medial and lateral femorotibial joint spaces and intracondylar notch are then visualized and examined for necrotic debris. The intercondylar notch frequently will have fibrous material present on the anterior and posterior cruciate ligaments. This material, as well as the overlying synovium, should be removed as completely as possible through the anterior portals. If significant scarring and evidence of loculated abscesses are present in

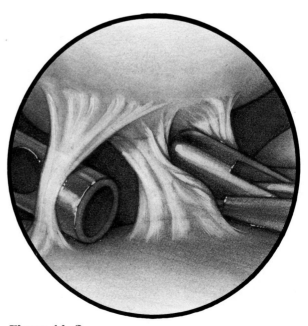

Figure 14–2
A basket punch may be used to excise dense fibrous adhesions.

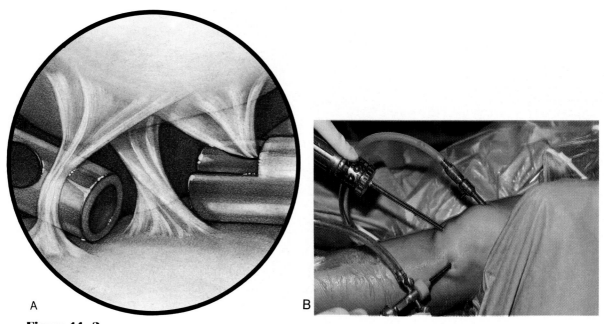

Figure 14–3

A and *B,* A rotary suction instrument can excise more friable adhesions and remove necrotic synovial tissue.

the posteromedial and posterolateral aspects of the knee, then posteromedial and posterolateral portals may be necessary to obtain adequate decompression of these areas. Care should be taken to avoid incising the medial and lateral collateral ligaments. These portals will enable the surgeon to visualize the posterior aspect of the femoral condyles and joint capsule

adequately. Usually these portals are necessary only in cases of chronic joint infection with multiloculated abscesses.

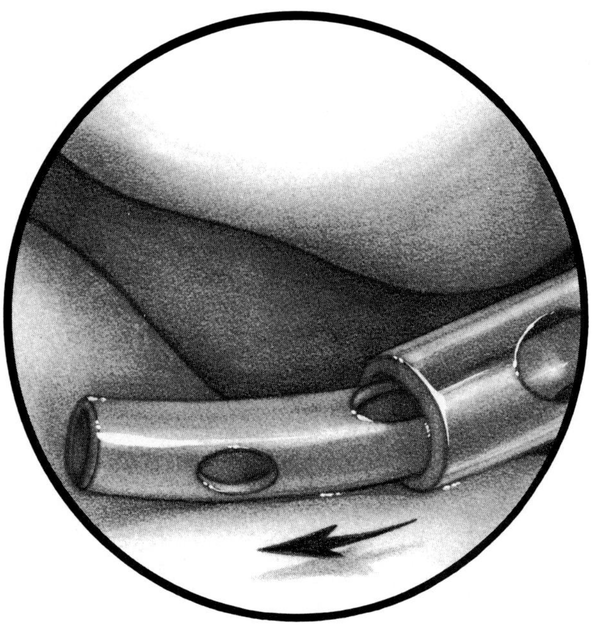

A minimum of 12 liters of saline solution is used during the procedure, and sometimes as many as 20 liters may be needed to afford complete, thorough irrigation of the knee joint. All necrotic debris and synovial tissues should be completely removed.

After the surgeon is comfortable that a complete debridement has been accomplished, suction drains are then placed into the knee under direct visualization (Fig. 14–4). The inflow cannula is disconnected from the saline solution, and a suction drain is inserted through the cannula. A grabbing forceps should be placed in the inferomedial portal to place the drain in the medial or lateral gutter (Fig. 14–5). The inflow cannula can be removed through the proximal aspect of the drainage tube, leaving the distal aspect in place within the knee (Fig. 14–6). This same technique can be used to place a second drainage tube through a superolateral portal. Alternatively, a drainage tube can be placed through the sheath of the arthroscope after it is removed (Fig. 14–7). The sheath is then withdrawn through the distal aspect of the drainage tube (Fig. 14–8). Direct visualization of this tube insertion, however, cannot be performed.

The position of the arthroscope should be freely changed from one portal to the other, if necessary, in order to carry out a complete debridement of the knee. The surgeon should not hesitate to do this if difficulty is met in obtaining full access to a particular area of the knee. The suction tubes are attached to continuous suction and are kept in place for 48 to

Figure 14–4

A suction drain is placed through the inflow cannula under arthroscopic visualization.

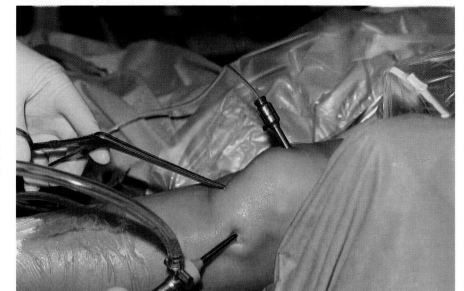

Figure 14–5
An alligator-toothed grabbing forceps is utilized through the inferomedial portal to place the drain in the medial or lateral gutter.

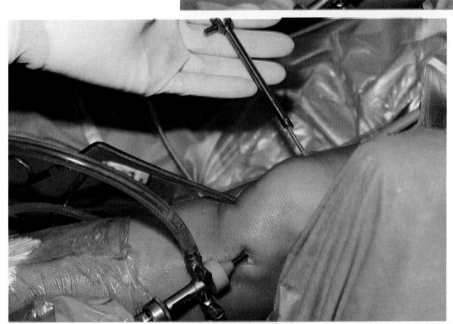

Figure 14–6
The inflow cannula is removed as the drain is kept in place.

Figure 14–7
A suction drain is placed through the sheath of the arthroscope.

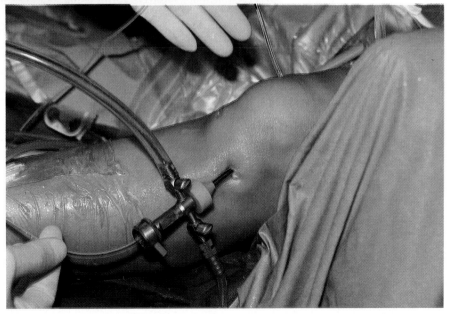

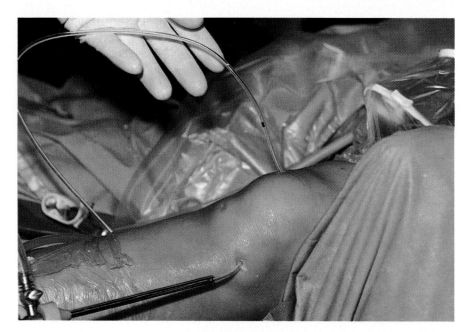

Figure 14—8
The sheath of arthroscope is removed and the drain is left in place through the inferolateral portal.

72 hours. Ingress/egress tubes with continuous antibiotic infusion are not utilized because there is a great risk of infecting the knee with a resistant organism that has gained entry to the knee by way of these tubes. A light, sterile dressing is applied and the knee is placed in a continuous passive motion (CPM) machine that is set to allow motion from 0 to 90 degrees. Partial to full weight-bearing with crutches commences when the suction tubes are removed, and active, assistive range of motion and isometric exercises are begun.

With the arthroscopic method of decompression of a septic knee, we rarely have found it necessary to do a formal arthrotomy and debridement on The Knee Service at The Hospital for Special Surgery. The two exceptions to this rule are a severely ankylosed knee with dense, fibrotic adhesions and abscess formation and an infected total knee replacement in which it is difficult to decompress adequately the medial and lateral femoral gutters and posterior aspect of the joint.

This procedure provides the surgeon with the ability to satisfy the three basic goals for treatment of a septic knee: (1) complete joint decompression, (2) debridement and irrigation, and (3) quick functional rehabilitation of the knee. The early results appear encouraging, since this procedure has minimal operative morbidity. Motion is preserved postoperatively, and functional recovery is fast. The surgeon should completely examine and record the appearance of the articular cartilage at the time of joint decompression so that the patient's prognosis for recovery may be assessed. If the diagnosis is made promptly and debridement and irrigation are performed immediately, the chance for full functional recovery of the knee and preservation of the joint articular cartilage is excellent.

References

1. Argen RJ, Wilson CH, Wood P: Suppurative arthritis. Arch Intern Med 113:117–661, 1966.
2. Ballard A, Burkhalter WE, Mayfield GW, Dehne E, Brown PW: The functional treatment of pyogenic arthritis of the adult knee. J Bone Joint Surg 57A:1119, 1975.
3. Bynum DK, Nunley JA, Goldner JL, Martinez S: Pyogenic arthritis: Emphasis on the need for surgical drainage of the infected joint. South Med J 75:1232, 1982.
4. Chartier Y, Martin WJ, Kelly PJ: Bacterial arthritis: Experience in the treatment of 77 patients. Ann Intern Med 50:1462, 1959.
5. Clawson DK, Dunn AW: Management of common bacterial infections of bones and joints. J Bone Joint Surg 49A:164, 1967.
6. Curtiss PH, Klein L: Destruction of articular cartilage in septic arthritis. J Bone Joint Surg 45A:797, 1963.
7. Daniel D, Akeson W, Amiel D, Ryder M, Boyer J: Lavage of septic joints in rabbits: Effects of chondrolysis. J Bone Joint Surg 58A:393, 1976.
8. Gainor BJ: Instillation of continuous tube irrigation in the septic knee at arthroscopy: A technique. Clin Orthop 183:96, 1984.
9. Gillespie R: Septic arthritis of childhood. Clin Orthop 96:152, 1973.

10. Goldenberg DL, Brandt KP, Cohen AS, Cathcart ES: Treatment of septic arthritis, comparison of needle aspiration and surgery as initial modes of joint drainage. Arthritis Rheum 18:83, 1975.
11. Goldenberg DL, Cohen AS: Acute infectious arthritis. Am J Med 60:369, 1976.
12. Hirsch HL, Feffer HL, O'Neil CB: A study of the diffusion of penicillin across the serous membranes of joint cavities. J Lab Clin Med 31:535, 1946.
13. Insall JN, Thompson FM, Brause BD: Two-stage reimplantation for salvage of infected total knee arthroplasty. J Bone Joint Surg 65A:1087, 1983.
14. Ivey M, Clark R: Arthroscopic debridement of the knee for septic arthritis. Clin Orthop 202:201, 1985.
15. Jackson RW, Dandy DJ: Arthroscopy of the Knee. New York, Grune & Stratton, 1976, p 81.
16. Jackson RW, Parsons CJ: Distension-irrigation treatment of major joint sepsis. Clin Orthop 96:160, 1974.
17. Jarret MP, Grossman L, Sadler AH, Grayzel AI: The role of arthroscopy in the treatment of septic arthritis. Arthritis Rheum 24:737, 1981.
18. Johnson LL: Diagnostic and Surgical Arthroscopy. 2nd ed. St. Louis, CV Mosby, 1981, p 370.
19. Kelly PJ, Martin WJ, Coventry MB: Bacterial (suppurative) arthritis in the adult. J Bone Joint Surg 52A:1595, 1970.
20. McGinty JB: Editorial. J Bone Joint Surg 65A:287, 1983.
21. Morrey BF, Bianco AJ, Rhodes KH: Septic arthritis in children. Orthop Clin North Am 6:973, 1975.
22. Morrey BF, Bianco AJ, Rhodes KH: Suppurative arthritis of the hip in children. J Bone Joint Surg 58A:388, 1976.
23. Nelson JD: Antibiotic concentrations in septic joint effusion. N Engl J Med 284:349, 1971.
24. Peltola H, Vahvanen A: Acute purulent arthritis in children. Scand J Infect Dis 15:75, 1983.
25. Rhodes KH: Antibiotic management of acute osteomyelitis and septic arthritis in children. Orthop Clin North Am 67:915, 1975.
26. Russell AS, Ansell BM: Septic arthritis. Ann Rheum Dis 31:40, 1972.
27. Salter RB, Bell RS, Keeley FW: The protective effect of continuous passive motion on living articular cartilage in acute septic arthritis: An experimental investigation in the rabbit. Clin Orthop 159:223, 1981.
28. Sharp JT, Lidsky MD, Duffy J, Duncan MW: Infectious arthritis. Arch Intern Med 139:1125, 1979.
29. Skyhar MJ, Mubarak SJ: Arthroscopic treatment of septic knees in children. J Pediatr Orthop 7:647, 1987.
30. Weissman G, Spilberg I, Krakauer K: Arthritis induced in rabbits by lysates of granulocyte lysosomes. Arthiritis Rheum 12:103, 1969.
31. Windsor RE, Insall JN, Urs WE, Miller D, Brause BD: Two-Stage Reimplantation for Infected Total Knee Replacements. Presented at The Annual Meeting of The American Academy of Orthopaedic Surgeons, Atlanta, Feb 1988.

15

John P. Reilly
Albert B. Accettola, Jr.

Arthroscopic Diagnosis and Treatment of Intra-Articular Fractures

Arthroscopic surgery has progressed rapidly over the last 15 years. Arthroscopy was employed initially as a diagnostic instrument but is now utilized in numerous therapeutic modalities. Meniscal, ligamentous, chondral, and synovial pathology have all become manageable as the sophistication of equipment and the originality of researchers expanded its use. The diagnosis of the closed intra-articular fracture does not require the use of the arthroscope; neither does its treatment, either by closed or open technique. However, this area can benefit from the operative use of the arthroscope, with the goal being to improve the functional results.[1,6,7,9,12,13,15]

Intra-articular fractures of the proximal tibia have always been troublesome to both the patient and the orthopedist because of the early and late complications of the articular surface, no matter how satisfactory the appearance of the initial reduction. Difficulties exist in determining the exact amount of displacement, in assessing articular cartilage comminution, and determining the presence of loose bodies. Loss of reduction, settling, condylar spreading, and traumatic arthritis with ensuing stiffness are also late concerns. Certainly, the potential benefits of the arthroscope in solving some of the pitfalls of these fractures can now be seen: (1) ability to provide a more anatomic reduction, (2) minimizing the extent of dissection into an area already traumatized, (3) concurrent repair of associated meniscal/ligamentous injuries, (4) early range of motion and physical therapy continuous passive motion (CPM), and (5) optional utilization of cancellous bone grafting.

The indications for this procedure must be clarified, since the types of fracture patterns that can benefit most from its use are limited. The classic literature must be reviewed in order to fully understand the mechanisms of fracture[8] and associated soft tissue injuries, as well as the biomechanical stresses on the weight bearing of the knee joint.[10] One must always take care not to fall into the proverbial "triumph of technique over reason."

This chapter provides a detailed and illustrative guide for the orthopedist who is familiar with both arthroscopy and fracture management to consider combining these techniques for the benefit of the patient. Percutaneous methods of reduction have long been available to treat plateau fractures but they lack the ability to confirm true articular congruity. Arthroscopy provides an optimal method to visualize the articular surfaces while reduction is performed and maintained. It is agreed that no matter what the treatment selected, varus or valgus deformity, joint incongruity, and associated untreated intra-articular soft tissue injuries (ligament, meniscus) will predict a less than optimal result.

CLASSIFICATION

Many authorities have categorized tibial plateau fractures.[3,4,11,14,16] The classic and most frequently used classification is that described by Hohl (Fig. 15–1).[3]

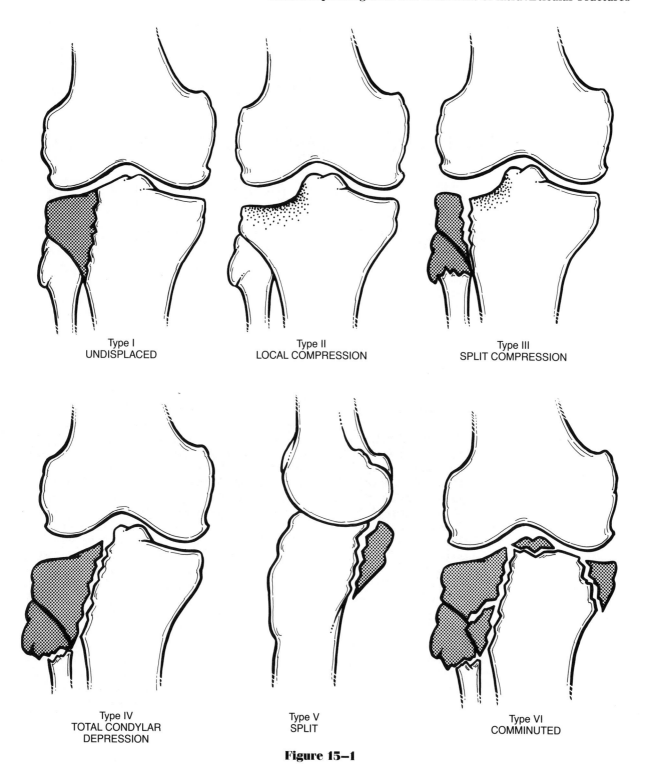

Type I
UNDISPLACED

Type II
LOCAL COMPRESSION

Type III
SPLIT COMPRESSION

Type IV
TOTAL CONDYLAR
DEPRESSION

Type V
SPLIT

Type VI
COMMINUTED

Figure 15–1

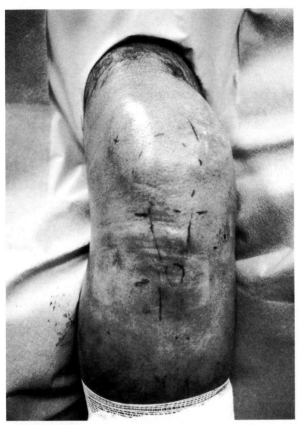

Figure 15–2

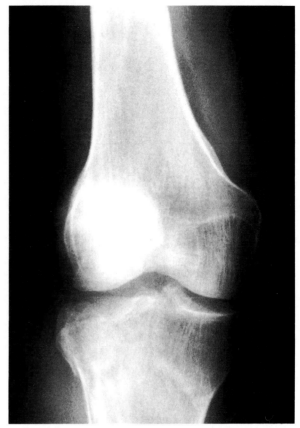

Figure 15–3

SURFACE/ARTHROSCOPIC ANATOMY (FIGS. 15–2 AND 15–3)

The positioning of the knee for operation is shown in Figure 15–2. Figure 15–3 is a preoperative radiograph for use in planning the approach and portal placement.

The surface anatomy and osseous landmarks of the *normal* knee should be reviewed and understood prior to considering arthroscopy. Normal articular relationships can be distorted due to the fracture, to soft tissue injuries, and to the associated intra-articular hematoma. When planning for introduction of arthroscopic portals, it is important to know how much depression exists, and whether there is an as-

sociated fracture of the tibial spine or interruption of the tibial tubercle–patellar tendon mechanism. With the surface anatomy thereby visualized, the underlying arthroscopic anatomy should be assessed in the same systematic fashion as in any other arthroscopic problem.

Clinical Examination

Although there is usually an effusion of the knee, an associated tear in the capsule may allow blood to pass into the periarticular soft tissues.

Under general anesthesia the knee may be aspirated and the ligaments examined.

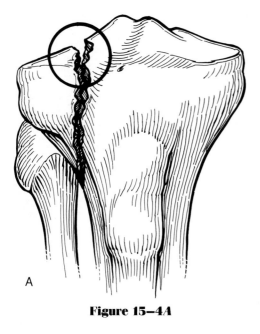

Figure 15–4A

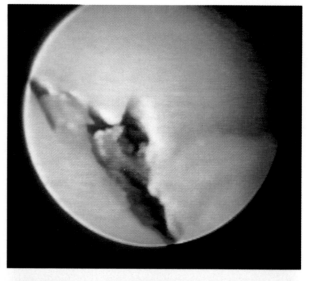

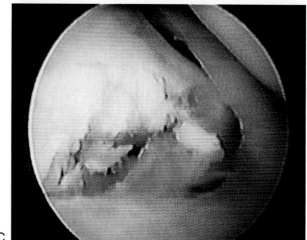

Figure 15–4B, C

ARTHROSCOPIC ANATOMY

Type I: Split Fracture (Fig. 15–4A)

Figure 15–4B is a small split fracture; C is a large fracture with blood clot in the gap.

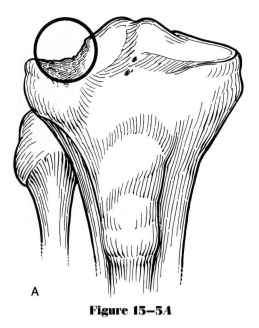

Figure 15–5A

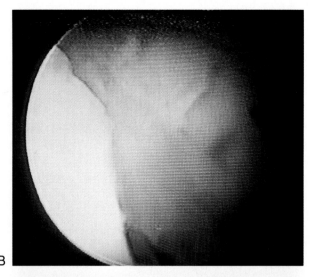

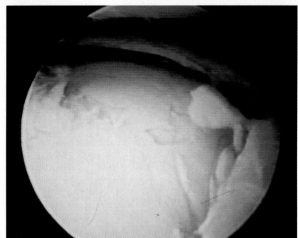

Figure 15–5B, C

Type II: Compression Fracture (Fig. 15–5A)

In Figure 15–5B, an arthroscopic view of a compression fracture, the tibial spine is to the left and an articular depression to the right. In C, a large area of depression is lying below the meniscus. Note the extent of articular damage.

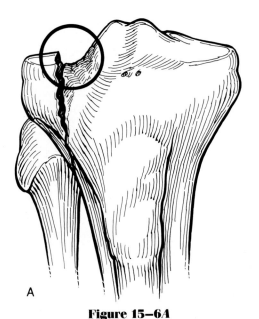

Figure 15–6A

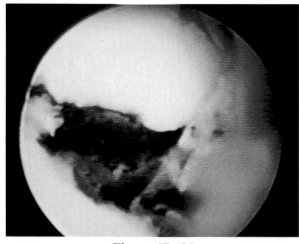

Figure 15–6B

Type III: Split Compression Fracture (Fig. 15–6A)

Figure 15–6B shows the tibial spine to the left and cancellous bone in the center with depressed articular cartilage above.

PREOPERATIVE WORK-UP

A patient with a suspected tibial plateau fracture will require an appropriate work-up before surgical intervention, regardless of what method is employed. The recommended plan of treatment includes (1) plain radiographs (AP, lateral, oblique, and tunnel projections); (2) tomograms; (3) computed tomography (with lateral reconstructions or 3-D reconstructions if available); (4) magnetic resonance imaging (MRI)[5]; and (5) arteriography (if indicated). Figure 15–7 is an arteriogram for a Type VI fracture.

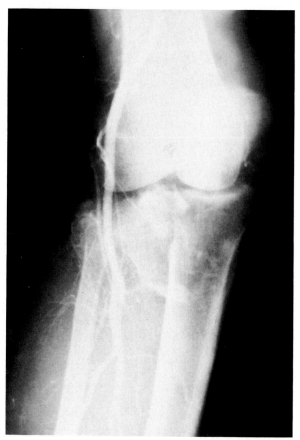

Figure 15–7

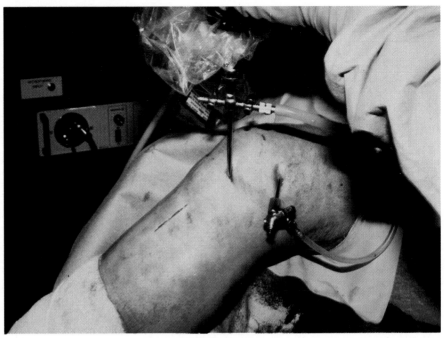

Figure 15–8

PATIENT POSITIONING

The patient is placed on the operating table in the supine position. Routine protection of all pressure points is assured with appropriate padding. A leg holder is recommended. A tourniquet may be applied to the upper thigh but is not inflated unless needed. The table is flexed at the patient's knee joint, and a routine surgical prep is given, with inclusion of the anterosuperior iliac crest if preoperative planning indicates the need for a possible bone graft. (Depending on the surgeon's preference, or the availability of assistants, the contralateral crest may be selected.)

Portals for the procedure include inflow and outflow with wide-bore cannulas, to provide sufficient irrigation and flow to clear the field of organized hematoma and evacuate clot from in between the fracture fragments. An arthroscopic set-up with portals in place is shown in Figure 15–8. Incision is made on the proximal shaft for elevation and bone grafting. Figure 15–9 provides an arthroscopic view of a fracture before (A) and after (B) clot is removed.

A constant pressure pump may be helpful in maintaining joint space distention. This will allow for the appropriate arthroscopic examination and permit determination of the extent and type of the fracture pattern. However, the risk of producing a compartment syndrome must be considered.

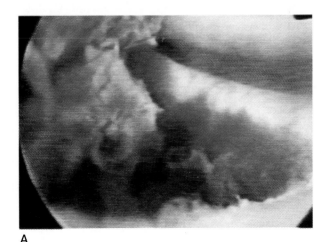
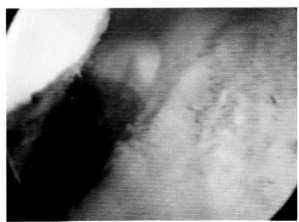

A   B

Figure 15–9

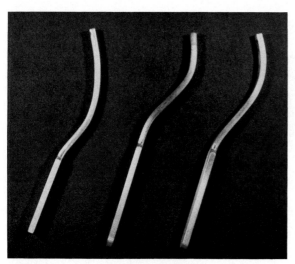

Figure 15–10

EQUIPMENT

For the optimal reduction and fixation of a fracture arthroscopically, a full complement of arthroscopic equipment and tools should be available. This includes biters, rongeurs, and other associated instruments to debride chondral or meniscal damage, and a high-speed suction instrument to irrigate and clean out the joint. Other necessary equipment includes K-wires to manipulate the fracture fragment and provide for temporary fixation. Various clamps and Richardson retractors may be helpful in the external closed reduction of the split fragment. Elevators are necessary to raise depressed sections of chondral surface and serve as a bone tamp. Straight and curved tamps of various radii and lengths should be available to anticipate different fracture patterns and different-sized tibias (Fig. 15–10).[2]

Radiographic equipment is also necessary for intraoperative documentation of fracture reduction, guide wire placement, and final screw fixation. This is best obtained with the fluoroscopic C-arm. Use of a radiolucent operating table would be beneficial.

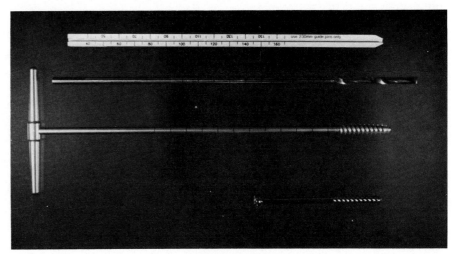

Figure 15–11

METHODS OF FIXATION

Initial treatment of tibial plateau fractures before the advent of internal fixation was by various means: cast immobilization, traction immobilization, or cast bracing. When internal fixation came into use, operative indications for surgical intervention were considered to be 3 to 4 mm of articular depression. The Swiss influence has pressed forward with this concept to obtain exact anatomic restoration. In order to accomplish this, a large dissection traditionally would be necessary in many cases, but the arthroscope can provide for anatomic reduction without extensive dissection.

In deciding the method of fixation and the approach, whether open or arthroscopic, the personality of the fracture must be considered. Lateral plateau fractures are more common because of the physiologic valgus. The most important factor is the amount of comminution. If there are too many pieces, or subchondral support is poor, the fracture will require an open approach and buttressing to avoid spreading of the plateau.

Percutaneous screw fixation is effective for the split and split depression types of fractures. The development of cannulated screws (Fig. 15–11) (Synthes) has simplified the arthroscopic placement of the percutaneous screws.

External fixation devices have been suggested in severe fractures, but complications such as pins cutting out of the soft metaphyseal bone and pin tract infections must be considered. A quadrilateral frame (Vidal) has been described.[6] From the more recent experience of external fixation from trauma centers, modifications can be made to incorporate an anteriorly designed frame.

If fixation is solid, the use of continuous passive motion might minimize the stiffness that often follows these injuries to the knee, and might improve the condition of the traumatized articular cartilage. It is necessary to keep the patient's weight off the injured extremity until adequate healing has occurred, to prevent the loss of reduction. The arthroscope can also be utilized for repeat examinations of the chondral surface.[1,13]

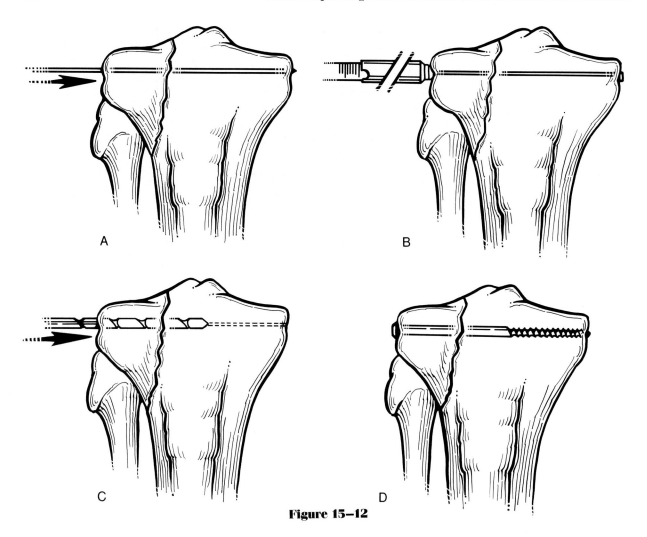

A

B

C

D

Figure 15–12

Method of Fixation—Type I *(Fig. 15–12)*

Visualize the split and evacuate the interfragmentary hematoma using intra-articular probes and irrigation.

Pass 1 or 2 K-wires.

Measure, using the cannulated depth gauge, and drill over the K-wires with a cannulated drill. Then tap the hole and tighten a cannulated, large fragment cancellous screw over the K-wire prior to removing it. A washer may be used in osteoporotic bone.

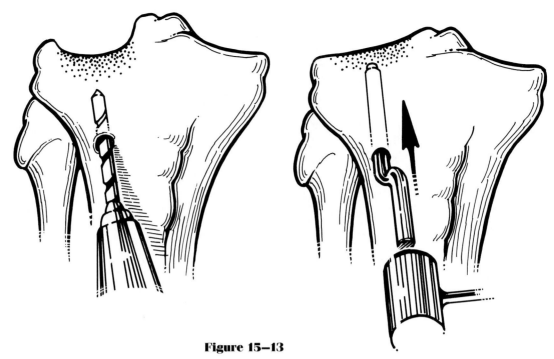

Figure 15–13

Method of Fixation—Type II (Fig. 15–13)

A 3/8-inch hole is drilled through the cortex of the tibia medially or laterally to the anterior tibial tubercle, on the side of the fracture. The 1-inch skin incision is planned so that its proximal end is at the level of the anterior tubercle, to permit angling the drill in a cephalad direction without catching the skin. This oval hole permits the passage of a curved bone tamp. The tamp forces the depressed fragment upward under direct vision through the arthroscope (Fig. 15–14 is a model of a pure depression fracture elevated from below). Tamps with several different arcs are needed to reach each part of the tibial plateau. Iliac bone graft can be packed in the subchondral void through the same opening.

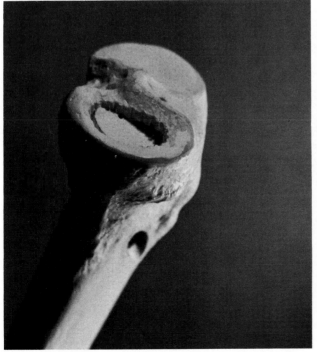
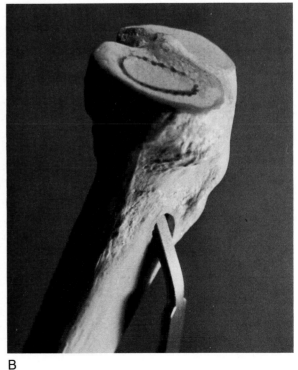

A   B

Figure 15–14

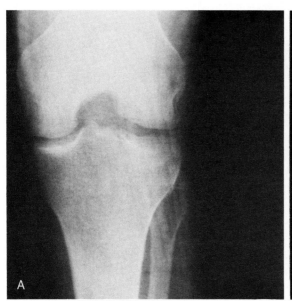

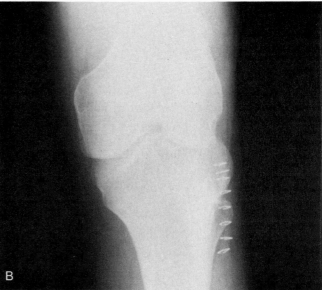

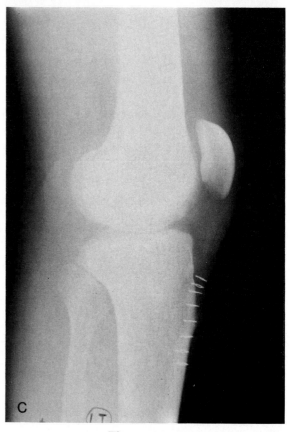

A preoperative radiograph showing simple depression of the lateral plateau can be seen in Figure 15–15A. B and C are radiographs of the same fracture after arthroscopic evaluation and bone grafting.

Method of Fixation—Type III
(Fig. 15–16. X-ray)

The fracture is visualized and clot removed using probes and irrigation.

A K-wire is placed percutaneously into the split fragment to serve as a handle for control of the fragment.

A 3/8-inch hole is drilled in the anterior cortex of the tibia; the skin is protected from the drill while it is directed in a cephalad direction. Curved bone tamps are then used to elevate the depressed articular fragment under direct vision (see Figure 15–14).

The split portion of the fracture is then reduced, using the K-wire. When arthroscopic examination shows an adequate reduction, the K-wire can be driven across the tibia. If the fragment is large enough, a second K-wire is placed, the depth measured, the holes drilled and tapped, and screws placed prior to removing the K-wires.

Cancellous bone graft from the iliac crest can be placed through the cortical hole to fill the subchondral void.

Figure 15–15

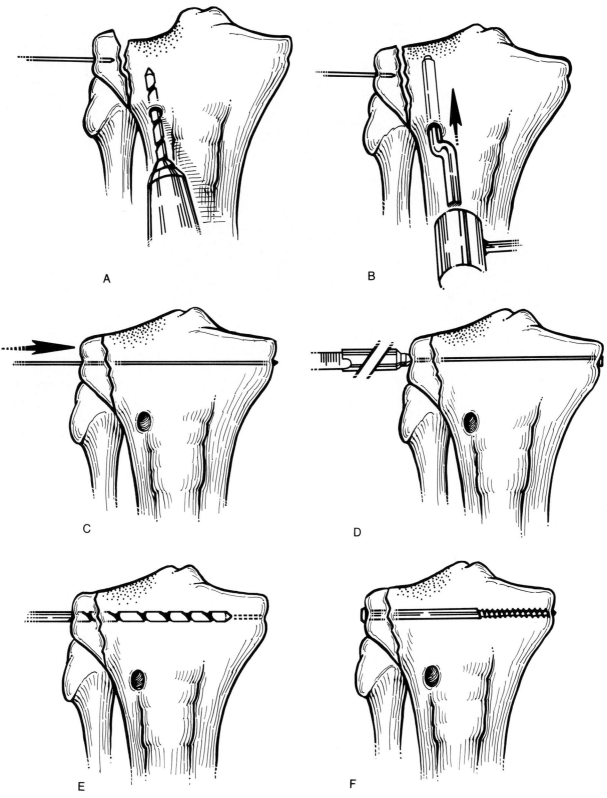

A

B

C

D

E

F

Figure 15–16

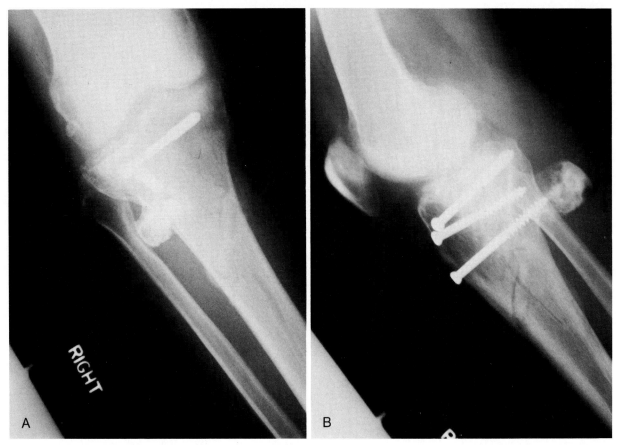

Figure 15–17

Postoperative radiographs for a Type III fracture
treated arthroscopically are seen in Figure 15–17.

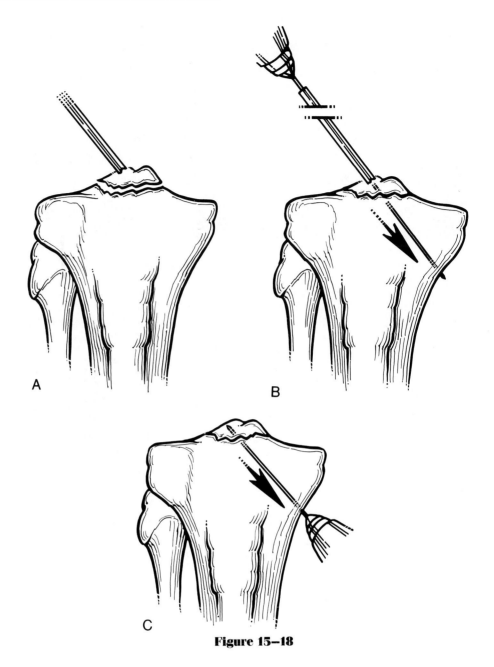

A

B

C

Figure 15–18

Method of Fixation—Tibial Spine Avulsion

Two different methods of fixation can be used, depending on the size of the avulsed fragment of bone.

Large Fragment (Fig. 15–18). The fracture is visu-alized and the hematoma removed with probes and irrigation. Reduction is obtained using a cannula with a serrated end to prevent slippage. The fragment is then fixed with a threaded K-wire, exiting from the skin distally, so that the wire can be advanced into the fracture fragment far enough to clear the femoral surface.

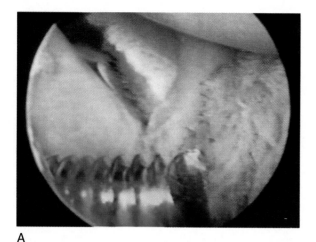

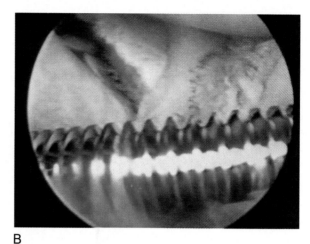

A   B

Figure 15–19

Figure 15-19*A* and *B* shows arthroscopic reduction of a tibial spine fracture with K-wire. The spine is on the left. Figure 15–20 is a postoperative radiograph of tibial spine avulsion.

Small Fragment (Fig. 15–21). The avulsed fragment and its bed are visualized and cleaned in the manner just described. If the fragment is too small to hold a fixation device, a nonabsorbable suture can be used. A 2-cm incision is made on the anterior surface of the tibia, medial to the tibial tubercle. By means of a jig designed for anterior cruciate replacement, two K-wires can be placed into the edges of the fracture bed. A wire loop is placed through one hole into the knee, and a heavy, nonabsorbable suture is passed through the other. Under arthroscopic control, the suture is passed through the base of the cruciate ligament and into the wire loop so that it can be drawn back out of the knee. It is then tied down over the tibial cortex while the fragment is held in its bed with an intra-articular probe.

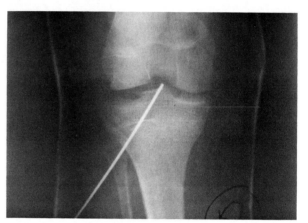

Figure 15–20

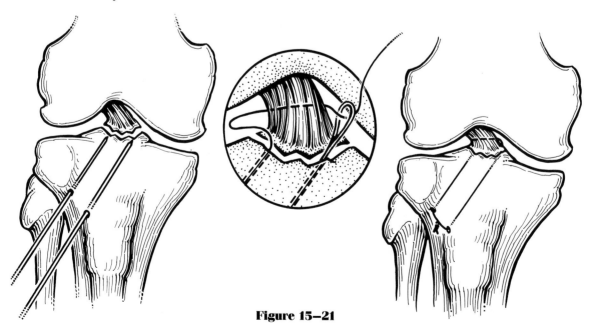

Figure 15–21

Bibliography

1. Caspari RB, Hutton PM, Whipple TL, Meyers JF: The role of arthroscopy in the management of tibial plateau fractures. Arthroscopy 1:76–82, 1985.
2. Edeland HG: Open reduction of central compression fractures of the tibial plateau. Preliminary report on a new method and device arrangement. Acta Orthop Scand 47:686, 1976.
3. Hohl M: Tibial condylar fractures. J Bone Joint Surg 49A:1455, 1967.
4. Hohl M: Fractures and dislocations of the knee. *In* Rockwood CA, Greene DP (eds): Fractures. Vol 2. 2nd ed. Philadelphia, JB Lippincott, 1984, p 1453.
5. Jackson DW, Jennings LD, Maywood RM, Berger PE: Magnetic resonance imaging of the knee. Am J Sports Med 16:29–38, 1988.
6. Jennings JE: Arthroscopic management of tibial plateau fractures. Arthroscopy 1:160–168, 1985.
7. Johnson LL: Practice of Arthroscopic Surgery. 3rd ed. St. Louis, CV Mosby, 1986, pp 677–685.
8. Kennedy JC, Bailey WH: Experimental tibial plateau fractures. Studies of the mechanism and a classification. J Bone Joint Surg 50A:1522, 1968.
9. Lennon RA, Bartlett DH: Arthroscopic-assisted internal fixation of certain fractures about the knee. J Trauma 25:355–358, 1985.
10. Maquet PC, VanDeBerg AJ, Simonet JC: Femoral tibial weight-bearing areas. J Bone Joint Surg 57A:766, 1975.
11. Moore TM: Fracture dislocations of the knee. Clin Orthop 156:128, 1981.
12. Pankovich AM: Arthroscopic management of tibial plateau fractures (letter). Arthroscopy 2:132, 1986.
13. Perry CR, Evans LG, Rice S, Fogarty J, Burdge RE: A new surgical approach to fractures of the lateral tibial plateau. J Bone Joint Surg 66A:1236, 1984.
14. Rasmussen PS: Tibial condylar fractures: Impairment of joint stability as an indication for surgical treatment. J Bone Joint Surg 55A:1331, 1973.
15. Reinor MJ: The arthroscope in tibial plateau fractures: Its use in evaluation of soft tissue and bony injury. J Am Osteopath Assoc 81:704, 1982.
16. Schatzker J, McBroome R, Bruce D: The tibial plateau fracture. The Toronto Experience, 1968–1975. Clin Orthop 138:94, 1979.

INDEX

Page numbers in *italic* type indicate illustrations; page numbers followed by t refer to tables.

Abrasion arthroplasty, 124, *126*
  results of, 125
Age, as factor in outpatient surgery, 38
Amici prism, 2
Anatomy, arthroscopic, 49–66
Andrew, J., magnesium filament of, 1
Anesthesia, in arthroscopy, 37–42
  epidural, advantages and disadvantages
    of, 37t, 41
    vs. other anesthetic techniques, 37t
  femoral, with and without sciatic, vs.
    other anesthetic techniques, 37t
  general, 39–40
    advantages and disadvantages of, 37t,
      39
      vs. other anesthetic techniques, 37t
    contraindications for, 38
    induction agents for, 40
    maintenance agents for, 40
    muscle relaxants in, 40
    postoperative pain after, 40
    problems in, 39
    recommendations for, 39–40
  local, advantages and disadvantages of,
    vs. other anesthetic techniques, 37t
    plus sedation, advantages and
      disadvantages of, vs. other
      anesthetic techniques, 37t
    technique of, 38–39
    with or without sedation, 38–39
  spinal, advantages and disadvantages of,
    vs. other anesthetic techniques, 37t
    for arthroscopic surgery, 40–41
  techniques of, grading of, 37t
Anterior cruciate ligament (ACL), anatomy
  of, *50–52*, 52
  chronic tear of, midsagittal MRI section of,
    27
  injuries to, 52
    attachment to posterior cruciate
      ligament in, 134, *135*
    evaluation of associated injuries in, 134
    intersubstance tear of, *134*
    magnetic resonance imaging of, 24–29,
      26–29
    midsubstance tear of, MRI image of, *27*
    normal, arthroscopic view of, 64, *64*, 134
    midsagittal MRI section of, *26*
    partial tear of, sagittal MRI images of, *28*
    prosthetic replacement of, 133
Anterior cruciate ligament (ACL)
  reconstruction, applied anatomy in,
    133–138
  arthrofibrosis following, 145
  decision making in, 132–133
  diagnosis and repair of associated
    pathology in, 133–134
  future developments in, 152–153
  guidewire placement in, 139, *139*
    device for, *140*
  isometry in, 136–137
    placing of guide pins for, 137, *138*

Anterior cruciate ligament (ACL)
  reconstruction (*Continued*)
  notchplasty in, 134–136
  osseous tunnel preparation in, 137
  pes tendons as graft in, 133, 141, *141*, *142*
  results of, 152
  role of extra-articular stabilization in,
    133
  semitendinosus/gracilis, technique of,
    138–143, *139–142*
  specific techniques of, 138–148
  technical aspects of, 133–138
  tensioning of graft in, 138
  using Gore-Tex, 147–148, *147–148*
  using patellar tendon, 143–146
Arcuate ligament, 51, *51*, *52*
Arthritis, 100–101. See also *Degenerative
  joint disease* and *Osteoarthritis.*
  rheumatoid, 101
    synovial changes in, 101, *102*, *103*
    synovial pannus from, on medial femoral
      condyle, *123*
    treatment of, 101
    vs. degenerative joint disease, 100–101
  septic, granulation tissue invasion of
    patellar articular surface in, *115*
Arthrofibrosis, after anterior cruciate
  ligament reconstruction, 145
Arthrography, of knee, 11–21
  early history of, 11
Arthroplasty, abrasion, 124, *126*
  results of, 125
Arthroscope, Burman, 3, *3*
  Grave, 3
  Selfoc, Watanabe and, 3, *4*
  Takagi, 2, *2*
  Wolf, 5, *6*
Arthroscopic anatomy, 49–66
Arthroscopic instruments, evolution of, 1–10,
  1–8
Arthroscopic knives, *8*
Arthroscopic lateral retinacular release
  (ALRR), 166–170
  complications in, 169
  indications for, 166
  patellar rotation after, *168*
  portal and instrument locations for,
    167
  postoperative program for, 169–170
  technique of, 166–169, *167–169*
    electrosurgical, 168
    Schreiber, 167, *169*
Arthroscopic microchip camera, 4, *6*
Arthroscopic probes, *8*
Arthroscopic shavers, *8*
Arthroscopic surgery, choice of anesthetic
  options for, 37t, 38
Arthroscopy, anesthesia in, 37–42
  evolution of, 1–10
  historical background of, 1–10
Articular cartilage, degeneration of, in
  hemophilia, *124*

233

Articular cartilage (*Continued*)
  disorders of, 113–130
  fragmentation of, *122*
  normal, 113–114
  response to injury of, 114–117
  softening and swelling of, *122*
  structure of, 113, *114, 115*
  zones of, 114, *115*
Articular cartilage injury, blunt probe
      evaluation of, 123, *124*
  by blunt trauma, repair process in, 117
  by repetitive trauma, repair process in, 117
  diagnosis of, 118
  effect of compression on, 117
  effect of immobilization on, 117
  effect of motion on, 117
  extrinsic repair of, 116, *116, 117*
  iatrogenic, 124, *125*
  intrinsic repair of, 116
  management of, 118–119
  mechanisms of repair in, 115
  osteochondral fractures and, 119–120
  perichondral grafts for, 118
  postoperative rehabilitation after, 117–118
Articular cartilage lesions, 120–123
  arthroscopic evaluation of, 123
  classification of, 121
  etiology of, 121
  treatment of, 123
Asystole, after epidural anesthesia, 41
  after spinal anesthesia, 40

Backache, after spinal anesthesia, 41
Baker's cyst, loose bodies in, *199*
Bircher, E., arthroendoscopy of, 2
Blumensaat's line, 158, *159*
Blunt trauma, response to injury of articular
      cartilage in, 117
Bone tumors, diagnostic imaging of, 31, *32*
Bozzini lichtleiter, 1, *1*
Bradycardia, after spinal anesthesia, 40
Bruch, J., 1
Bullet fragments, in knee, 195, *196*
Burman arthroscope, 3, *3*

Calcium pyrophosphate crystals, microscopic
      appearance of, *106, 107*
  radiographic appearance of, *106*
Calcium pyrophosphate deposition disease
      (CPDD), 105. See also *Pseudogout.*
Carbon dioxide, as irrigation medium, in
      arthroscopy, 123, *125*
Cartilage, articular. See also *Articular
      cartilage.*
  anatomic features of, 56
  degeneration of, 56, *56–58*. See also
      Chondromalacia.
  disorders of, 113–130
  normal, 113–114
Cartilage transplantation, 126, *127*
  allografts vs. autografts in, 126
  results of, 126
Chondral fracture(s), articular cartilage
      injury and, 119–120
  response to injury of articular cartilage in,
      115
  to subchondral bone, of medial femoral
      condyle, *115*
Chondrocalcinosis, 105. See also *Pseudogout.*

Chondrocytes, in articular cartilage, 113
  in response to injury of articular cartilage,
      114
Chondromalacia, arthroscopic treatment of,
      166
    by local excision of defect, 166
    by patellar and femoral groove shavings
      and débridement, 166
  classification of, 162
  conservative treatment of, 163–164
  diagnosis of, 163
  Grade I, 56, *56, 57,* 162, *163*
  Grade II, 56, *57,* 162, *164*
  Grade III, 56, *57, 58,* 162, *164*
    abrasion chondroplasty for, 56, *58*
  Grade IV, 162, *164*
  Kerlan-Jobe rehabilitation protocol for, 163
  malalignment and, surgical indications for,
      164
    treatment flow chart for, *165*
  patellofemoral, 162–166
  phases of, 163
  with abnormal plicae, *88, 90*
Chondromatosis, synovial, 105–107
  loose bodies of, 106, *108, 109, 194, 195*
Chondrosarcomas, diagnostic imaging of, 31
Collateral ligament(s), anatomy of, 50,
      50–52
  fibular, anatomy of, 29
    MRI imaging of, 29
  medial, acute tears of, MRI imaging of, 29
    chronic tears of, MRI imaging of, 29, *30*
    MRI imaging of, *23, 28*
  tears of, arthrographic evaluation of, 17,
      18
Congruence angle, of patellofemoral joint,
      159, *160*
Coronary ligament (meniscotibial), *51, 52*
Compartment(s) of knee, arthroscopic
      anatomy of, 62–66, *63–66*
  lateral, arthroscopic anatomy of, 62–63,
      63, 64
    loose bodies in, *201*
  medial, arthroscopic anatomy of, 64–65,
      65
    loose bodies in, *200*
    removal of osseous body from, *204*
  posterior, loose bodies in, *201*
  posterolateral, arthroscopic anatomy of, 66
Computed tomography, high-resolution. See
      *High-resolution computed tomography
      (HRCT).*
  of patellofemoral joint, 161–162
Cruciate ligament(s), anterior. See *Anterior
      cruciate ligament (ACL).*
  arthrography of, reliability of, 19
  injuries to, arthroscopic diagnosis and
      treatment of, 131–154
  normal, arthroscopic view of, *134*
  posterior. See *Posterior cruciate ligament.*
  tears of, arthrographic evaluation of, 18
Cruciate ligament reconstruction. See also
      *Anterior cruciate ligament
      reconstruction* and *Posterior cruciate
      ligament reconstruction.*
  arthroscopic, advantages of, 131
    vs. "mini-arthrotomy," 131
  choice of graft materials for, 132
  contraindications for, 132
  decision making in, 132–133
  future developments in, 152–153
  indications for, 132
  results of, 152

Crystal(s), in synovial fluid, types of, 46
Crystal synovitis, *53*, 102–107, 103t
Cystoscope, introduction of, by Desormeaux, 1, *2*
    Leiter, 2

Débridement, arthroscopic, 124, *126*
    in articular cartilage lesions, 123, 124–126
    in septic knee, 209
    in treatment of chondromalacia, 166
    results of, 125
    open, 124
Degenerative joint disease, chondroid metaplasia in, *109*
    involvement of knee joint in, 101, *101*
    loose bodies in knee in, 194, *194*
    secondary, calcium pyrophosphate deposition in, *123*
    synovial hyperplasia in, 100, *101*
    vs. rheumatoid arthritis, 100–101
Desormeaux, A. J., introduction of cystoscope by, 1, *2*
Drill guide, for femoral holes, 139, *140*
Dural puncture, in spinal anesthesia, 40
Dwarfism, osteochondritis dissecans and, 183

Electrocautery, cartilage injury due to, 124, *125*
Electrosurgery, cartilage injury due to, 124, *125*
Enchondral dysostoses, osteochondritis dissecans and, 183
Endocrine abnormalities, in osteochondritis dissecans, 182
Endoscope, Nitze, 2, *2*
Epidural anesthesia, for arthroscopic surgery, advantages and disadvantages of, 37t, 41
    total spinal anesthesia in, 41
Epiphyseal abnormalities, in osteochondritis dissecans, 183
Epiphyseal dysplasia, multiple, osteochondritis dissecans and, 183
Excessive lateral facet compression syndrome, 166

Familial occurrence, of osteochondritis dissecans, 182
Femoral condylar osteochondral fractures, loose bodies and, 193, *193*
Femoral condyle(s), anatomy of, 49, *50*
    articular defect of, with separation of osteochondral fragment, *19*
    lateral, osteochondral fracture of, arthroscopic appearance of, *119*
        radiographic appearance of, *119*
        screw repair of, *121*
        regenerative fibrocartilage of, after abrasion arthroplasty, *126*
    medial, blister formation on, *122*
        cartilage transplantation to, *127*
        fibrocartilaginous repair of, *116, 117*
        giant cell tumor of, MRI scans of, *32*
        osteoarthritis of, calcium pyrophospate deposition in, *123*
        osteochondral fracture of, bone peg repair of, *121*

Femoral condyle(s) (*Continued*)
    medial, osteochondritis dissecans of, arthroscopic appearance of, *120*
        defect due to, *178*
        MRI imaging of, 31, *31*
        reduction and fixation with Kirschner wires of, *120*
        synovial pannus on, in rheumatoid arthritis, *123*
Femoral epiphyses, distal, irregular ossification of, osteochondritis dissecans and, 180
Femoral gutter, lateral, 65
Femoral nerve block, with or without sciatic nerve block, for anesthesia, 39
Fibrocartilage, after abrasion chondroplasty, 56, *58*
Fibrosarcomas, diagnostic imaging of, 31
Finkelstein, H., 3
Fluoroscopic double-contrast spot filming, 11
Forceps, for removal of loose bodies in knee, 201, *202*
Fractures, intra-articular, 215–231. See also *Intra-articular fracture(s).*
    osteochondral. See *Osteochondral fracture(s).*

Gazogene lamp, 1, *2*
Giant cell(s), multinucleated, hypertrophy of synovial cells and, 98, *98*
Giant cell tumor(s), diagnostic imaging of, 31, *32*
    of medial femoral condyle, MRI scans of, *32*
Gore-Tex, in anterior cruciate ligament reconstruction, 147–148, *147–148*
Gout, 102–105
    bone erosion in, radiographic appearance of, *104*
    sodium urate crystals in, 103, *104, 105*
    tophi in, appearance of, 103, *104*
        microscopic appearance of, *104*
    vs. pseudogout, characteristics of, 103t
Grafts, perichondral, for articular cartilage injury, 118
Grant's notch, *50, 52*
Grave arthroscope, 3
Grimley-Sokoloff giant cells, *98*

Ham F12 solution, as irrigation medium, in arthroscopy, 124
Headaches, after spinal anesthesia, 40
Hemarthrosis, iron synovitis in, 99–100, *100*
    synovial appearance in, *100*
Hemophilia, articular cartilage degeneration in, *124*
    iron synovitis in, 99–100, *100*
    pseudotumor of, 100
Hemorrhagic synovial fluid (Group IV), characteristics of, 45t, 48
Hemostat, for removal of loose bodies in knee, *203*
High-resolution computed tomography (HRCT), advantages of, 20
    combined with double-contrast arthrography, 20
    of meniscal tears, 19, *20–22*
    vs. double contrast arthrography, 20, *21*

Hughston's sulcus angle, *159*
Hypotension, after epidural anesthesia, 41
    after spinal anesthesia, 40

Iatrogenic injury, to articular cartilage, 124,
    125
Inflammatory synovial fluid (Group II),
    characteristics of, 45t, 47
Infrapatellar plica (ligamentum mucosum),
    54, 55, 84, 157
Instruments, arthroscopic, evolution of, 1–10,
    1–8
        for removal of loose bodies in knee, 201,
        202, 203
Intercondylar notch, anatomy of, *50,* 51–52
        arthroscopic, 63–64
        loose bodies in, 201
Intra-articular fractures, 215–231
    arthroscopic anatomy of, 217–220, *217–
        220*
    arthroscopic treatment of, equipment for,
        222, *222, 223*
        patient positioning for, 221, *221*
    classification of, 215, *216*
    clinical examination for, 217–220
    methods of fixation for, 223–230
    positioning knee for operation in, *217*
    preoperative work-up for, 220
    role of arthroscopy in, 215
    surface anatomy of, 217–220, *217–220*
    tibial spine avulsion and, method of
        fixation for, 229–230, *229, 230*
    Type I, split fracture, *216, 218*
        method of fixation for, 224, *224*
    Type II, compression fracture, *216, 219*
        method of fixation for, 225, *225, 226*
    Type III, split compression fracture, *216,
        220*
        method of fixation for, 226, *226, 227,
        228*
    Type IV, total condylar depression, *216*
    Type V, split, *216*
    Type VI, comminuted, *216, 220*
Iron synovitis, 99–100, *100*
Irrigation medium, in arthroscopy, carbon
    dioxide as, 123, *125*
        Ham F12 solution as, 124
        Ringer's lactate as, 124
        saline as, 124, *125*
Ischemia, as cause of osteochondritis
    dissecans, 182
Isometry, in anterior cruciate ligament
    reconstruction, 136–137

Jackson, R., 4

Knee, anterior view of, anatomic features in,
    54
    arthrography of, 11–21
    compartments of, 62–66. See also
        Compartments of knee.
    diagnostic imaging of, 11–35
    embryonic development of, 83, 97, *97*
    flexed, anterior view of, anatomic features
        in, *50*
        lateral view of, anatomic features in, *51*
    inflammation of. See *Osteochondritis
        dissecans of knee.*

Knee (*Continued*)
    loose bodies in, 193–205. See also *Loose
        bodies in knee.*
    magnetic resonance imaging of, 11, 20
    septic, arthroscopic diagnosis and
        treatment of, 207–213. See also *Septic
        knee.*
Knives, arthroscopic, *8*
Kreucher, P., 3
Kurosaka screw, 144, *146*
Kutner, R., photocystoscope and, 2

Labelle and Laurin line, 158, *159*
Lateral compartment, arthroscopic anatomy
    of, 62–63, *63, 64*
    loose bodies in, *201*
Lateral ligaments, MRI imaging of, 29
Leiter, J., cystoscope of, 2
Lichtleiter, Bozzini, 1, *1*
Ligament(s), collateral. See *Collateral
    ligament(s).*
    cruciate. See *Cruciate ligament(s).*
    prosthetic, development of, 153
Ligament of Humphry, 50, *51*
Ligament of Wrisberg, 50, *51*
Ligament surgery, arthroscopic, history of, 7
Ligamentum mucosum (infrapatellar plica),
    54, 55, 84, 157
Lino's band. See *Mediopatellar plica.*
Loose bodies in knee, 193–205
    arthroscopic grasping of, 199–201
    arthroscopic removal of, 196–205, *196–
        205*
        from medial compartment, *204*
        instruments for, 201, *202, 203*
        motorized shaver for, *203*
        planning procedure for, 196–197
        techniques of, 197–204
    arthroscopic search for, 197–199
    diagnosis of, 195–196
        physical examination in, 195
        radiography in, 196, *196–199*
    foreign materials as, 195, *196*
        arthroscopic removal of, *197,* 204–205
    in Baker's cyst, *199*
    in intercondylar notch, 201
    in lateral compartment, *201*
    in lateral recess, *200*
    in medial compartment, *200*
    in posterior compartment, *201*
    in prepatellar bursa, *199*
    origin of, 193–195
    osteoarthritis and, 194, *194*
    osteochondral fractures and, 193, *193*
    osteochondritis dissecans and, 194
    osteochondromatosis and, 195, *195, 196*

Magnetic resonance imaging (MRI), 21–23
    in diagnosis of articular cartilage injury,
        118–119
    of knee, 11, 20
    of osteochondritis dissecans, *175, 176,* 178,
        178
McGinty, J., 4
Medial compartment, arthroscopic anatomy
    of, 64–65, *65*
    loose bodies in, *200*
    removal of osseous body from, *204*
Mediopatellar (medial) plica(e), 85, *85, 86*
    abnormal, clinical parameters of, 91t
        Grade III articular changes due to, *90*

Mediopatellar (medial) plica(e) (*Continued*)
  abnormal, resection of, superolateral
    portal, *93*
  above medial femoral condyle, *85*
  anatomic location of, *84*
  double, *87*
  in 15 degrees of flexion, *86*
  in 30 degrees of flexion, *87*
  in 60 degrees of flexion, *87*
  in 90 degrees of flexion, *87*
    with erosions and chondromalacia, *88*
  in full extension, *86*
  thickened, from chronic trauma, *86*
  types of, 85, *85*
  Type A, *89*
  Type B, *89*
  Type C, *89*
  with patella contact, and chondromalacia
    and displacement, *88*
  with spur formation, *88*
Meniscal cysts, arthrography of, 15, *16*
Meniscal disorders, 67–82
Meniscal injuries, arthrography of, single- vs.
    double-contrast, 19
  high-resolution computed tomography of,
    19, *20–22*
Meniscal repair(s), 76–81
  contraindications for, 81–82
  indications for, 80, *81*
  inside-out technique for, 78–79, *78–81*
  lateral, incisions for, *79*
  medial, incisions for, *79*
  open technique for, 78
  outside-in technique for, 78, *78*
Meniscal surgery, history of, 5
Meniscal tear(s), abnormal biomechanics
    associated with, 68
  arthrography of, 12, *14–16*
  arthroscopic partial meniscectomy for, 72–
    76
  arthroscopic principles for, 70–72
  arthroscopic repair of, 77–81
    contraindications for, 82
    indications for, 81–82
    inside-out technique for, *78–80*, 80–81
    open technique for, 78–79
    outside-in technique for, *78*, 79–80
  arthroscopy for, patient positioning in, 71,
    71
  bucket handle, *69, 70*
    arthroscopic partial meniscectomy for,
      72, *72–74*
    arthroscopic repair of, *80, 81*
    hemorrhagic, *72*
  classification of, 12
  common patterns of, 68, *69*
  degenerative and complex, arthroscopic
    partial meniscectomy for, 75–76, *76–77*
  degenerative flap, *69*
  excision vs. repair of, 69–70
  "fish-mouth," *74*
  flap, *69, 70*
    arthroscopic partial meniscectomy for,
      74–75, *74–75*
  horizontal, arthrogram of, *14*
    cleavage, *69, 70*
      arthroscopic partial meniscectomy for,
        75, *75–76*
  of posterior horn, arthrogram of, *15, 16*
  medial, bucket handle, sagittal MRI
    sections of, *26*

Meniscal tear(s) (*Continued*)
  medial, complex radial, sagittal MRI
      images of, *25*
    parrot beak, coronal MRI image of, *24*
    Type III, parasagittal MRI sections of,
      24
  MRI evaluation of, 23–24
  MRI grading of, 23
    system for, 24
  parrot beak, arthrogram of, *14*
  radial, *69, 70*
    arthroscopic partial meniscectomy for,
      74, *74*
    double, *69*
  "root," 73
  vertical, arthrogram of, *14*
Meniscectomy, arthroscopic electrocautery
    for, cartilage injury due to, 124, *125*
  degenerative changes following, 67
  early history of, 5
  "Fairbank's" changes following, 67, *68*
  medial, articular cartilage erosion after,
    122
  partial, arthroscopic, for meniscal tears,
    72–76
    vs. total, 68
Meniscocapsular attachment, double-contrast
    arthrogram of, *12*
Meniscocapsular junction, double-contrast
    arthrogram of, *12–13*
Meniscus(i), anatomy of, 49–51, *51, 52*
  arthrography of, 11–21
  blood supply in, 70, *71*
  discoid, tears of, arthroscopic repair of,
      76, *77*
    double radial, *69*
  functions of, 67
  lateral, discoid, arthrogram of, *18*
    normal, *67*
      capsular attachments of, *16–17*
      coronal MRI arthrogram of, *23*
      HRCT arthrogram of, *22*
      serial arthrographic views of, 15, *16–
        17*
  medial, extrusion of, resembling plica, *94*
    incomplete vertical tear of, *69*
    normal, buckling of free edge of, *69*
      coronal MRI arthrogram of, *23*
      high-resolution CT arthrogram of, *20*
      MRI medial parasagittal view of, *23*
      sequential views of, on double-
        contrast arthrogram, *12–13*
    peripheral separation of, arthrogram of,
      18
    vertical tear of posterior horn of, CT
        arthrogram of, *21*
      double-contrast arthrogram of, *21*
  normal, through medial compartment, *65*
  probing of, 68, *69*
"Mini-arthrotomy," vs. arthroscopic
    reconstruction, of cruciate ligaments,
    131
MRI. See *Magnetic resonance imaging (MRI)*.
Multiple myeloma, diagnostic imaging in, 31
Muscle relaxants, in general anesthesia for
    arthroscopic surgery, 40

Needlescope, Selfoc, 3, *3*
Nitze, M., endoscope of, 2, *2*

Noninflammatory synovial fluid (Group I),
    characteristics of, 45t, 47
Notchplasty, in anterior cruciate ligament
    reconstruction, 134–136

O'Connor, R., 5
Olecranonization, 150, *152*
Osteoarthritis, chondroid metaplasia in, *109*
    involvement of knee joint in, 101, *101*
    loose bodies in knee in, 194, *194*
    secondary, calcium pyrophosphate
        deposition in, *123*
    synovial hyperplasia in, 100, *101*
    vs. rheumatoid arthritis, 100–101
Osteochondral fracture(s), articular cartilage
        injury and, 119–120
    blunt probe evaluation of cartilage damage
        in, *124*
    etiology of, 120
    of femoral condyles, loose bodies and, 193,
        193
    of lateral femoral condyle, arthroscopic
        appearance of, *119*
        radiographic appearance of, *119*
        screw repair of, *121*
    of medial femoral condyle, bone peg repair
        of, *121*
    patellar dislocation and, radiograph of, *122*
Osteochondritis dissecans of knee, 175–191
    bone grafting for, 186, *186*
    bone peg fixation for, 186, *186*
    classification of, anatomic, 179, *180*
        by age of patient, 179
    constitutional factors as cause of, 182–183
    defect of medial femoral condyle due to,
        178
    definition of, 30, 175
    detached lesions in, surgical treatment of,
        185
    diagnosis of, 177–179
        arthroscopy in, 178, *178*
    direct trauma as cause of, 181
    endocrine abnormalities in, 182
    epiphyseal abnormalities and, 183
    etiology of, 31, 175, 181–183
    familial occurrence of, 182
    fixation with Kirschner wires in, 186, *187*
    fixation with Smillie pins in, 185, *185*
    genetic factors in, 182
    indirect trauma as cause of, 181–182
    ischemia as cause of, 182
    location of, 177, 177t
    loose bodies in knee and, 194
    magnetic resonance imaging (MRI) of, 30,
        31, 175, *176*, 178, *178*
    multiple epiphyseal dysplasia and, 183
    of medial femoral condyle, arthroscopic
        appearance of, *120*
        MRI imaging of, 31, *31*
        reduction and fixation with Kirschner
            wires of, *120*
    pathology of, 179–180, *180*
    physical findings in, 177, 177t
    radiography of, 19
    retrograde drilling of, arthroscopic, 184,
        184
    revascularization for, 185
    symmetric lesions of, in adolescent, *181*
    Stage I, bone grafting for, 184, *185*
    staging of, 179–180, *180*
    "tissue laxity" and, 183

Osteochondritis dissecans of knee
        (*Continued*)
    treatment of, 183–187
        conservative, 183
        surgical, 184–187
    vs. osteonecrosis, 175, *176*
Osteochondromas, diagnostic imaging of, 31
Osteochondromatosis, loose bodies in knee
        in, 195, *195*, *196*
    synovial, 105–107
Osteochondrosis, synovial, osseous bodies in
        knee from, *204*
Osteochondrosis dissecans, 175. See also
    Osteochondritis dissecans of knee.
Osteomas, diagnostic imaging in, 31
Osteonecrosis, 29–33
    causes of, 29
        ischemia as, 182
    classification of, 30
    magnetic resonance imaging (MRI) of, 30,
        176
Osteosarcoma, diagnostic imaging of, 31
Outpatient surgery, anticipated postoperative
        pain after, 38
    eating and drinking before, 38
    factors influencing ability to perform, 38
    limits of extent of surgery in, 38
    postoperative instructions for, 38
    preoperative testing before, 38

Paget, Sir James, on osteochondritis
        dissecans, 175
Pain, postoperative, after general anesthesia,
        40
    after outpatient surgery, 38
Patel's (midpatellar) portal, *58*, *59*, 61
Patella(s), acute dislocation of, arthroscopic
        repair of, 170
    anatomy of, 55–56, *55*
    articular defect in, HRCT arthrogram of, *22*
    classification by shapes of, 161, *161*
    everted, after medial arthrotomy, *55*
    facets of, *155*
    functions of, 156
    medial subluxation of, after arthroscopic
        lateral retinacular release, *170*
    osteochondral fracture of, blunt probe
        evaluation of cartilage damage in, *124*
    quadriceps attachments to, 157, *157*
    subluxed and tilted, CT scan of, *163*
Patella alta, Blumensaat's line and, 158, *159*
    vs. normal patellofemoral joint, 158, *158*
Patella baja, Blumensaat's line and, 158, *159*
Patellar dislocation, acute, arthroscopic
        repair of, 170
    loose bodies in knee and, 193, *194*
    osteochondral fracture and, radiograph of,
        122
Patellar disorders, medial patellar plica in,
        171, *171*
Patellar index, 159, *159*
Patellar pain, diagnosis and treatment of,
        algorithmic chart for, *165*
Patellar plicae, 157
Patellar tendon, as graft, harvesting of, 143,
        143
    in anterior cruciate ligament
        reconstruction, 143–146, *143–146*
Patellofemoral angle, 159, *160*
Patellofemoral articulation, patellar contact
        areas in, 156, *156*
    tangential view of, *156*

Patellofemoral disorders, arthroscopic diagnosis and treatment of, 155–173
Patellofemoral index, 160, *161*
Patellofemoral joint (suprapatellar pouch), arthroscopic anatomy of, *63,* 65
    computed tomography of, 161–162
    fibrous band in, *93*
    functional anatomy and biomechanics of, 155–157
    loose body in, radiograms of, *198*
    malalignment of, definition of, 162
        types of, by CT scan, 161, *162, 163*
    radiographic anatomy and evaluation of, 157–161
        on anteroposterior film, 157–158, *158*
        on lateral film, 158, *159*
        on tangential film, 158–161
    static ligamentous stabilizers of, 156, *157*
    transverse fibrous band across, *94*
Patellofemoral ligaments, 156, *157*
Patellofemoral syndrome, 56
Patellofemoral tracking, arthroscopic determination of, 162
Patellotibial ligaments, 156, *157*
Patient condition, as factor in outpatient surgery, 38
Patient positioning, for intra-articular fractures, 221, *221*
Perichondrial grafts, for articular cartilage injury, 118
Phagocytes, synovial, function of, 99, *99*
Pigmented villonodular synovitis (PVNS), 107–111
    clinical types of, 108
    diagnostic imaging of, 31, *32*
    diffuse type of, gross appearance of, 111
        synovial hypertrophy in, *111*
    medial capsular, MRI scans of, *33*
    MRI scans of, *32*
    radiologic appearance of, *111*
    villous nodules of, *109, 110*
Plica(e), abnormal, 87–89
    diagnosis of, 91
    in suprapatellar pouch, resection of, *92*
    range of symptoms in, 91t
    symptomatology of, 89–91, 91t
    treatment of, 91
        arthroscopic techniques for, 91–94
        results of, 92t
        role of arthroscopy in, 91
        with fibrosis and thickening from inflammation, *89, 90*
    anatomy of, 54–55, *54*
    infrapatellar. See *Ligamentum mucosum.*
    mildly thickened, *54*
    small, HRCT of, *22*
    symptomatic, arthroscopic diagnosis and treatment of, 83–95
    synovial. See *Synovial plica(e).*
Plica alaris elongata. See *Mediopatellar plica.*
Plica syndrome, 90
    etiology of, 88
    patellofemoral disorders and, 171, *171*
Plica synovialis patellaris. See *Mediopatellar plica.*
Plica synovialis suprapatellaris. See *Suprapatellar plica.*
Popliteal hiatus (recess), *51,* 62, *64*
Popliteal tendon, 50, *52*
    arthrogram of, *16–17*
Popliteal tendon sheath, *66*
Popliteus muscle, anatomy of, 50, *51*

Portal(s) (puncture sites), 57–62
    anterior, *59*
    anterolateral, *60,* 61
        advantages of, 61
        disadvantages of, 61
    anteromedial, 60, *60*
        advantages of, 60
        disadvantages of, 61
    central (Swedish), *58,* 61
        disadvantages of, 61
    lateral, *59*
    medial, *59*
    medial auxiliary, *58, 59,* 61
    midpatellar (Patel's), *58, 59,* 61
    posterolateral, *58, 59,* 62
    posteromedial, *60,* 61–62
    primary, 58–62, *58*
    superolateral, 60
    superomedial, 58–60, *58, 59*
Posterior compartment, loose bodies in, *201*
Posterior cruciate ligament, acute tears of, MRI imaging of, 27
    anatomy of, *50–52, 52*
    arthroscopic view of, 134, *135*
    avulsion from femoral origin of, 134, *135*
    chronic tears of, MRI images of, 27, *29*
    injuries to, 53
    normal, arthroscopic view of, *134*
    sagittal MRI image of, 27, *28*
Posterior cruciate ligament reconstruction, 133
    arthroscopic, 148–151, *149–152*
    attachment site on femur in, 149, *149*
    femoral and tibial tunnels in, *149*
Preoperative testing, for outpatient surgery, 38
Prepatellar bursa, loose bodies in, radiogram of, *199*
Probes, arthroscopic, *8*
Prosthetic ligaments, development of, 153
Proteoglycans, in structure of cartilage, 113
    structure of, *114*
Pseudogout, vs. gout, characteristics of, 103t
Puncture sites, 57–62. See also *Portal(s).*

Quadriceps, components of, angles of insertion on patella of, 157, *157*

Retinaculum, lateral, arthroscopic release of. See *Arthroscopic lateral retinacular release (ALRR).*
    medial, arthroscopic repair of, 170
Rheumatoid arthritis, 101
    synovial changes in, 101, *102, 103*
    synovial pannus from, on medial femoral condyle, *123*
    treatment of, 101
    vs. degenerative joint disease, 100–101
Rheumatoid factor, in synovial fluid, 47
Rheumatoid variants, 101
Rice bodies, synovial, in rheumatoid arthritis, 101, *103*
Ringer's lactate, as irrigation medium, in arthroscopy, 124

Sarcomas, diagnostic imaging of, 31
Sciatic nerve block, with femoral nerve block, for anesthesia, 39

Sedation, with local anesthesia, 38–39
Segalos, P. S., 1
Selfoc arthroscope, Watanabe and, 3, *4*
Septic arthritis, granulation tissue invasion
    of patellar articular surface in, *115*
Septic knee, arthroscopic débridement and
    drainage for, 208
      technique of, 208–212, *209–212*
    arthroscopic decompression of, advantages
      of, 212
    arthroscopic diagnosis and treatment of,
      207–213
    diagnosis of, 207
    excision of fibrous adhesions by basket
      punch in, 209, *209*
    principles of treatment of, 207
    suction drain placement in, *210–212*
    use of rotary suction instrument for, *210*
Septic synovial fluid (Group III),
    characteristics of, 45t, 48
Shavers, arthroscopic, 8
Sodium urate crystals, of gout, 103, *104, 105*
Spinal anesthesia, for arthroscopic surgery,
    advantages and disadvantages of, 37t,
    40–41
Sulcus angle, Hughston's, *159*
Suprapatellar plica, 84, *84, 85,* 157
    anatomic location of, *84*
    common appearance of, *84*
    thickened and fibrotic, *85*
Suprapatellar pouch (patellofemoral joint),
    arthroscopic anatomy of, *63,* 65. See
    also *Patellofemoral joint.*
    loose body in, radiograms of, *198*
Suture placement device, 152, *152, 153*
Synovial chondromatosis, 105–107
    loose bodies of, 106, *108, 109,* 194, *195*
Synovial disorders, 53, *53,* 97–112
Synovial fluid, abnormal, 43–44
    characteristics of, 45t
    classification groups of, 45t, 47–48
    conditions associated with, 45t
    hemorrhagic (Group IV), characteristics
      of, 45t, 48
    inflammatory (Group II), characteristics
      of, 45t, 47
    noninflammatory (Group I),
      characteristics of, 45t, 47
    septic (Group III), characteristics of,
      45t, 48
    analysis of, 43. See also *Synovianalysis.*
    contraindications for, 43
    cell counts in, 46
    characteristics of, 43–48
    chemistry of, 47
    clarity of, 45–46
    color of, 46
    crystals in, 46–47
      types of, 46
    microbiology of, 47
    normal, 43
      characteristics of, 43, 43t
    serology of, 47
    viscosity of, 44–45
    volume of, 44
    white cell count in, 46
Synovial plica(e), abnormal, 87–89
    classification of, 84–86
    historical background of, 83t
    incidence of, 83t
    infrapatellar, anatomic location of, *84*

Synovial plica(e) (*Continued*)
    medial, anatomic location of, *84*
    sites of, *84*
    suprapatellar, anatomic location of, *84*
Synovial shelf. See *Mediopatellar plica.*
Synovianalysis, 43
    contraindications for, 43
    technique of, 44–47
    volume of fluid aspirated in, 44
Synoviocytes, 98, *98*
Synovitis, chronic, *53*
    crystal, *53,* 102–107
      characteristics of, 103t
    iron, 99–100
    pigmented villonodular. See *Pigmented
      villonodular synovitis (PVNS).*
    with abnormal plicae, 87
Synovium, anatomy of, 53–54
    embryonic formation of, 97, *97*
    hyperplastic, *98*
      in degenerative joint disease, 100, *101*
    intima of, iron accumulation in, *100*
    mucinous hypertrophy of, 98, *98*
    normal, appearance of, 97, *98*
      function of, 99, *99*
      intima and subintima of, *98*
      microanatomy of, 97–99, *98, 99*
      phagocytic function of, 99, *99*
      rice bodies in, in rheumatoid arthritis, 101,
      103
    subintima of, as source of tumors, 99

Takagi, K., introduction of arthroscope by,
    2, *2*
Tendon passer, plastic (DePuy), 143, *146*
Tibial plateau, anatomy of, 49, *50*
    superior view of, *51*
Tibial spine(s), anatomy of, 49, *50*
Tibial spine avulsion, method of fixation for,
    229–230, *229, 230*
"Tissue laxity," osteochondritis dissecans
    and, 183
Tophi, in gout, gross and microscopic
    appearance of, 103, *104*
Transplantation, of cartilage, 126, *127*
Trauma, as cause of loose bodies in knee,
    193
    as cause of osteochondritis dissecans, 181–
    182
    blunt, response to injury of articular
      cartilage in, 117
    chondroid metaplasia in, *109*

Urinary retention, after epidural anesthesia,
    41
    after spinal anesthesia, 41

Van Dittel, L., 2

Wappler, R., arthroscope of, 3
Watanabe, M., 3
    arthroscopic instruments of, *4, 5*
Wolf arthroscope, 5, *6*